Eating Clean

for dummies®
A Wiley Brand

2nd edition

**by Jonathan Wright, MD, and
Linda Larsen, BS, BA**

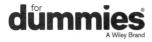

for
dummies®
A Wiley Brand

Eating Clean For Dummies®, 2nd Edition

Published by: **John Wiley & Sons, Inc.,** 111 River Street, Hoboken, NJ 07030-5774, www.wiley.com

Copyright © 2016 by John Wiley & Sons, Inc., Hoboken, New Jersey

Published simultaneously in Canada

No part of this publication may be reproduced, stored in a retrieval system or transmitted in any form or by any means, electronic, mechanical, photocopying, recording, scanning or otherwise, except as permitted under Sections 107 or 108 of the 1976 United States Copyright Act, without the prior written permission of the Publisher. Requests to the Publisher for permission should be addressed to the Permissions Department, John Wiley & Sons, Inc., 111 River Street, Hoboken, NJ 07030, (201) 748-6011, fax (201) 748-6008, or online at http://www.wiley.com/go/permissions.

Trademarks: Wiley, For Dummies, the Dummies Man logo, Dummies.com, Making Everything Easier, and related trade dress are trademarks or registered trademarks of John Wiley & Sons, Inc., and may not be used without written permission. All other trademarks are the property of their respective owners. John Wiley & Sons, Inc., is not associated with any product or vendor mentioned in this book.

LIMIT OF LIABILITY/DISCLAIMER OF WARRANTY: THE CONTENTS OF THIS WORK ARE INTENDED TO FURTHER GENERAL SCIENTIFIC RESEARCH, UNDERSTANDING, AND DISCUSSION ONLY AND ARE NOT INTENDED AND SHOULD NOT BE RELIED UPON AS RECOMMENDING OR PROMOTING A SPECIFIC METHOD, DIAGNOSIS, OR TREATMENT BY PHYSICIANS FOR ANY PARTICULAR PATIENT. THE PUBLISHER AND THE AUTHOR MAKE NO REPRESENTATIONS OR WARRANTIES WITH RESPECT TO THE ACCURACY OR COMPLETENESS OF THE CONTENTS OF THIS WORK AND SPECIFICALLY DISCLAIM ALL WARRANTIES, INCLUDING WITHOUT LIMITATION ANY IMPLIED WARRANTIES OF FITNESS FOR A PARTICULAR PURPOSE. IN VIEW OF ONGOING RESEARCH, EQUIPMENT MODIFICATIONS, CHANGES IN GOVERNMENTAL REGULATIONS, AND THE CONSTANT FLOW OF INFORMATION, THE READER IS URGED TO REVIEW AND EVALUATE THE INFORMATION PROVIDED IN THE PACKAGE INSERT OR INSTRUCTIONS FOR EACH MEDICINE, EQUIPMENT, OR DEVICE FOR, AMONG OTHER THINGS, ANY CHANGES IN THE INSTRUCTIONS OR INDICATION OF USAGE AND FOR ADDED WARNINGS AND PRECAUTIONS. READERS SHOULD CONSULT WITH A SPECIALIST WHERE APPROPRIATE. NEITHER THE PUBLISHER NOR THE AUTHOR SHALL BE LIABLE FOR ANY DAMAGES ARISING HEREFROM.

For general information on our other products and services, please contact our Customer Care Department within the U.S. at 877-762-2974, outside the U.S. at 317-572-3993, or fax 317-572-4002. For technical support, please visit https://hub.wiley.com/community/support/dummies.

Wiley publishes in a variety of print and electronic formats and by print-on-demand. Some material included with standard print versions of this book may not be included in e-books or in print-on-demand. If this book refers to media such as a CD or DVD that is not included in the version you purchased, you may download this material at http://booksupport.wiley.com. For more information about Wiley products, visit www.wiley.com.

Library of Congress Control Number: 2016941727

ISBN 978-1-119-27221-2 (pbk); ISBN 978-1-119-27222-9 (ebk); ISBN 978-1-119-27223-6 (ebk)

Manufactured in the United States of America

10 9 8 7 6 5 4 3 2 1

Contents at a Glance

Recipes at a Glance

Entrees

Side Dishes and Toppings

Desserts

Smoothies

Table of Contents

Introduction

Clean eating isn't a new idea, although it has been outshone by other, less healthy eating plans over the years. Coming out of World War II, in the space age during the race to space, packaged and processed foods started crowding the supermarket shelves. Just look at cooking and baking trends in the Pillsbury Bake-Off, which has been around for more than 40 years, and you can literally see the transformation from cooking and baking with whole foods to depending on convenience foods. But then the health-food craze began in the 1960s and 1970s, and health foods, promoted by experts like Adele Davis, became the next big thing.

Of course, many people scoffed at what they called "hippie food," which they perceived as nuts, roots, and twigs eaten by people wearing hemp necklaces and hand-woven shirts. But Ms. Davis was right. The "modern" diet of processed, quick, artificially flavored convenience foods isn't good for the body.

In this book, we break down the scientific reasons for eating whole foods and avoiding processed and refined foods, and we show you how the eating clean plan can help you and your family live a healthier life. Along the way, we give you plenty of options so that you can design a plan that fits your lifestyle, tastes, and budget.

About This Book

Nutrition is an art and a science. The art comes from mixing different foods to create recipes that tempt the senses and satisfy the soul. The science comes from all the nutrients the foods provide and the complicated ways those nutrients interact in the body. Not to mention science is a pretty big part of baking and cooking, too!

To help you understand the art and science (and the many benefits) of the eating clean lifestyle, we've arranged this book in a practical format. First, we look at what *eating clean* really means and explain why you should avoid processed food, fast food, and junk food. We offer tips for how to handle cravings and feelings of deprivation and explain why you really are what you eat.

We look at the basics of nutrition, explaining why proteins, fats, carbohydrates, vitamins, and minerals are essential to daily life. Then we discuss the other nutrients in whole foods that can make a big difference in your overall health and well-being.

We show you how you can accomplish different goals with the eating clean plan. For example, we tell you which foods to eat (and which ones to avoid) to help prevent heart disease, lower cholesterol, reduce cancer risk, and prevent diabetes. And we explain how eating clean can help you manage these diseases if you already have them.

Understanding the physical science underpinning nutrition and healthy eating is all well and good, but working through the practical aspects of transforming your diet is just as important. To help you get the most out of your new lifestyle, we give you plenty of tips for how to get your family on the eating clean bandwagon, how to prepare and stock your newly clean kitchen, how to incorporate organic foods, and how to prepare delicious clean foods to maintain as many nutrients as possible.

But what if you eat out a lot? And what do you do when you're at a party? Don't start stressing yet! We offer lots of tips and tricks to help keep you on the right track in any social situation. And just in case you have any special dietary needs, we tell you how to handle food allergies and gluten intolerance, as well as how to adapt the clean eating plan to fit a vegetarian or vegan lifestyle.

Finally, we include a plethora of delicious recipes! These recipes cover your whole day from morning to night with easy breakfast choices, delicious (and packable) lunch recipes, and satisfying dinner entrees. We even include snack and dessert recipes for those of you with a case of the munchies or a strong sweet tooth!

Like with all cookbooks, we recommend that you read through each recipe before you start making it. If you jump right in, you may not account for the refrigerating time, standing time, or freezing time in your schedule (and, as a result, your recipe may not be ready to eat when you are!). Reading the recipe's directions beforehand also clues you into any special tools or materials, like food processors or cheesecloth, you may need to complete that particular recipe.

Here are a few other guidelines to keep in mind about the recipes in this book:

>> All butter is unsalted. Margarine is not a suitable substitute for butter unless we state you can use either one.

>> Unless otherwise noted, all eggs are large.

>> All onions are yellow unless otherwise specified.

>> All pepper is freshly ground black pepper unless otherwise specified.

>> All salt is kosher unless otherwise specified.

>> All dry ingredient measurements are level. To make sure your measurements are level, use a dry-ingredient measuring cup, fill it to the top, and scrape it even with a straight object, such as the flat side of a knife.

>> All temperatures are Fahrenheit.

>> All lemon and lime juice is freshly squeezed.

>> ♨ This little tomato symbol designates vegetarian recipes.

Feel free to skip the sidebars that appear throughout the book; these shaded gray boxes contain interesting info that isn't essential to your understanding of meditation.

Within this book, you may note that some web addresses break across two lines of text. If you're reading this book in print and want to visit one of these web pages, simply key in the web address exactly as it's noted in the text, pretending as though the line break doesn't exist. If you're reading this as an e-book, you've got it easy — just click the web address to be taken directly to the web page.

Foolish Assumptions

As we wrote this book, we assumed the following about you:

>> You want to change your diet, lose weight, or manage some type of medical condition and have heard about the eating clean plan.

>> You're the head of a household, and you want your family to change their eating habits and eat food that will help them live longer, happier lives — with as little fuss and fighting as possible.

>> You want to get off the fast-food/processed food/refined food treadmill and eat to live longer and just plain feel better, but you're not quite sure how to start.

>> You're interested in knowing more about how food and the body interact — without having to wade through all the jargon of a scientific text.

Icons Used in This Book

To make this book easier to navigate, we include the following icons that can help you find key ideas and information about the eating clean lifestyle:

REMEMBER

Whenever you see this icon, you know that the information that follows is so important it's worth reading twice. Or even three times!

TIP

This icon appears whenever the information next to it can help you in your quest for better health or in your progress in the eating clean lifestyle.

WARNING

This icon highlights information that could be dangerous to you if you ignore it. So pay attention whenever you see this icon!

Beyond the Book

In addition to the material in the print or e-book you're reading right now, this product also comes with some access-anywhere goodies on the web. Check out the free Cheat Sheet for the basic principles of eating clean, information on how whole foods and eating clean help you stay healthy, and tips on using spices to, well, spice up your meals. To get this Cheat Sheet, simply go to www.dummies.com and type **Eating Clean For Dummies Cheat Sheet** in the Search box.

Where to Go from Here

We've organized this book so that you can go wherever you want to find complete information. You can use the table of contents to find the broad categories of subjects or use the index to look up specific information.

Do you want to know more about getting your family to embrace this new eating lifestyle? Check out Chapter 13. Do you need to know how to plan and stock your kitchen for your new diet plan? Turn to Chapter 9. Do you want to know how foods can help you manage conditions and diseases that may already be present in your family? Take a look at Chapter 8. Are you just itching to try your hand at some delicious clean recipes? Go to Chapters 15 through 18, which include lots of choices for everyday meals and snacks.

If you're not sure where to start, read Part 1. It gives you all the basic information you need to understand the eating clean lifestyle and tells you where to go to get the details.

1

Eating Clean: It Does a Body Good

IN THIS PART . . .

Get an understanding of the dangers in processed foods and the benefits of eating clean.

Explore how the eating clean principles apply to your daily life.

Explore the multicultural history of meditation to understand how it evolved.

Discover what your body needs, how vitamins and minerals keep you healthy, and the foods you should avoid.

Learn about the Paleo diet and who should follow it.

Chapter 1

Eating Clean for a Healthier Body, Mind, and Soul

Eating clean has been getting a lot of press lately — in books, websites, seminars, and various other media outlets. But what exactly is eating clean? Is it a diet? If so, what kinds of foods can you eat (and not eat) on the plan? And what is "clean" food, anyway?

You may be turning to this book because you've tried just about every other diet on the planet and you're tired of counting calories, carbs, and fat grams. If that's the case, you've come to the right place! One of the best things about the eating clean plan is that after you get the basics down pat, you don't have to keep track of your fat or protein intake or add up any points. After all, the plan's main focus is eating whole foods, which are naturally nutrient dense and low in calories.

Like most other diets, the eating clean plan offers several guidelines for following it, but another one of the great things about this plan is that you get to decide how much of your diet will be clean (and how much won't). You're in control, so if you decide that 90 percent of your diet is going to be clean, you can still fit some processed foods into your diet. If you decide to start out with a 50-50 mix, half of your diet will consist of clean foods while the other half includes the foods you already eat and enjoy.

In this chapter, we define clean eating and look at the differences between whole foods and processed foods. We look at some of the dangers of processed and refined foods and list the benefits of eating clean. Finally, we look at food's effect on your body, mind, and soul and explain how following the eating clean lifestyle can improve all three!

What Clean Eating Really Is

Clean eating is the act of basing your diet on whole, unprocessed, preferably organic foods. In other words, when you eat clean, you try to eat as low on the food chain as possible; choose foods that are not processed, but just as they are harvested. By focusing on whole foods, your diet automatically becomes higher in vitamins, minerals, and phytochemicals and lower in refined sugar, bad fats, and food additives.

In this section, we take a closer look at what *clean* really means and cover the difference between whole and processed foods. Then we give you six degrees of clean eating so that you can decide what's right for you.

Eating clean doesn't mean cleaning your food before eating it

Eating clean doesn't mean washing all your food, although you certainly do need to rinse produce before adding it to a recipe or eating it raw. The basic principle of this plan is eating whole foods, which include unprocessed fruits and vegetables, lean meats, nuts, seeds, legumes, and whole grains. The *clean* part simply means that the food is unprocessed. In other words, clean, whole foods don't have ingredient labels because they consist of only one ingredient!

TIP

Think of eating clean as cleaning up your life. Just as you'd like to live life in a house free of clutter, you need to remove the clutter from your diet. What makes up the clutter in your diet? Junk foods, refined sugar, additives, preservatives, trans fats, white flour, artificial flavors, and toxins — just to name a few! (Check out Chapter 2 for more details on how to apply eating clean principles to your daily life.)

But following the eating clean plan is more than just choosing to eat whole foods. You get to eat more often, too! Because people will eat anything within reach when they're so hungry it hurts, the eating clean plan involves eating smaller meals plus at least two snacks throughout the day. Spreading out your food intake helps keep your blood sugar stable, which evens out your mood, improves your concentration on tasks during the day, and can even help reduce the risk of some diseases!

REMEMBER

Essentially, the eating clean plan calls you to do the following:

>> Eat the foods made by nature, not man.

>> Plan to eat five or six meals and snacks throughout the day.

>> Avoid processed foods (in other words, anything in a box with a label).

>> Use healthy cooking methods.

>> Eat before you become super hungry.

>> Stop eating when you're satisfied, not stuffed.

>> Don't count your calories, fat grams, or points.

>> Enjoy your food and appreciate its flavor.

The difference between the eating clean plan and other diets is that this plan is a lifestyle, not a complicated regimen that restricts entire categories of food. With fewer chemicals to deal with, your body becomes better able to concentrate on keeping you healthy.

In Chapters 3 and 4, we explain how eating clean can improve your body on the cellular level. Don't be scared; you don't need a degree in science to use this book and eat clean. But you do need to understand that you literally are what you eat. Your cells, tissues, organs, and entire body will be happier when you eat a great diet.

Comparing whole versus processed foods

To really get a feel for the difference between whole and processed foods, take a look at the following ingredient list. Can you guess what this product is just by reading the ingredients in it?

Water, xylitol, modified food starch, cocoa processed with alkali, milk protein concentrate, hydrogenated vegetable oil, salt, sodium alginate, sucralose, acesulfame potassium, artificial flavor, artificial color

We don't blame you if you have no clue what this food is. It's full of ingredients you don't recognize and can't pronounce, and it's a perfect example of why the eating clean diet is so good for you. After all, why eat this sugar-free instant chocolate pudding mix when you could make your own chocolate pudding with chemical-free, whole ingredients, like milk, eggs, and bittersweet chocolate?

Whole foods are foods that grow in the garden, roam freely on farms, or swim in the sea. Think about the food chain you learned about in science class. Single-celled animals, plants, and plankton are at the bottom. Small fish and other tiny animals eat the single-celled animals, and bigger animals eat the small fish and other tiny animals, and so on up the chain. People (and sharks) are at the top, so everything eaten by the creatures lower on the chain becomes part of the creatures at the top.

To understand all the health benefits of eating clean, you need to consider another food chain: the processed food chain. A plain apple, a handful of chickpeas, or an organic egg are at the bottom. As you move further up the chain, manufacturers manipulate the food until it becomes more artificial ingredients than real food. The foods at the top of this chain include traditional snack foods, fast food, and foods packed with additives, preservatives, and artificial flavors.

Manufacturers end up stripping processed foods of many of their nutrients either to make them easier to combine with other ingredients or to change their characteristics. In contrast, whole foods come to you just as nature intended — bursting with flavor, color, texture, and nutrients.

The foods that are part of the eating clean plan are at the bottom of the processed food chain. They don't have labels, they don't carry preparation instructions, and they certainly don't have ingredient lists. These are the foods that should fill your shopping basket each time you go to the supermarket. (See Chapter 9 for tips on how to stock a clean kitchen and Chapter 20 for a list of clean foods you should always put in your shopping cart.)

TIP

Of course, some processed foods are perfectly acceptable on the eating clean plan. Whole-grain pasta is obviously processed, but it's minimally processed. Read the label; if it lists whole grains, water, and perhaps salt, it's a pretty clean food. Cheese is another processed food, but if you choose a natural cheese that doesn't come loaded with additives and artificial colors, it still fits into the eating clean plan.

Gaining control with six degrees of clean eating

One of the best things about the eating clean plan is that you're in control. In other words, you get to choose how much of the eating clean plan you implement. You can go all out and make 100 percent of your diet clean. Or you can choose to eat an occasional fast-food meal or include some processed foods in your diet. The choice is yours!

Table 1-1 shows the six degrees of clean eating. Take a look at what each degree entails, and think about which one best fits your life.

TABLE 1-1   The Six Degrees of Clean Eating

Degree	What You Eat When Following This Degree
20%	At the beginning of your eating clean adventure — or if you're trying to wean kids (or a reluctant spouse) off of a junk food diet — start by changing one meal in a five-day week into a clean meal.
40%	Add another clean meal a week to your plan to continue the eating clean journey. You can also start at this level.
50%	If you want to live an eating clean lifestyle, 50% is really the minimum degree to shoot for. At this level, you get some of the benefits of the eating clean diet plan but can still eat a few fast-food meals and the occasional junk food. Just try to make the nonclean 50% of your diet a bit healthier! Make homemade potato chips instead of eating processed, flavored chips; use multigrain pasta in place of white; and enjoy just one brownie rather than five.
60%	Now you're getting more serious! At this level, most of your foods are clean and unprocessed, but you still eat processed foods two or three days a week. You have to do more cooking, but you're also saving money because you're eating out less and buying fewer processed (and expensive) foods.
80%	Many people stop at this level of clean eating. The vast majority of your meals are clean, using whole, unprocessed foods, but you can still include some bottled pasta sauce and bakery bread in your diet.
100%	Not many people can follow a true clean eating plan all the time, but if you can, bravo! If you've been diagnosed with a serious illness, this level may be the best option for you. Or if you're sick and tired of feeling sick and tired, the pure eating clean plan may help you feel better.

Of course, you can set your target somewhere in between these six degrees. Heck, your plan may vary between 100 percent clean and 60 percent clean within the same day! If you're serious about living the eating clean lifestyle, though, aim for making whole foods the basis for at least 50 percent of your diet. Don't worry about backsliding or falling off the eating clean wagon; just focus on the big picture and enjoy your food and your life. (See Chapter 2 for tips on how to deal with backsliding and get back on the eating clean wagon.)

Considering the Dangers in Processed Foods

Are processed foods really as bad as some people think? In a word, yes. Consider just one example: trans fats. Manufacturers make these fake fats by bubbling hydrogen through liquid oils. Although this process (called *hydrogenation*) sounds like something out of a Frankenstein movie, it's not that complicated. The hydrogen simply transforms the oil into a solid substance. Hydrogenation is a very inexpensive way to make solid fats, which is why food processors love it.

For years, doctors (yes, doctors!) recommended that people eat margarine made with this method rather than butter or simple oils. Now, of course, researchers know that trans fats may be one of the culprits behind America's skyrocketing heart disease rates. The fake fats literally become part of your cell walls, making them flabby and changing their ability to interact with other parts of your body. Nobody wants flabby arms, let alone flabby cell walls!

In this section, we look at some of the preservatives and additives packed into processed foods and explain why you should avoid them. We also consider whether fortified foods are really any better than unfortified foods and explain why breaking the junk food habit is so important to your health.

Preservatives and additives

Surprisingly enough, the U.S. Food and Drug Administration (FDA) and U.S. Department of Agriculture (USDA) haven't tested many of the preservatives and additives used in processed foods because they're on the Generally Recognized as Safe (GRAS) list. A chemical's presence on this list means that it has been used for so long (since before 1958) — with no known harmful side effects attached to it — that the FDA allows manufacturers to use it in food without any required testing.

The FDA defines *safe* as "a reasonable certainty in the minds of competent scientists that the substance is not harmful under its intended conditions of use." That's not exactly a ringing endorsement! And the phrase *intended conditions of use* needs some further explanation; see the nearby sidebar "How many chemicals do you consume?" for details.

The FDA has developed four different classifications of chemicals that manufacturers add to processed food:

>> **Food additives:** This category includes preservatives, flavor enhancers, emulsifiers (calcium stearoyl di laciate, polyglycerol ester, and monoglycerides, among others), vitamins and minerals, and chemicals that control the pH of a product.

>> **GRAS substances:** These products are the ones that have "existing evidence of long and safe use." These substances have not been tested by the FDA or USDA.

>> **Prior-sanctioned substances:** The FDA or USDA tested and approved these products before the government developed the GRAS list.

>> **Color additives:** This category includes color enhancers and additives.

The FDA doesn't guarantee that the chemicals included in the GRAS list and the prior-sanctioned substances list are safe, but it doesn't test them unless some new evidence shows that they may be unsafe. You may have heard of the artificial sweetener cyclamate. It was in the GRAS list until testing found that it caused cancer in animals; then the FDA removed it from the list.

WARNING

The FDA has removed some chemicals from the market. Red Dye #2 and Violet #1, for example, were removed from the market after Congress passed the 1960 Color Additive Amendment. Before the amendment passed, manufacturers used 200 food dyes; less than 35 of those dyes passed the testing process and were declared safe. So how much damage was done by the 165 unsafe food dyes? Think of it this way: Some manufacturers used to put lead in butter to give it that beautiful yellow color or chalk in milk to make it look thick and creamy!

Many people, especially those who eat clean, don't want to wait for some food additive, pesticide, or preservative to be declared dangerous retroactively. They'd rather take control of what they put into their bodies and consume as few of these chemicals as possible — through the eating clean diet, of course! (Find out more about these chemicals in Chapters 2 and 9.)

Of course, a few preservatives and additives may be perfectly safe if consumed in small amounts. But many people really don't like the phrase *may be*. Do you really want to be a guinea pig in a huge experiment conducted on the population? If you want to gain more confidence about the safety of the foods you eat, give the eating clean plan a try and avoid processed, refined, and packaged foods as much as you can.

HOW MANY CHEMICALS DO YOU CONSUME?

One of the problems connected with the chemicals in your food is how much of each particular food you consume. If your diet consists mainly of fast food and the amount of hormones in that beef burger you love is considered "safe in a reasonable diet" but you eat 400 hamburgers a year, you're going to ingest more than the amount of hormones the FDA approved. Similarly, if you love asparagus, eat it three times a week, and can't afford to buy organically grown produce, you'll be getting more than the studied dose of pesticides used to grow that particular product.

To reduce your exposure to preservatives, additives, and other chemicals added to food, vary what you eat. Don't subsist on fried chicken and roasted potatoes. Add different types of fresh fruits and vegetables, even if they aren't grown organically, and you can reduce your exposure to many chemicals. (See Chapter 10 for everything you need to know about incorporating organic foods into your diet.)

Label claims (also known as marketing hype)

Many processed foods have lots of claims plastered all over their labels. "Fortified with calcium!" "Strengthens your immune system!" and "Made with real fruit!" are just some of the banners you see on packaged foods these days. But what, if anything, do these claims mean?

Many fortified foods have only some (key word *some*) of the nutrients that manufacturers removed during processing added back in. For instance, a cereal made from white flour may have vitamins and fiber added back in. But the amounts added back in aren't even close to 100 percent of what was removed in the first place. The process to turn the wheat grain into white flour permanently strips out many of those nutrients.

Although eating fortified foods is better than eating unfortified foods, it's not as good as eating the whole foods in the first place. Unfortunately, many people blissfully put these fortified products in their shopping baskets, unaware that many of the claims on the packages have no real meaning.

The FDA does regulate some label claims, but many companies change a word or two to get around these regulations. Then the claim becomes misleading. For example, most flavored strawberry juices don't actually contain strawberries. The "real fruit" you see on the label claim is actually pear concentrate, and the "strawberry" is present only in the form of artificial flavoring.

The following list presents some common label claims and explains what they actually mean:

>> **Made with organic ingredients:** Only 70 percent of the ingredients in the food must be grown organically. (See Chapter 10 for a lot more details about organic foods.)

>> **High or rich in . . . :** These food products must have 20 percent of the Recommended Dietary Allowance (RDA) of the nutrient in question per serving.

>> **Zero trans fats:** The product can contain up to 0.5 grams of artificial trans fats per serving. But be aware that if you eat more than one serving, those partial grams can add up fast.

>> **More, fortified, enriched:** For this designation, the product must contain 10 percent of the RDA of the nutrient in question per serving or more than a similar product contains.

>> **Natural:** This claim means the product can't contain anything synthetic. But it can still be high in sodium, fats, and sugars.

>> **Made with whole wheat:** This claim doesn't mean that the food contains no refined grain products. In fact, the food has to contain only a tiny amount of whole wheat to legally use this label.

Understandably, these claims can confuse consumers. The claims don't tell you about substances that you may need or want to avoid; you have to read the ingredient list for that information. Funny how these claims, when clearly explained, don't seem as wonderful as you'd think! If a food has "more vitamin A" but the "more" is only 10 percent of your RDA and the food has enough sodium to put you over your limit for the day, is it really a healthy choice?

Overall, eating foods without labels is less complicated and better for you. When you buy whole, unlabeled foods, you can be pretty sure that what you see is what you get.

Junk food addiction

The term *junk food junkie* used to be pretty popular in the American lexicon. People used it as a joke, but unfortunately, that term is very accurate because junk food is actually quite addictive.

Consider this: A study published in *Nature Neuroscience* found that your brain reacts to junk food just like it does to addictive drugs like heroin. Kind of scary, right? You've likely seen pictures of heroin addicts, who will do anything for that next hit.

One of the most dangerous things about addiction is that over time, the addict has to consume more and more of the addictive substance to create the same amount of pleasure in the addict's brain. That fact is what causes the death of many drug addicts; eventually they overdose.

That fact is also what can cause the illness and death of junk food junkies; eventually the ever-increasing consumption of empty calories, lots of sugar, refined ingredients, sodium, and artificial additives wear out the body. With little or no vitamins, minerals, and phytochemicals to help the body repair itself, junk food junkies eventually come to the end of the line and develop a disease. To think that manufacturers actually develop junk foods to be as addictively appealing as possible!

REMEMBER

The eating clean plan helps remove your addiction to junk food simply by substituting whole foods that are healthy and nutritious for the unhealthy, addictive junk foods. This process takes time, though, so don't think you'll find an easy way out of the junk food maze. But you can get out of it, and with some thought and effort, you can get your family off the junk food treadmill, too. One of the best things about the eating clean lifestyle is that the more you follow it, the better you feel, so you get on an upward spiral toward good health rather than a downward spiral into sickness.

Surveying the Benefits of Eating Clean

So other than containing clean, natural ingredients rather than artificial chemicals, what can clean, whole foods do for you? Eating a clean diet can help you live longer, make you stronger, prevent disease, and maybe even treat some diseases. These claims may sound like one of those late-night infomercials, but they're all true — backed up with scientific research conducted by real doctors wearing lab coats!

In this section, we look at how you can use the eating clean lifestyle to obtain and maintain good health. We discuss how to eat clean to lose weight, to prevent disease, and to lead the longest, most active life you can. (See Chapter 6 for more on losing weight and living a longer, healthier life and Chapters 7 and 8 for more on disease prevention and management.)

Overall good health

If you've been blessed with good health, you're lucky. After all, your genes do play a part in whether or not you develop disease. But scientists estimate that 310,000 to 580,000 deaths in the United States every year are caused by an unhealthy diet and lack of physical exercise. After all, your diet has a very real effect on your health:

>> Diet causes up to one-third of all cancers.

>> Poor diet causes most cases of obesity.

>> A diet based on processed foods, junk foods, and refined foods is a major risk factor for developing heart disease.

>> Not getting enough vitamins, minerals, and phytochemicals in your diet puts you at greater risk for catching infectious diseases.

>> Eating too much sugar, alcohol, and bad fat can reduce the efficiency of your immune system.

JUNK FOODS: FAKE EVERYTHING

You know that junk foods contain artificial colors and flavors, along with sugar and salt to increase their addictive qualities. But do you know that junk food manufacturers also manipulate texture? Texture and flavor are the two big players in food's appeal. Emulsifiers, two or three trips into the frying pan, thickeners, fats, and stabilizers increase the *mouthfeel,* or texture, of processed foods. In other words, manufacturers artificially manipulate their foods to make them more pleasing to your mouth. This artificial mouthfeel gives junk food an advantage over regular food, so you tend to crave it more than whole foods. After you realize that the whole mouthfeel is just as artificial as the ingredients, you may be able to say no the next time you crave a triple-fried cheese doodle. Try a crisp apple or some cauliflower instead.

The eating clean plan can help you stay as healthy as you can be by putting your dietary focus on whole foods that pack a nutritional punch. No matter what the current state of your health is, you can feel better and get healthier if you ditch the refined, overly processed foods and start concentrating on eating healthy foods.

The characteristics of overall good health are

>> Stamina

>> Normal body weight

>> Normal blood pressure

>> Good blood cholesterol counts and other normal blood parameters

>> A healthy heart

>> Good digestion

>> Clear skin

>> Mental acuity

Overall good health has many more markers, of course, but the point is that good health isn't perfection. It isn't about achieving a model's body or looking like your favorite movie star. Good health means that your body is able to do what you want it to do, whether that's to hike Mount Annapurna or take a walk around the block.

Weight loss and disease prevention

More than 60 percent of all Americans are overweight. Even with messages about nutrition being blasted all day long, through every form of media, Americans are getting more and more overweight. What's going on?

Many nutritionists think the problem is what's in the food most people eat. Your body wasn't made to use all the chemicals and artificial ingredients packed into much of the American diet. And it certainly wasn't made to consume as much sodium, fake fat, and sugar as many people do today. Plus, your body was made to efficiently process food and store fat since your ancestors couldn't guarantee that they'd get three square meals a day. When Americans are faced with unlimited quantities of food available 24 hours a day, something has to give. Often, that something is their waistbands.

REMEMBER

The key to healthy, sustained weight loss is to gradually lose weight by eating a nutrient-dense diet of filling foods, which is exactly what the eating clean plan is all about. On the plan, you eat more often and you eat foods that are satisfying and very nutritious. After you get into the clean eating plan, you really won't have any more room in your life (or your stomach) for the junk food that made you overweight in the first place!

Remember the thousands of deaths caused every year by poor diet and lack of exercise that we talk about in the preceding section? Well, people don't die because of a poor diet; they die because of the diseases caused (or exacerbated) by that poor diet. Those diseases include

>> Heart disease

>> Cancer

>> Diabetes

>> Hypertension

>> Stroke

>> Autoimmune diseases

>> Osteoporosis

Disease occurs when something goes wrong in your body. Cells grow too fast, and your body is so busy filtering toxins that it takes longer to respond to infection. Over time, these factors can lead to a serious disease.

In Chapter 7, we focus on how to eat to reduce your risk of developing certain diseases. After all, what you eat has a direct impact on your disease risk. Then in

Chapter 8, we discuss how to eat to help manage certain diseases after you already have them.

The eating clean diet really is the model for eating to prevent disease. One of its main focuses is on getting plenty of phytochemicals, which help prevent inflammation, keep your immune system strong, and keep your cardiovascular system running smoothly. The only way to get your phytochemicals is to eat lots of whole fruits, vegetables, nuts, seeds, and grains.

A longer, more active life

A good motto for the eating clean life is "It's not only the years in your life, but the life in your years!" Everyone wants to live a long life, of course, but if that life is full of preventable pain, disease, and suffering, all bets are off. Living a long life should mean being able to easily walk up stairs, walk around the block, and participate in active hobbies well into your 80s and 90s.

Fortunately, the eating clean diet can help you do just that! If you're blessed with basically good health, eating whole foods prepared in a clean way is one of the best ways to keep yourself healthy. Of course, no diet can guarantee good health or a long life. But you can tip the odds in your favor with the eating clean plan.

Chapter 2

Applying Eating Clean Principles to Daily Living

E ating clean isn't just about the food you put in your mouth; it's a total life-style. By buying, preparing, and eating whole foods, you're affecting far more than your waistline and your health. You're making a positive impact on the world around you.

The eating clean lifestyle doesn't restrict you from eating any foods except processed foods. So you don't have to become a vegan or vegetarian (although you can if you want to!), and you don't have to count carbs, fat grams, or calories. By eating lower on the food chain, you save money and improve your health while making the world a better place to live.

One of the main benefits of this lifestyle is its simplicity. Because you don't have to keep track of calories, fat grams, or carbohydrates, planning meals is a lot less complicated than it is for other diets. Plus, the eating clean diet includes every food group, so you don't have to feel deprived. You don't have to worry about going hungry, either, because you get to eat satisfying meals and snacks through-out the day.

In this chapter, we look at the principles of clean eating, including eating for your health, consuming whole foods, avoiding processed foods, and figuring out how to enjoy healthy foods. We also show you how to handle feelings of deprivation and cravings that may undermine your clean eating efforts. Finally, we look at how supporting local farms, buying organic produce and free-range meats, going meatless one day a week, and reducing packaging waste can mean a healthier world for everyone.

The Principles of Clean Eating

Depending on who you talk to, different clean eating plans have different principles. This flexibility is another reason why so many people find this lifestyle rewarding and doable. As long as you eat whole foods and avoid processed foods, you can create the clean eating lifestyle that works best for you.

In this section, we look at the overall eating clean platform. You can pick and choose which facets appeal to you and your family. Then we explain how to make clean changes in your diet. Finally, we look at the real flavor of real food and show you how to appreciate it.

REMEMBER

The reason we're stressing *lifestyle* rather than *diet* is that most diets fail. Only 5 percent of all dieters stay on their diets and keep the weight off for more than a few years. Because clean eating is a lifestyle choice, the benefits you reap from it last a lifetime.

Getting your footing on the eating clean platform

The eating clean movement really started in the 1960s thanks to the efforts of Adele Davis and other health food authors. At that time, health food stores started springing up around the country, and people told jokes about tofu eaters who dressed in natural fibers and sandals and ate nuts and berries. In 1987, Ralph Nader wrote the book *Eating Clean: Overcoming Food Hazards,* which focused on the hazards of processed foods. But then Corporate America started pushing convenience foods and time-saving products above everything else. Mixes, frozen dinners, and junk foods started crowding whole foods off grocery store shelves.

After decades of Americans' eating processed foods and, not coincidentally, watching their population become more obese, fad diets became more and more popular. But they weren't successful, because following a really restrictive diet for long periods of time is nearly impossible. Everyone falls off the wagon, and many people have a hard time getting back on — which is why, after losing weight, more than 90 percent of overweight people eventually put the weight back on. On the other hand, the clean eating lifestyle has become more popular as more people realize how simple it really is. It's a lifestyle you can live with for the rest of your life.

REMEMBER

The basic planks of the eating clean platform are

» **Eat whole, unrefined, and unprocessed foods that are low on the food chain.** Buy bunches of broccoli, whole heads of lettuce, corn on the cob, cantaloupe, whole chickens, and unrefined grains rather than processed foods, like broccoli in sauce, packaged salads, canned corn, and lunch meat.

» **Eat a wide variety of unprocessed foods.** Today's markets and grocery stores offer many more fruits and vegetables today than they did a few years ago. Try unusual foods like passion fruit, salsify, or broccoli rabe. Experiment with unfamiliar foods to help make mealtime more interesting.

» **Avoid artificial substances, including artificial flavors and colors, preservatives, and artificial sweeteners.** These items can harm your health by literally becoming part of your body's cell structure and changing some basic biological mechanisms. These changes weaken your body's ability to stay healthy.

» **Cut back on sugars, especially processed sugars like high fructose corn syrup and artificial sweeteners.** That means no more soda pop or other sugary drinks. Your body processes these ingredients differently, and they provide nothing but empty calories.

» **Avoid trans fats and artificial fat substitutes.** The trans fatty acids found in shortening, lots of baked products, and snack foods may be behind the skyrocketing heart disease rates in this country, so don't eat them. Two more reasons why you should avoid artificial fats are that they cause unpleasant side effects and no one really knows about their long-term safety.

» **Choose low-fat, not nonfat, dairy products.** Nonfat products use processed and artificial substances, like additives and starches, to mimic the texture and flavor of fat.

» **Choose foods that are nutrient dense.** In other words, for every calorie a food provides, it should also provide vitamins, minerals, protein, carbs, fiber, and good fats. Good fats include the fats found in nuts, olive oil, and lean meats, especially seafood. On the other hand, you find empty calories, which are calories with little or no nutritional value, in snack foods, cookies, candies, and soda.

» **Combine protein, complex carbohydrates, and healthy fats at every meal for the most satisfaction.** This combination helps stave off hunger and gives you more energy than you get from consuming something that's sugary or salty.

>> **Drink lots of water.** Try to drink several glasses of water a day. If you don't enjoy the taste of plain water, you can also drink unsweetened tea. Drinking plenty of water helps keep your digestive system running smoothly. Avoid drinking fruit juices, because they can be high in sugar and calories.

>> **Eat five or six minimeals a day rather than three large meals.** Make breakfast your largest meal, with whole-grain cereal or toast with butter or peanut butter and some form of protein, like a hard-boiled egg. Your other meals need to include protein, carbs, and fat, like celery sticks with nut butters and dried fruits or sandwiches made with sliced chicken and vegetables such as avocado and tomatoes.

>> **Practice portion control, especially when you eat more than three meals a day.** Each meal should be about 300 to 400 nutritious calories. Figure out what ½ cup of brown rice or other whole grain or fruits and vegetables looks like, because that's how big a typical serving is. A serving of bread is one slice; a serving of meat is 3 ounces, or about the size of a deck of cards. With time, eating proper portions will become second nature. Depending on which meal schedule works best for your day, you can adjust the amounts accordingly. For more information about portion sizes, see `www.niddk.nih.gov/health-information/health-topics/weight-control/just-enough/Pages/just-enough-for-you.aspx`.

Making clean changes in your life

Clean changes in your life aren't difficult to make, but they do take some gumption, perseverance, and practice. When you make a concentrated effort to eat lower on the food chain, notice how this decision affects other areas of your life. To be successful, you have to think about food and eat differently, which will no doubt prompt changes in other areas of your life.

REMEMBER

As you adopt an eating clean lifestyle, you may also

>> **Lose weight and gain more energy.** Eating healthy foods with lots of vitamins, minerals, fiber, protein, complex carbohydrates, and good fats automatically makes you healthier. Of course, adding exercise to your new lifestyle is also important. As you feel stronger and gain more energy from the foods you eat, exercising will be much easier.

>> **Add fun exercise to your life.** Go for a walk with your kids, play on a jungle gym, take up a new sport, or invest in a gym membership. The combination of

healthy eating with regular exercise can improve all parts of your life. With more confidence in how you look and feel, who knows what you can achieve?

» **Improve your skin condition and overall appearance.** People who eat clean food also enjoy clear and smooth skin, thick and shiny hair, and bright eyes. The saying "you are what you eat" is absolutely true. Do you really want to be a nacho cheese chip?

» **Spend more time cooking at first.** Before you can eat whole, unprocessed foods, you need to, well, process them. Don't panic. Cooking whole foods doesn't have to be difficult. After all, making simple meals, like baked chicken with a chopped salad, isn't time-consuming. Plus, you're learning a valuable skill.

» **Spend more time planning meals at first, now that you aren't relying on fast food or convenience foods to feed your family.** As you get into the eating clean lifestyle, you accumulate more recipes and ideas for clean foods, so the planning gets easier.

» **Spend more time shopping for food and reading labels.** Especially at first, allow more time for shopping. Picking out the ingredients for a chopped salad takes longer than buying a frozen dinner. Keep reminding yourself that the health and life benefits are well worth the extra time and effort.

» **Shop more often.** Because the foods you're buying aren't laced with preservatives, their shelf life is shorter. So shop more often and buy a bit less each time you shop.

» **Produce less waste.** You can compost most food waste (except meats). Plus, you no longer buy foods that are wrapped and sealed in many layers, so you use less packaging. That's good for the earth and your garbage bill.

» **Make preparing and eating food an event.** Use the time to talk to your family and teach them skills. Let each family member plan out a meal or two in a week or a month, and take the time to find out more about the food and the cuisine behind each meal.

Discovering real flavor

Flavor in food is what makes eating enjoyable. But flavor doesn't come only from the reaction between foods and the taste buds on your tongue. Taste is only a small part of the flavor equation. The other important characteristics of flavor include aroma, color, temperature, and something called *mouthfeel*, which is the texture of food.

Processed foods are infamous for including artificial flavors and colors, along with tons of added sugar and salt. These ingredients interfere with your body's natural appetite centers, spurring you to eat more and crave more of these unhealthy foods. When you embark on your clean eating lifestyle, you'll notice some changes in how food tastes.

REMEMBER

Your tongue has five different types of taste receptors that are bundled into buds and that react with the ions and molecules in food and then send messages to your brain through chemical reactions. Sour and salty taste receptors detect ions, while the others detect molecules. The five types of taste receptors are

>> **Sour:** The acid in foods stimulates these taste receptors, which have channels that pick up the hydronium ions found in foods like lemon juice and balsamic vinegar.

>> **Salty:** The sodium ions in food stimulate these taste receptors.

>> **Bitter:** G-protein receptors on specialized taste buds perceive alkaloids (certain amino acids or proteins) in food, which cause bitter flavors, and directly activate neurons in the brain. Human bodies are hard-wired to detect bitter taste because many poisonous plants are bitter.

>> **Sweet:** Hydroxyl groups on sugar molecules stimulate your sweet taste receptors by using a protein called *gustducin,* which prompts reactions on the tongue that the brain recognizes as sweet.

>> **Umami or meaty:** The glutamic acid salts, which are part of the amino acids found in meats, cheeses, and some vegetables, stimulate these taste receptors.

Note: Spicy or hot flavors don't stimulate any of the taste receptors. The so-called spicy flavor is actually the perception of pain, which the nerve endings just below the taste buds detect. That's why your tongue takes a few seconds to register the spiciness and heat when you bite into a jalapeño pepper.

A single taste bud has dozens of taste-receptor cells that include all five of the basic taste sensations. (Contrary to popular belief, they aren't grouped around the tongue in separate sections.) With the addition of salt, sugar, and flavor enhancers, processed foods are formulated to stimulate salty, sweet, and umami taste receptors, which are collectively called *appetitive tastes.* The threshold for tasting these substances is very low.

Clean foods activate your taste receptors without any help from artificial ingredients. Their flavors are much more pure. After just a short period of time on the eating clean diet, you'll start to recognize the clean taste of natural foods. Table 2-1 lists some clean foods with the five basic taste attributes plus spicy.

TABLE 2-1   **Flavorful Clean Foods**

Food	Sweet	Sour	Salty	Bitter	Umami	Spicy
Bananas, mangos, melons, honey, agave nectar	X					
Yogurt, pomegranates, tamarind		X				
Kelp, pickled foods			X			
Spinach and dark greens, broccoli, Brussels sprouts, celery, eggplant, grapefruit				X		
Mushrooms					X	
Peppers, herbs, spices, ginger, radishes, raw onions and garlic, horseradish						X
Apples, oranges, strawberries	X	X				
Cooked onions and garlic, carrots, tomatoes	X				X	
Lemons, limes		X	X			
Tea, vinegar		X		X		
Mint		X				X
Kale, asparagus			X	X		
Meat stocks, lean meats, soy products, nuts, shellfish			X		X	
Kohlrabi				X		X
Miso					X	X
Natural cheeses		X	X		X	

Combining the foods in Table 2-1 and choosing foods that incorporate more than one flavor can enhance your eating experience. (Now, that sounds like a restaurant commercial, doesn't it?) Think about an apple: It's both sour and sweet. The sweetness makes the sour flavor more pronounced, and vice versa. Plan your meals using this concept. Include some clean foods that have several flavors to enhance every meal.

Even though junk foods are designed to hit all the right taste buds, you can use a biological advantage to appreciate clean and healthy whole foods: More than 80 percent of what you perceive as flavor is actually aroma. Processed foods include artificial ingredients that mimic aromas of clean foods. But clean foods are full of natural aromas that make their flavors much more complex and satisfying than their artificial counterparts.

Don't forget the important impact that color, texture, and temperature have on the flavor experience. To use your natural flavor–detecting abilities to fully appreciate clean foods, pay attention to these three flavor factors and try out the following tips:

>> **Eat more slowly.** When you chew your food slowly, you give your taste buds time to detect the different flavors and aromas being released. Not only is gulping down food bad for your digestion, but it also keeps you from experiencing all the flavors natural foods have to offer. Chewing also releases vapors into the back of your mouth, which stimulate your sense of smell. Chewing food for a longer period of time releases more flavor.

>> **Put away the salt shaker.** Many people have become used to the flavor of salt. As a result, they need more and more salt to satisfy the salty appetite center of the brain. Foods may taste bland at first on the eating clean plan, but your taste buds will gradually adjust to less sodium and the natural flavors of the foods will become more prominent.

There is an exception to this rule: If your blood pressure is low (100/60 or less on either reading), you may have weak adrenal function and need salt. These people feel better and are healthier with more added salt, not less. If that's you, check with a physician skilled and knowledgeable in natural, nutritional medicine before making a decision to cut back on salt.

>> **Smell your food before you taste it.** We're not saying you should sniff each bite before you put it in your mouth, a practice that can be construed as rude in some cultures. But breathe in over your plate before you start eating. Notice the rich smell of meats, the clean spiciness of a vegetable salad, and the sweet, complex aroma of herbs and spices.

>> **Plan meals with different textures.** Texture is an important part of flavor assessment. For example, if you make a whole meal of foods with soft textures, it will seem less interesting and more bland. Try to incorporate crisp, chewy, smooth, soft, and hard textures in your meals.

>> **Incorporate as many colors as possible on your plate.** You eat with your eyes before you eat with your mouth! No wonder your meal seems more appetizing when it contains reds, greens, browns, and yellows than when it's all beige or brown. Biting into a deep-red strawberry is more satisfying than biting into one that's pale and anemic-looking. As an added bonus, eating more colorful foods means giving your body more nutrients.

>> **Plan meals with different temperatures.** The contrast between hot and cold enhances the eating experience. Think about eating some warm grilled bread topped with a cold tomato salsa.

REMEMBER

Appreciating your food's natural flavors is easy to do on a clean diet because clean, whole foods hit all the flavor points that are built right into your anatomy. Foods that are less processed take more time to eat, forcing you to slow down and really notice the flavor and aroma of your food. The natural flavors of clean foods are more pleasing than artificially flavored and colored foods, especially when you get used to eating foods without so much added salt and sugar. Whole foods offer different textures and colors, making the meal much more appetizing. And you can serve clean, whole foods at any temperature or mix of temperatures, which adds interest to meals.

Managing Cravings and Feelings of Deprivation

For many people, just the thought of switching to a healthy eating plan is depressing. After all, life without chocolate chip cookies or nacho cheese chips seems pretty sad to a lot of people. To deal with these types of thoughts, you need to unleash your natural taste sensors and reprogram your brain so you start craving good foods.

In this section, we look at the biological factors behind cravings and feelings of deprivation, and we show you what you can do to rewire your brain so that you enjoy eating (and even crave) healthy foods.

Understanding cravings

Did you know that the cravings you feel are real and not the result of low will-power and that they may actually be food addictions? Food companies understand the relationship between cravings and addiction, which is why they load processed food with salt, sugar, unhealthy fats, food colorings, and additives.

Food cravings and hunger have both psychological and physical facets. True hunger is a physical response to low blood sugar. But stress, boredom, aromas wafting through the air, and tempting television commercials can trigger food cravings. Unlike the actual need for food, however, a craving diminishes over time. If you give yourself some time and space to process what you're actually feeling, the craving will probably subside. Plus, the only way to satisfy cravings is by eating one particular food; you can satisfy true hunger with any nutritious food.

In a 2010 study published in *Nature Neuroscience*, scientists at the Scripps Research Institute showed that you can activate the same biological mechanisms that drive addiction to tobacco, cocaine, or heroin to create food addictions. A constant diet of foods like cheeseburgers, chips, and candy can turn into a vicious cycle of addiction and cravings. As the body becomes obese, reward and pleasure centers in the brain deteriorate, requiring more and more processed junk foods to satisfy them. This phenomenon is called *sensory overload,* and it creates a vicious cycle of cravings for junk food that result in more weight gain, which increases cravings, which result in more weight gain . . . you get the picture. If you don't break this cycle — by changing your eating habits — you'll likely end up suffering from obesity, type-2 diabetes, and other diseases.

REMEMBER

Refined carbohydrates like those found in cakes, cookies, and white bread cause insulin levels to spike. The rapid rise in blood glucose levels causes the release of insulin, which plays an important role in cravings by

>> Storing refined carbs by converting them to fat

>> Slowing down production of fat-burning hormones

>> Telling your body to hold on to its stored fat

>> Making you hungry more quickly

REMEMBER

Eating a lot of junk food, or foods high in sugar and refined carbohydrates, may literally rewire your brain, creating a chemical imbalance. This imbalance occurs in the area of the brain that creates feelings of reward and satiety. When this change occurs, compulsive eating habits and addiction usually follow.

The main problem with food addiction is that people need to eat to live. While cocaine addicts can change their lives to avoid the addictive substance, people can't avoid food. But you can take control of this cycle by applying the clean eating principles we discuss in the earlier section "The Principles of Clean Eating."

Your brain also associates many of the foods you crave with pleasurable events. For example, if your mother always made chocolate cake on cold, snowy days or baked some fabulous chocolate chip cookies when you had a bad day at school, you may have come to associate those foods with comfort and warmth. So you're probably not craving the food; you're craving the feelings the food engenders! To overcome these types of psychological cravings, look for other ways to create the feelings you long for: Snuggle up next to a fire in the fireplace, wrap yourself in a blanket with a good book, or play a quiet board game with your family.

TIP

Although fighting cravings and food addiction takes a lot of effort and hard work, you can be successful by following these tips:

>> **Keep food that tempts you out of the house.** If that candy bar isn't readily available but some sweet grapes or crunchy baby carrots are, you'll be much more inclined to reach for healthy snacks when you're hungry.

>> **Go for a walk or get some exercise.** These activities stimulate the production of feel-good chemicals in your brain, which give you feelings of well-being and satisfaction.

>> **Delay satisfying your cravings for 20 minutes.** Research shows that if you can wait 20 minutes to eat what you crave, the feeling will usually subside. If you're still hungry after that period of time, have a clean and healthy snack.

>> **Take chromium supplements to help you get rid of the sugar and carb cravings.** This crave-control process can take months, but a recent controlled study found that chromium supplementation can significantly reduce carbohydrate craving and improve depression in women. However, many individuals need as many as 1,000 micrograms of supplemental chromium daily to achieve this effect. Fortunately, chromium supplementation is very safe; the Environmental Protection Agency (EPA) says that 70,000 micrograms daily is the upper limit.

>> **Have a small portion of the food you're craving, especially when you're just starting your new lifestyle.** Have a few spoonfuls of that ice cream you love rather than a bowlful and then distract yourself by partaking in a pleasant activity, such as a walk or a game. By satisfying the craving in small ways, you can head off a larger binge later.

>> **Stick with your eating clean plan and feel your cravings diminish.** When you eat clean, whole foods, you feel better and stronger and have more energy. Compare these feelings to the feelings you have after bingeing on chocolate candy or a fat-laden, heavy fast-food meal. You don't need much more motivation to stay the course!

>> **Cravings intensify when you think you're hungry, but you may just be thirsty or tired.** Have a drink of water, brush your teeth, and go to bed!

DO CRAVINGS SIGNAL NUTRIENT DEFICIENCIES?

Some people think that cravings are a sign that you're deficient in the nutrient that the food you crave provides. This theory may have some truth to it, but the types of foods that people crave usually aren't nutrient dense; they're full of sugar, fat, and salt. And you likely aren't deficient in any of those food components. Rather, if you crave sweets or chocolate, you may be deficient in nutrients like the vitamin B complex, chromium, zinc, and magnesium. But eating a chocolate bar isn't a good way to satisfy this deficiency since it contains only about 50 mg of magnesium; the recommended daily allowance (RDA) for that mineral is at least 300 mg per day. Snacking on foods like nuts, seeds, and legumes provides more of the needed minerals and other nutrients along with fiber and protein.

One real biological craving, called *pica,* is when people who are deficient in iron or other minerals crave nonnutritive things like soil, flour, raw rice, and chalk. After they fix their iron deficiency, those cravings subside. So you can't blame your craving for double chocolate chip ice cream on a calcium deficiency!

Dealing with deprivation

Human beings are complex creatures that are trained to respond to emotions by eating. When babies get hungry, they feel uncomfortable and cry; the parent responds with food and cuddles. You don't have to be a rocket scientist to see the connection that can build up between love, comfort, and food.

When you eliminate the foods you've relied on for comfort throughout your life, you're naturally going to feel deprived at first. Several factors cause feelings of deprivation, and, fortunately, you can address all of them with a clean eating plan. In Chapter 5, we discuss emotional eating and eating because of cues other than hunger, but you can feel deprived for other reasons, too.

The following list describes some of the reasons why you may feel deprived when you first start your eating clean plan and offers some tips for how to deal with those feelings:

>> **You don't consume enough calories.** Because you're eating more whole foods, more foods with fewer calories, and more fiber, you may not be getting enough calories, especially if you live a very active lifestyle. Unless you're obese and continue to gain weight, consider adding more high-calorie foods to your diet, especially foods high in protein and good fats, like lean meats, cheeses, and nuts.

- » **You eat a bland diet.** Make sure to season your food well (but not with salt!) and use condiments, herbs, and spices to keep the food interesting. Experiment with recipes from different ethnic cuisines and don't be afraid to try new foods to spice up your plate.

- » **You miss foods you're used to eating.** If you're used to eating lots of chips and dip, you don't have to eliminate those types of foods completely. Think of ways to incorporate the same flavors and textures by using clean foods. Instead of eating processed chips with a luridly orange artificially-flavored cheese dip, make some kale chips and eat them with a spiced edamame dip. Instead of eating chocolate chip cookies, have a small bar of dark chocolate, maybe chopped and sprinkled over yogurt flavored with fresh fruit. (See Chapter 18 for some delicious snack and dessert recipes.)

- » **You focus too much on food.** Food is only part of your life. Yes, you do need to eat to stay alive. But if food occupies most of your consciousness, think of ways to make it a smaller part of your life. Try to add more interest and stimulation to your daily routine. Take up a hobby. Learn something new. Make new friends and interact with other people in your life.

REMEMBER

Don't forget to be kind to yourself! You're attempting a complete life makeover, which is an honorable and responsible thing to do. Just trying something new can be very rewarding. Think about how you're really feeling and try to address emotional issues honestly without burying them in food.

Understand that you're not going to stick perfectly to this plan and resolve to enjoy the process. If you can involve your family in this new lifestyle, all the better. By getting your family and friends involved, you create a built-in support system with people who will support you in your journey to improve your life.

REMEMBER

Learn to trust your body's signals. A feeling of deprivation means your brain is trying to tell you that something isn't right. Whether you're dealing with stress or you have unresolved emotional issues, numbing yourself with food isn't the answer. Listen to your body and try different ways to soothe and tame bad feelings. Food is only the solution to hunger — nothing else.

Living with lapses and backsliding

One guarantee in any diet or lifestyle change is that you will fall off the wagon. No one can eat a perfect diet forever. Life is full of too many temptations. So accept that you won't eat clean 100 percent of the rest of your life and figure out how to deal with your lapses.

TIP

To deal with lapses and missteps, try these ideas:

» **Build lapses and breaks into your eating plan.** Aim to eat clean 50 to 70 percent of the time, especially when you're first getting started. In other words, let yourself have a few potato chips or a reasonable serving of ice cream occasionally. By doing so, you curb feelings of deprivation, which can cause backsliding. Plus, if you know that you can have a treat later in the day, you'll be more likely to pass up that tray of baked goodies at lunch.

» **Set aside some fairly clean foods that are better for you than the typical junk food.** For instance, if you find yourself craving a chewy candy bar in the afternoon, make some Dark Chocolate Bark (Chapter 18) and keep it handy for a treat. If you really enjoy a creamy, cold, sweet bowl of ice cream, sweeten some yogurt with agave nectar and fruit and freeze it for a clean treat. You have infinite possibilities for creatively satisfying cravings without reverting to old bad habits.

» **Recognize that you strayed from your clean eating plan and get back on track.** Many people simply give up when they give in to the cravings for junk food or sweets. Don't give up! Just resume your clean eating plan. Try to recognize what event or emotion triggered your lapse and write about it in a food journal (see Chapter 5 for details). Then think of ways to deal with that issue instead of turning to junk food.

After you've been on the clean eating plan for a month or two, you'll find that eating a clean diet is actually more satisfying than eating your old diet ever was. You'll feel better and have more energy. Just as you can get stuck in a vicious downward spiral of eating and craving junk, you can achieve a healthy upward spiral of eating and craving clean!

Eating Clean for a Healthier World

When you eat clean, you not only make your body healthier but also help make the world healthier for your children, grandchildren, and future generations. Yes, really! Clean foods are usually green foods, which means that they're grown with fewer potentially toxic chemicals, are produced locally, use less packaging, and produce less waste. Because producing clean, whole foods requires less energy-burning industrial processes and machinery, the *carbon footprint* of these foods, or amount of pollution produced, is smaller than that of processed foods. Eating with an eye on the environment is called *eating green*.

Sustainability is a buzzword in the clean eating movement. It means making an effort to meet the current needs of society without weakening future generations' abilities to meet their needs. Reducing packaging, pollution, and reliance on chemicals are all part of the sustainability movement. And clean foods fit right into that goal.

In this section, we look at how eating a clean diet benefits the environment. We consider the effects waste and excess packaging have on your body and the planet and explain how eating clean translates to less pollution. We look at the "cides" that eating organic foods keeps out of your body. And we examine the Meatless Monday trend, which Catholics have adhered to for centuries.

Reducing waste and packaging

Eating green enhances your clean eating lifestyle, helps you stay healthier, and has many other benefits. Because you don't have to open a package made of cardboard, cellophane, or plastic to get to the edible parts of the food you buy, you produce less garbage, which, in turn, helps reduce the amount of stuff in landfills (and the huge number of floating garbage islands in the ocean). Plus, in a few cases, less garbage may help reduce your garbage collection bill. Almost 33 percent of the waste collected in the United States comes from excess packaging. Eating a clean diet can help reduce this staggering stat and others like it.

Here are a few more shocking stats related to the amount of garbage being created today:

>> Americans throw away enough garbage every day to fill more than 60,000 garbage trucks, which equals 56 tons of trash per person per year.

>> Countries all over the world dump more than 14 billion pounds of garbage into the ocean each year. All this garbage can't be healthy for the fish or the people who eat those fish!

>> Americans throw out more than 40,000 tons of food every day.

>> Americans throw away more than 2.5 million plastic bottles and millions of glass bottles every day.

Staying local and in season

Locally grown and produced food has a smaller carbon footprint than most processed food because the food requires less effort and energy to get to your table.

The whole foods grown in your area are fresher, too. Many nutrients in harvested foods break down because of exposure to heat or light or because the foods had to sit around while being shipped for thousands of miles. Because locally grown foods are usually picked the day they're sold or the day before, you get them when they're ripe and at their peak of flavor and nutrition. No one has to treat them with preservatives and additives to keep them wholesome until they end up on your table. Plus, a tomato (or any other whole food) picked in the morning and sold to you in the afternoon doesn't need to be aseptically packaged or heat treated to keep it safe, fresh, and wholesome.

In addition to eating locally grown foods to keep your family green and healthy, you can also choose to eat only the foods that are in season in your area. Out-of-season vegetables and fruits are often tempting, but they must be either transported thousands of miles (which degrades nutrient content for you) or grown in local hothouses, which use more energy and run up energy bills.

Avoiding BPA

Another reason to avoid packaged and processed foods is that foods packed in plastic and plastic-lined cans are most likely riddled with bisphenol A (BPA). This chemical is an organic compound that mimics the function of estrogen in the body. Manufacturers use it to make shatter-proof plastic. Scientists are concerned that this chemical may affect the brain of infants and children and could be a key factor in the increasing obesity rate in the United States. BPA can increase sensitivity to the addiction centers in the brain, contributing to the spiral of junk food-craving/obesity behavior. It also has an effect on thyroid function.

PESTICIDES AND CROP YIELDS

Farmers first used pesticides, which include insecticides and fungicides, to help increase crop yields. Insects can damage crops and reduce yields, so it made sense that reducing the number of harmful insects would result in increased harvests. But scientists are finding that pesticides may actually reduce crop yields. A 2007 study published in the *Proceedings of the National Academy of Sciences* found that pesticides and herbicides have actually reduced crop yields by 33 percent. These chemicals reduce nitrogen fixation in the soil. Nitrogen is a critical component in the soil, and its reduction results in anemic plants with poor yields. Plus, some insects are becoming resistant to pesticides, which means farmers have to use more of these chemicals — and more lethal combinations of them — to be effective.

The *Journal of the American Medical Association* published a study in 2008 that found that people with higher BPA levels in their urine had higher rates of heart disease and diabetes. Most clean, whole foods aren't packed in cans or plastic, so eating clean minimizes your exposure to this chemical. If you read labels carefully, you can find BPA-free cans in some grocery stores and health food stores.

Staying away from "cides"

You don't have to go organic to eat clean, but doing so certainly doesn't hurt. Since you're reducing or eliminating exposure to artificial chemicals, preservatives, colorings, and flavorings, why not reduce or eliminate your exposure to poisons like pesticides, fungicides, and herbicides while you're at it?

Large farms use pesticides and herbicides because pulling up weeds and killing plant-eating bugs by hand is too expensive and time-consuming.

WARNING

Imported fruits and vegetables are often produced with chemicals that are banned in the United States because other countries have more lax food-safety standards. The U.S. Environmental Protection Agency (EPA) receives many complaints about the export of unregistered pesticides every year. Other countries aren't required to label the foods they export with the chemicals used to grow them, and the EPA doesn't test for these chemicals. Therefore, those grapes grown in Chile may look delicious in the grocery store, but they could contain unacceptably high amounts of toxic chemicals. So even if you don't look for organically produced foods, purchasing locally produced foods can reduce your family's exposure to harmful pesticides and herbicides.

Eating clean, organically produced foods also limits your exposure to genetically modified foods (often called *GMOs*), which are foods that have been altered in laboratories to include DNA from other plants or even animals. These alterations can pose threats to biodiversity and human health.

See Chapter 10 for more information about which foods to buy organic and which ones are still clean and safe to eat even though they aren't organic. You also find more information about GMOs in that chapter.

Meatless Monday and sustainability

Meatless Monday is a fairly new concept often mentioned on Facebook and Twitter. All it means is that one day a week you choose to eat vegetarian or vegan. Not only can Meatless Monday save money (because meats are expensive), but the plan helps the environment (because large beef, pork, and chicken facilities create nitrate pollution and generate almost 20 percent of greenhouse gas emissions that accelerate climate change). Livestock also uses a tremendous amount of precious fresh water: Every pound of beef takes around 2,000 gallons of water to produce.

So, on Mondays, think about eating meatless for breakfast, lunch, and dinner. Enjoy meals made with lots of vegetables, whole grains, beans, and cheese. Your wallet and the planet will thank you!

REMEMBER

Even if you're on a Paleo diet, you can still eat a meatless meal or two. Your body doesn't need to consume all nine of the essential amino acids every single day to stay healthy. Recipes using eggs and cheese are a good choice. Or you can just eat meals rich in veggies and nuts. Don't worry — your protein needs are still being met by your diet.

Chapter 3

Nutrition Basics: You Really Are What You Eat

Everyone has heard the phrase "you are what you eat," but did you know that it's literally true? Your body uses everything you put into it for some particular purpose: It uses proteins to build muscles and repair injuries; carbohydrates to create energy; fats to make cell membranes supple and to lubricate joints; and vitamins and minerals to keep your cells alive and healthy.

Getting the right amounts and combinations of these nutrients isn't easy. But the eating clean diet is one of the best ways to achieve the perfect balance of nutrients, calories, and taste. After all, whole foods automatically provide more nutrients, especially micronutrients, than any supplemented or enhanced processed food.

In this chapter, we look at what your body needs to perform at its peak capacity. We explain how your body uses food, and we look at what your body doesn't need. We break down the roles of proteins, carbohydrates, fats, vitamins, and minerals, and we explain how your body uses them. Finally, we show you how to find the best nutrient-dense foods to get the most bang for your buck.

Figuring Out What Your Body Needs (And What It Doesn't Need)

Without food, you would die. How long you could survive depends on your fat stores and overall health, but most people can only survive for a few months without food.

Consider this: Your body is an amazing machine. It efficiently extracts nutrients from the food you eat, processes that food, storing essential nutrients to ensure survival over a long period of time, and heals itself by using the nutrients it gets from food. In this section, we look at how your body uses food, what happens when you take in more calories than you need, and what happens when you don't get the nutrients essential to good health.

How your body uses food

Your body's digestive system breaks down everything you put into your mouth and then uses what the body needs for basic functions.

Your digestive tract includes your mouth, esophagus, stomach, intestines, rectum, and anus. Your mouth starts breaking down food, and your esophagus takes the food to your stomach, which breaks it down further. The intestines further digest and absorb nutrients, and the rectum and anus dispose of the solid material you don't need.

Other organs in the digestive tract include the liver, gallbladder, and pancreas. The liver produces bile (which is stored in the gallbladder) to aid in your body's digestion, particularly of fats and oils. The liver itself starts the process of "reassembling" fully digested food into a form useful to the human system, and it processes toxins for disposal. The pancreas produces digestive enzymes that work on fats and carbohydrates, as well as on the proteins that the stomach hasn't completely digested. A complex system of nerves, blood vessels, enzymes, and hormones keeps everything working smoothly.

From one end to the other

Here's a step-by-step look at how your body uses food:

>> **Your mouth starts the digestive process.** Your teeth break down the food you eat, and digestive enzymes from your salivary glands start to break down starch. You swallow, thus moving the food through the esophagus. Although the action of swallowing is voluntary and you control it, you give up control as the food starts moving down the esophagus. From that point on, nerves and muscles control the food's path.

» **Your stomach is the food's next stop.** A normal stomach, when empty, has a very acidic pH of 1.5 to 3.5, which makes sense because it produces hydrochloric acid (HCl) to digest your food. Depending on its dilution, hydrochloric acid can have a pH from 0 or below to 3.0. (At those concentrations, it can burn through your clothes in seconds!) With the aid of *pepsin,* a protein-digesting enzyme produced almost exclusively in the stomach, your stomach starts processing protein and, to some extent, fats, carbohydrates, and fiber. Your stomach contracts to mechanically break down the food and mix it with pepsin. The stomach's muscle movements also move the food into the small intestine.

» **Your small intestine continues the digestive process.** Enzymes from the pancreas and bile from the liver and gallbladder enter the small intestine to digest the food as it leaves the stomach.

The small intestine absorbs many nutrients through small fingerlike projections called *villi* and even smaller projections called *microvilli.* These projections increase the surface area of the intestine so that your body can quickly and efficiently absorb nutrients into the bloodstream. Any food that your body can't digest in the small intestine goes onto the large intestine.

» **The blood that has absorbed nutrients from your small intestine goes to the liver.** The liver acts as a processing plant by filtering out harmful toxins. It then reassembles some of the digested nutrients and passes them on to the rest of your body, where your cells use them for energy and tissue repair and replacement.

» **Your large intestine is the final step on the digestive journey.** Fiber, water, bacteria, and other foods your body can't or won't digest travel through the large intestine, which is your body's last chance to retrieve nutrients from the food you ate. Your body expels whatever's left.

The macronutrients of food

The three main components, or *macronutrients,* that make up food are carbohydrates, proteins, and fats (including oils). Your body uses each component in different ways. (For more about these nutrients, see the later section "Considering the Roles of Proteins, Carbs, and Fats.")

» **Carbohydrates:** Your body uses carbohydrates for energy. It breaks them down into individual sugars, which your cells then transform into energy. A very small proportion of the carbohydrates you consume aren't used for energy.

» **Proteins:** Your body uses proteins for repair and muscle function. It breaks them down into amino acids, which the body then uses to repair cells, improve muscle function, and make certain hormones that originate from cholesterol, neurotransmitters, and enzymes.

>> **Fats:** Fats are an essential component in every diet because they provide your body with energy, heat, and essential fatty acids. Plus, your body stores fat to fight against future starvation.

Your body uses vitamins and minerals to process macronutrients and to regulate growth and metabolism. These substances promote health by increasing efficiency of cell repair and production. They also prevent illness and keep your body running at maximum efficiency. (See the later sections "Getting the Vitamins You Need to Stay Healthy" and "Incorporating Minerals into Your Daily Diet" for more details.)

What happens to additives and chemicals

Eating processed foods means consuming preservatives, additives, and artificial ingredients. What happens to these chemicals? How does your body process them?

Put bluntly, your body isn't designed to process and incorporate preservatives, additives, stabilizers, and other artificial ingredients. Because many of these ingredients are fat–soluble, your body stores them in its fat instead of using them for energy or cell repair. Unfortunately, however, they don't just sit benignly in your body's fat. They can change cell structure and metabolize. Some even become carcinogens, which can, over time, cause cancer.

Here are just some of the artificial ingredients used in processed foods, along with a quick summary of what happens to them after they enter the body:

>> **Antibiotics:** Farmers feed many animals, particularly poultry and pigs, antibiotics to reduce the death rate from infection, which occurs in very crowded conditions, and to enhance growth and weight gain. The residues of these chemicals remain in the processed meat that humans eat. Overuse of antibiotics creates super bacteria that evolve to resist every antibiotic, which, as you can imagine, isn't good for the human population. Unfortunately, consuming small amounts of antibiotics in food is the best way to help these superbugs evolve. Antibiotic-resistant bacteria are becoming a huge problem in the medical field. There may come a day when a simple cut or scrape could lead to a life-threatening infection we can no longer treat.

>> **Aspartame:** This artificial sweetener becomes a neurotransmitter during digestion, meaning that it can cross the blood-brain barrier. After it crosses that barrier, it can damage and kill brain cells. The body quickly processes aspartame and breaks it down into methanol, which the body can then

convert into formaldehyde. This particular conversion can cause changes in cell structure, leading to disease and chronic health conditions.

TIP

Anecdotal evidence has revealed that aspartame is a good ant poison. When this product is damp, often — but not always — ants will carry it back to the nest, and within a few days, all the ants disappear.

Aspartame accounts for more than 75 percent of the adverse reactions to food additives reported to the FDA. Many of these reactions are very serious, including seizures and death. A few of the 90 documented symptoms listed in the FDA adverse reaction reports include

- Breathing difficulties
- Depression, anxiety attacks, fatigue, and irritability
- Dizziness
- Headaches/migraines
- Hearing loss
- Heart palpitations
- Insomnia
- Joint pain
- Memory loss
- Muscle spasms
- Nausea
- Rashes
- Seizures
- Tachycardia
- Vision problems
- Weight gain

» **Caffeine:** Caffeine is a quickly processed and relatively safe psycho-active stimulant, which is why so many people consume it in the morning. It raises your blood pressure and blocks adenosine receptors in your brain, thus reducing drowsiness. It also increases dopamine production, stimulating your brain's pleasure centers and reinforcing feelings of addiction. Caffeine is a *diuretic,* which means it removes water (as well as minerals such as calcium, zinc, and magnesium) from your blood and cells. But with long-term caffeine use, this diuretic effect lessens or disappears completely.

» **High-fructose corn syrup (HFCS):** The body partially processes this chemically concentrated sugar and stores it as fat. In fact, the body metabolizes it into fat very quickly. High-fructose corn syrup doesn't suppress the body's production of *ghrelin,* a molecule that stimulates the appetite, so your brain doesn't get the message that you've eaten enough food. Plus, the liver converts high-fructose corn syrup into triglycerides, which, when present in excess, can increase the risk of heart disease.

>> **Hormones:** Most factory farms feed hormones and *pseudo-hormones* (unnatural molecules that imperfectly mimic real human hormones) to the animals they raise for meat so that they grow bigger faster. The animals store the chemicals in their fat, which humans then eat. These hormones and pseudo-hormones can affect human growth and development. For example, too much estrogen and pseudo-estrogen increases breast and prostate cancer risk.

>> **Monosodium glutamate (MSG):** This ubiquitous additive, which is also known as *free glutamic acid,* is present in many processed foods and affects the body in many ways, including the following:

- MSG is an *excitotoxin,* which means it overstimulates and damages brain cells.

- MSG may be addictive, so you may crave foods that have MSG and eat more of them, creating a vicious cycle.

- MSG stimulates the umami taste bud, fooling your body into thinking that the food you're eating is nutritious.

- MSG changes the diameter of your blood vessels, which is why some people feel warm and develop headaches after ingesting it.

- MSG stimulates the pancreas, causing it to produce more insulin, so blood sugar levels drop and you get hungry sooner.

- MSG intake has been implicated in the development and exacerbation of diseases such as Parkinson's, multiple sclerosis, stroke, obesity, and depression.

MSG does occur naturally in meats and other foods, but it's bound up in the protein complexes of those foods and has less of an effect than the added MSG.

>> **Nitrates and nitrites:** These chemicals are used in processed meats such as hot dogs and bacon. They can bind with *hemoglobin,* the molecule in your blood that carries oxygen throughout your body, thus causing dizziness, headaches, and rapid heartbeat. Your liver converts nitrates into *nitrosamines,* which are carcinogenic in animals and probably humans, too. Nitrites are carcinogenic in humans.

>> **Olestra:** You find this artificial fat in snack foods. At first, snack-food manufac- turers touted olestra as a simple way to lose weight because the body doesn't

digest it, meaning that it travels right through the body. Unfortunately, this indigestible property causes some severe and unpleasant physical reactions, which can keep you chained to the bathroom. Plus, the fake fat binds to fat-soluble vitamins your body needs and takes them right out of your body.

>> **Trans fats:** These fake fats, made by hydrogenating polyunsaturated fats such as corn oil, are one of the most dangerous artificial ingredients. They raise your risk of heart attack, stroke, diabetes, high blood pressure, and cancer.

Because your body doesn't recognize that trans fats are artificial, they become part of your cell membranes, making the cells weaker. Consuming trans fats increases the level of LDL cholesterol (the bad stuff) in your blood. Your body easily stores trans fats but can't easily retrieve them for fuel, so they cause weight gain.

Keep in mind that the FDA says most of these ingredients are safe for human consumption, at least in tiny amounts. (A big change on the regulation of trans fats happened in 2015.) After all, some of them do help preserve food, keeping it safe for long storage periods and long transit times from the factory to the grocery store. But knowing what you know now, you can be the judge of what you want to ingest. Just remember that whole foods don't need artificial chemicals to stay safe, look better, or taste better.

One of the best things about the eating clean plan is that you avoid processed foods, chemicals, and additives that can harm your body, and you eat whole foods, which contain all the protein, fat, carbohydrates, vitamins, and minerals that your body needs, in the correct amounts and proportions.

What happens to excess macronutrients and calories

It's too bad your body doesn't discard the excess carbs, protein, fat, and calories you consume like it discards waste, fiber, and too much liquid. Human bodies evolved to hang on to fuel simply because starvation was part of life for early humans. If you eat only once a week or once a month, your body will hold on to all the calories it can as a hedge against starvation. Of course, now that you have 24-hour supermarkets and pizza delivery, starvation is the least of your worries.

Your body is extremely efficient. It extracts and uses the energy it needs from the food you eat and converts the excess into fat, which it then stores in your body. Too many calories equal excess fat. But all calories are not equal (the laws of thermodynamics aside). After all, human bodies aren't machines made out of metal and moving parts; every body is different. For example, simple carbs and sugars trigger insulin responses in the body, which tell it to store fat. In some people, this response is very easy to trigger; as a result, a high-carbohydrate diet makes them put on weight. On the other hand, for most people, the body has to work harder to digest proteins than it does to digest carbs, which means they gain less weight on a high-protein diet.

Understanding how your body processes excess nutrients

When you consume too many carbohydrates, proteins, and fats, your body processes the excess nutrients in different ways:

» **Carbohydrates:** The body breaks down carbohydrates into glucose, which it then uses for fuel. The body converts excess glucose into glycogen and sends it to muscles and the liver. If your body has too much glycogen, your liver converts it into fat and stores it in fat cells.

» **Proteins:** The body processes proteins into individual amino acids and peptides, which your liver sends into your bloodstream to maintain and repair cells, and make some hormones, neurotransmitters, and enzymes. The body converts excess proteins into fat and stores it in fat cells.

» **Fats:** The body breaks down fats into fatty acids, cholesterol, glycerol, and triglycerides in a process called *lipolysis*. Because fats are a rich source of energy, the body uses them in cell production. Oils are also fats; they contain fatty acids that the body uses in the metabolism process to keep your cells healthy and strong and to help move oxygen through your bloodstream. Some fatty acids (omega-3 and omega-6) are essential nutrients. The body stores excess fat and oil as fat (go figure!).

REMEMBER

You can eat too much of each of these macronutrients. For example, if you consume too much protein and not enough carbohydrates, you put stress on your kidneys and throw your body into ketosis — when your body burns fat rather than carbs for energy. The strain on your kidneys can lead to kidney disease, kidney stones, osteoporosis, and eventually ketoacidosis, a condition that's dangerous for diabetics. In addition, too much protein can cause gout in some people. Consuming high-fructose corn syrup can induce higher levels of uric acid, which also leads to gout. Researchers are finding that higher levels of uric acid are particularly damaging to the kidneys.

Eating too many carbohydrates can be problematic for most people. Compared with individuals who do *not* have a genetic predisposition to type-2 diabetes (approximately two-thirds of all Americans), individuals with this genetic predisposition (the other one-third) have considerably more insulin secretion after eating the very same amount of carbohydrates. This "over-the-top" insulin secretion leads to insulin resistance. To overcome this resistance, even more insulin is secreted, which leads to even more insulin resistance. This never ending loop ultimately "crosses over" to type-2 diabetes, with its higher risk of further complications including heart disease, kidney failure, and many others.

People *without* the genetic predisposition to type-2 diabetes will still gain excess weight when they consume too many carbohydrates, but have much less chance of actually developing type-2 diabetes with all its possible complications.

Eating too much fat can lead to obesity, which puts strain on your organs and bones and can lead to diseases like heart disease, cancer, diabetes, and arthritis. Some people, however, can eat as much fat as they want on the Paleo diet and still lose weight, if they have a certain metabolism that predisposes them to type-2 diabetes. Read more about this in Chapter 5.

REMEMBER

When you eat clean, you eat whole foods that contain good proportions of fat, carbs, protein, vitamins, minerals, and fiber. Whole foods take longer to eat and digest, which means you feel satisfied longer. As a result, you're less likely to overeat and your body's energy input and output stay in balance, keeping you at a healthy weight.

Examining the connection between excess calories and weight gain

If you eat the same number of calories that you burn, your weight stays the same. If you don't take in enough calories, you lose weight. And if you eat more calories than your body burns, you gain weight. Seems pretty straightforward, right?

As with many so-called rules, you need to consider some exceptions. For instance, for people with type-2 diabetes and people whose families have a history of this disease (about 36 percent of the population), eating large amounts of proteins, fats, and oils and very few, if any, calories from carbohydrates can lead to weight loss — which is why high-protein/low-carb diets are so popular, and why those 36 percent should follow this diet for better health. Read more about this in Chapter 5 on the Paleo diet, and learn if you should follow that plan.

But these diets are very acid-forming, causing your blood pH to lower and forcing your body to take calcium from bones and teeth, thus leading to the development of gout or osteoporosis. For these reasons, be sure to work with a physician who is knowledgeable in nutritional and natural medicine before you try a low-carb diet.

Each pound of fat contains 3,500 calories. To lose a pound of fat a week, you need to burn 500 more calories a day or eat 500 fewer calories a day. The number of calories you need in a day depends on your sex, age, weight, and activity level. Younger people, men, and more active people need more calories. Older people, women, and people who lead more sedentary lifestyles need fewer calories.

SO WHAT'S A CALORIE?

So what is this ubiquitous calorie? Here's the scientific definition: A *calorie* is the energy needed to raise the temperature of 1 cm^3 of water by 1 degree Celsius. In other words, a calorie is stored energy. Your body stores energy in the form of fat, which your body keeps in fat cells for quick access if needed. Your body converts the fat to glucose, which your cells use to create energy.

The macronutrients you consume have different numbers of calories per gram:

- Proteins have four calories per gram.
- Carbohydrates have four calories per gram.
- Fats have nine calories per gram.

Your body uses calories (or energy) to

» **Keep you alive:** Respiration, brain function, and muscle activity all require energy. Just being alive burns up a certain number of calories every day. The specific number of calories burned varies from person to person and is called your *basic metabolic rate,* or BMR. People with so-called high metabolisms usually have less efficient bodies that burn up more calories than most just to stay alive.

» **Repair damage:** Cells in your body die every day, and your body must replace them. You need energy to make new cells. You also need energy to repair or discard cells that free radicals and oxidation damage.

» **Keep you active:** Even sleeping and resting require energy. But if you move around, run, or exercise, your body uses more energy. You burn calories through metabolism to provide energy to your cells so you can move your muscles.

What happens if you don't get the micronutrients you need

Did you know that you can be overweight and malnourished at the same time? Overweight people don't lack access to macronutrients (proteins, carbs, and fats); they lack access to micronutrients — vitamins and minerals. A serious deficiency in some micronutrients can lead directly to disease. For example, beriberi develops when you don't get enough vitamin B1 in your diet, and scurvy can develop when you don't get enough vitamin C. A minor deficiency in micronutrients can lead to conditions such as high blood pressure, depression, and a weakened immune system.

Here are just a few things micronutrients (vitamins and minerals) do for your body:

>> Help maintain a proper oxygen level in your brain

>> Fight *free radicals,* which are unstable forms of oxygen that damage cells

>> Keep your red blood cells healthy so that they can transport oxygen to your body's cells

>> Keep your nerve cells healthy so that your body can react to stimuli and stay healthy and so that you can maintain a regular heartbeat and calm mood

>> Regulate your hormone balance so that diseases such as diabetes don't develop

>> Keep bones and teeth healthy by regulating calcium and phosphorus balance

>> Create and maintain enzymes so that your body can digest food and transform it into energy and cell components

REMEMBER

By eating whole foods, especially fruits and vegetables, you can provide your body with the micronutrients it needs, including the micronutrients no one knows about! Scientists don't know every single micronutrient your body needs. But whole foods contain them, in just the right proportions. And organically grown foods contain even more of these nutrients.

FOOD DESERTS (THINK HOT SAND, NOT CAKE AND PIE)

In the United States, nutritionists are discovering that literal food deserts exist in certain areas of the country, especially in inner cities. A *food desert* is a geographical area where few healthy whole foods are available. Many poor urban areas just don't have supermarkets that offer fresh produce and other wholesome foods. Instead, fast-food joints, pizza parlors, and convenience stores proliferate in those areas. For people who live there, the easiest way to satisfy hunger is by buying a burger for 99 cents; they don't have the time or money to travel miles to a supermarket where fresh food is available, purchase that more expensive food, and then travel home to cook it. These areas are rich in macronutrients but starved for micronutrients, and the people living there can be overweight and malnourished.

Missing out on micronutrients hurts your body. Diseases may not develop for months or years, but they will develop. Providing your body with a constant supply of vital micronutrients is one of the best ways to get healthy and stay healthy.

Considering the Roles of Proteins, Carbs, and Fats

All food is made up of proteins, carbohydrates, and fats. These macronutrients provide energy for your body, building blocks for cell maintenance and repair, and compounds such as hormones and enzymes that help your cells function properly.

In this section, we look at the composition of proteins, carbs, and fats and explain why you need all of them in your diet. We also look at what roles the macronutrients play in your body's function and show you how to find the best clean sources for each one.

Clean proteins: Amino acids, the building blocks of life

Proteins should comprise about 30 percent of your diet. (But if you have type-2 diabetes or you're overweight and type-2 diabetes runs in your family, you may need to eat more protein in a diet such as the Paleolithic diet; talk to your doctor for details.)

Proteins are made up of *amino acids*, which are individual molecules that are literally the building blocks of your body. Amino acids come in dozens of varieties. Nine of them are called *essential amino acids*, meaning that you must get them from a food source because your body can't make them — not even from other amino acids. The Protein Digestibility Corrected Amino Acid Score (PDCAAS) evaluates the quality of protein sources and the body's ability to digest them. Eggs have a score of 100 on this scale, which means they're a perfect source of protein.

As your body breaks down food, the proteins travel to the liver, which converts them into amino acids. The body uses these amino acids to build and repair tissue, provide energy, and produce enzymes, neurotransmitters, and certain hormones. If you don't eat enough protein, your body will start to break down the protein in your muscles to use for cell repair and other functions. You don't need to combine proteins at every meal, but you should try to combine proteins over a week.

Most Americans get more than enough protein. Unless you're an elderly person who doesn't eat enough or you have a special dietary need, or you have significant low stomach acid and don't digest enough protein into enough amino acids, you don't need protein supplements or shakes to get the protein your body requires. And people with hidden gluten sensitivity don't absorb enough amino acids for good health. Clean protein comes from meats, dairy, eggs, and whole foods such as whole grains, legumes, nuts, seeds, and beans. On the clean eating plan, you consume the right amount of good-quality protein.

Complete proteins: Everything you need

Some foods contain *complete proteins*, which are proteins that contain all nine essential amino acids. These foods include

>> Meat, such as beef, chicken, fish, lamb, pork, and shellfish

>> Dairy products, such as cheese, milk, and yogurt

>> Quinoa, soybeans, and amaranth, which are complete proteins that may have a score of less than 100 on the PDCAAS

>> Eggs, which are an excellent source of protein, in terms of both value and digestibility

If you eat these protein sources, you don't have to worry about whether you're getting enough protein because you definitely are. But if you eat a vegetarian or vegan diet, eating the right kind of protein is something you need to think about. This is easy to remember: Just eat all the plant foods available to you, including vegetables, fruits, nuts, seeds, and legumes.

Incomplete proteins: Combining to get what you need

Foods that don't contain all nine essential proteins are called *incomplete proteins*. If you don't eat enough complete proteins, you need to combine different incomplete proteins (making them *complementary proteins*) to get the essential amino acids your body needs. Here are the incomplete proteins you need to eat:

>> **Grains and legumes:** Eat a meal of vegetarian lentil soup with whole-grain bread or a meal of beans with rice.

>> **Grains and nuts or seeds:** Consume whole-grain breads with almond or peanut butter.

>> **Legumes and nuts or seeds:** Eat chickpeas with walnuts, blended together into hummus.

Carbohydrates: Energy for your body

You hear a lot of buzz about carbohydrates (or *carbs*, as they're often called) in the media these days. Proponents of high-protein diets claim that carbs are bad for you. Well, eating too much of any one food component is bad for you, but carbohydrates in and of themselves aren't bad. In fact, carbohydrates should comprise about 40 to 50 percent of your diet (less, in fat, much less if you're concerned about type-2 diabetes and should follow the Paleo diet plan).

Carbohydrates come in two types: complex and simple. *Complex carbohydrates* are the kind you want to include in your diet. They're long chains made up of *simple carbohydrates* (or sugars), such as glucose, sucrose, lactose, and fructose.

You find complex carbohydrates in the following foods:

>> Whole grains, such as wheat, barley, buckwheat, oats, quinoa, brown rice, wild rice, and amaranth

>> Vegetables, such as carrots, potatoes, corn, cabbage, asparagus, cauliflower, dark greens, zucchini, broccoli, celery, cucumbers, garlic, and onions

>> Fruits, such as apples, grapefruit, pears, strawberries, plums, oranges, berries, and dried fruits

>> Legumes, such as pinto beans, chickpeas, lentils, kidney beans, and split peas

Focus on these foods when you're planning the carbohydrate part of your diet. Because they've been minimally processed (and fit into the eating clean lifestyle!), they offer more to your body than simple carbohydrates. For example, complex carbohydrates provide fiber, vitamin B, and minerals, such as iron, magnesium, and selenium. Plus, your body digests them slowly, which can help stabilize your blood sugar levels. Fortunately, whole foods included in the clean eating plan contain lots of complex carbohydrates.

Unlike complex carbohydrates, simple carbohydrates raise blood sugar quickly and provide instant energy, especially in those genetically pre-disposed to type-2 diabetes. However, the quick spike of energy you get from foods with simple carbs soon leads to a slump in blood glucose, which means you get hungry quickly, your mood drops, and your energy lags. Foods that contain simple carbohydrates include the following:

>> Table sugar

>> Corn syrup and other syrups

>> Fruit juices

>> Candy

- » Sweetened beverages such as pop and soda
- » White rice and pasta
- » Baked goods made with white sugar and white flour
- » Sweetened processed cereals

REMEMBER

Always read the labels on food packages! Foods high in simple carbs are usually also highly processed and contain additives and preservatives (which means you need to avoid them if you're eating clean). Be sure to avoid any product that contains added simple carb ingredients like glucose, fructose, dextrin, maltodextrin, galactose, maltose, or anything with the suffix *-ose*.

Although complex carbohydrates are made up of chains of simple carbohydrates, the foods that contain complex carbohydrates also have fiber and lots of vitamins and minerals. You don't find fiber, B vitamins, and potassium in a lemon drop! But you do find those nutrients in a slice of whole-wheat bread.

Essential and clean fats

Fats are the third macronutrient in food. Despite the popularity of low-fat diets, you need to incorporate essential fats (omega-3 and omega-6 fatty acids) into your daily diet. In fact, fat should comprise about 30 percent of your diet. Many nutritionists recommend eating a diet higher in protein, higher in fat, and lower in carbs.

Fats provide the following benefits to your body:

- » Provide insulation and padding for your organs and skeletal system
- » Aid in metabolism and become part of your cellular structures
- » Aid in growth and reproduction
- » Allow the fat-soluble vitamins (A, D, E, and K) to travel through your body

But the type of fat you eat is important. You need to avoid trans fats and restrict the amount of saturated fats you eat (the following section explains why). To get the most benefits from the fats you eat, stick with the clean fats you find in foods such as nuts, avocados, olive oil, fatty seafood, and seeds.

Taking a look at what fats are made of

Fats consist of chains of fatty acids and glycerol. The fatty acids have long chains of carbon atoms bound to hydrogen atoms. They're classified according to the number of hydrogen atoms attached to the carbon atoms. If a fat is missing a hydrogen atom, it uses a double bond to join two carbon atoms and to replace the hydrogen atom.

The three kinds of fats are

>> **Saturated fats:** When all the carbon atoms in the fatty acid chain are paired with hydrogen atoms, the fat is *saturated*. Saturated fats are solid at room temperature. They include butter, hydrogenated shortening (note the name — hydrogen is added to oil to make it solid), and animal fats.

>> **Monounsaturated fats:** These fats have one double bond in their fatty acid chain. They're liquid at room temperature. Monounsaturated fats occur in avocados, olives, coconuts, and nuts, especially macadamia nuts. These stable fats are the best for your health.

>> **Polyunsaturated fats:** These fats have two or more double bonds in their fatty acid structures. They're liquid at room temperature. Polyunsaturated fats come from vegetable sources and include sunflower, safflower, and corn oil. (Canola oil is also polyunsaturated, but you should avoid eating it because it comes from a genetically modified, or GMO, plant. For more about GMO foods, see Chapter 10.) The problem with polyunsaturated fats is that they're unstable and can easily oxidize, causing inflammation in the body.

Getting more omega-3s and fewer omega-6s

Like the essential amino acids that are so important to your body's health, essential fatty acids play an important role in your body. Essential fatty acids consist of a straight chain of hydrocarbons with a carboxyl group on one end. They're classified by their length and by where the double bond, which is a bond between carbon atoms in molecules, exists in their chain.

>> *Omega-3 fatty acids* have the double bond in the number 3 position and include alpha-linolenic acid (ALA), eicosapentaenoic acid (EPA), and docosahexaenoic acid (DHA).

>> *Omega-6 fatty acids* have the double bond in the number 6 position and include linolenic acid (LA) and gamma-linolenic acid (GLA).

You must consume these nutrients in the food you eat because your body can't make them on its own. Your body can manufacture omega-9 (with the double bond in the number 9 position) as long as you consume enough omega-3 and omega-6 fatty acids. You need to keep these different fatty acids straight because the ratio of fatty acids in your diet is crucial to good health. Fatty acids play a role in the following bodily processes:

>> Functioning of the central nervous system — brain, nerve endings, and spinal column — which can help prevent depression and other mental problems

>> Production of hormones called *eicosanoids,* which monitor and regulate the activity of your cells

>> Regulation of insulin sensitivity, which can help prevent diabetes

>> Production of prostaglandins, which regulate your heart beat, blood pressure, clotting, and immune system

>> Increasing HDL cholesterol (the good stuff) and reducing LDL cholesterol (the bad stuff) in your blood

REMEMBER

The tricky part about fatty acids is that the ratio of omega-3s to omega-6s in your diet plays a critical role in your health. Nutritionists say that you should consume these two fatty acids in a ratio from 1:1 to 1:4 (omega-3s:omega-6s). But most American diets consist of foods that place the omega-3s:omega-6s ratio at 1:25. This unbalanced ratio may be a prime cause of many of the diseases that affect today's population.

In ancient times, the Paleolithic men and women ate a diet that included meats and fish, both of which are high in omega-3 fatty acids. Even though their lifespans were shorter (roaming wild animals and no antibiotics certainly played a part in this fact), they had fewer diseases like heart disease and cancer.

As civilization developed, grains, such as corn and wheat, became the basis of much of the human diet. Even the animals humans use for meat today are fed corn and wheat rather than the grasses they eat naturally. And guess what? Those foods are higher in omega-6 fatty acids. The modern diet of processed foods, especially highly refined carbohydrates, is messing with the essential fatty acid ratio necessary for good health.

If you consume too many omega-6s in relation to omega-3s, your body develops inflammation much more quickly and easily. When you consume too many omega-6s, your body breaks them down into compounds that destroy proteins and promote inflammation.

The foods that are higher in omega-3 fatty acids include

>> Fatty fish, including salmon, tuna, krill, and mackerel

>> Seeds, such as flaxseed and sesame seeds

» Nuts, such as walnuts, Brazil nuts, and pistachios

» Dark-green vegetables, including broccoli, collard greens, and spinach

» Legumes, such as kidney beans and navy beans

The foods that are higher in omega-6 fatty acids include

» Refined vegetable oils, including corn, soybean, and cottonseed oil

» Meats from animals fed a diet high in corn and wheat

» Foods cooked in vegetable oils

» Processed foods, including commercially fried foods and frozen foods

» Fast foods

TIP

When choosing the types of fats you consume, try to include more foods rich in omega-3 fatty acids. (The American diet is rich in omega-6 fatty acids, so you don't have to worry about not getting enough of that particular type of fat.) To get enough omega-3 fatty acids, many people consume fish oil supplements (which we recommend!). But if you follow the eating clean diet plan, you'll automatically reduce your intake of many of the foods high in omega-6 fatty acids and increase your intake of omega-3s. As a side note, older men should avoid consuming too much flaxseed because excess omega-3 fatty acids from plant sources (not from fish) can increase the risk of prostate cancer.

Getting the Vitamins and Minerals You Need to Stay Healthy

The right amount of carbohydrates, fats, and proteins keeps your body running and helps it repair cells. But how exactly do they do so? The answer is vitamins and minerals. Where macronutrients are the fuel your body needs to work properly, micronutrients (that is, vitamins and minerals) are the workers that help your metabolism go.

Your body can't manufacture vitamins or minerals, so you need to get them in the foods you consume. Eating whole foods is the perfect way to get just the right amount of these valuable micronutrients.

In this section, we look at what role vitamins and minerals play in your body, which are important to good health, the recommended daily allowance (RDA) for each, and which foods are the richest in these micronutrients.

Recommended daily allowances and reference intakes

The government has set minimum amounts of nutrients you need every day to prevent disease; these amounts are called *recommended daily allowances* (RDAs). The government established these numbers during World War II when the government found that many recruits for the army and navy were malnourished. You see RDA numbers on the labels of supplements and on many foods.

Another important nutrient-related number, or set of numbers, is the *DRI*, which stands for *dietary reference intakes*. The National Academy of Sciences developed the DRI in 1997 to address some nutritional concerns, such as the amount of non-essential nutrients everyone needs to consume and the safe upper limits of supplements. The Department of Agriculture is currently reviewing the DRI to see whether it should replace the RDA. The DRI includes the following four numbers:

- >> **Recommended daily allowance (RDA):** The amount of nutrients that 98 percent of healthy adults need to meet their dietary needs

- >> **Adequate intake (AI):** The recommended daily amount of nutrients that have no established RDA

- >> **Tolerable upper levels (UL):** The maximum amount of nutrients (such as fat-soluble vitamins) that can be harmful when taken in large doses

- >> **Estimated average requirement (EAR):** The amount of nutrients that meets the needs of 50 percent of a population

Don't worry if you're not much for numbers. Unless you're a dietician, you really don't need to know any of these terms except the RDA. Just remember that the RDA values are set at a minimum value necessary to prevent diseases, including scurvy and rickets. For optimum health, you probably need more than the RDA in many circumstances. Check with a physician skilled and knowledgeable in natural medicine if you're uncertain. Also, the RDA values are set for healthy adults. If you're ill, you need more vitamins.

REMEMBER

The best way to get plenty of nutrients is, of course, to eat whole foods in a good variety. But you may want to supplement your diet with vitamins and minerals. In that case, you also need to know the UL values so that you don't get sick from vitamin or mineral overdose.

The role of vitamins

Vitamins play a key role in metabolism: They assist the enzymes that break down the macronutrients you eat so that your body can use them. They also assist in building new molecules in our bodies. Without vitamins, you would die. And although a lack of vitamins can cause disease, too many of some types of vitamins can also be harmful to your health.

The two kinds of vitamins are water-soluble and fat-soluble. Each type plays a different role in metabolism, growth, and repair. The following sections explain these two types of vitamins in more detail.

REMEMBER

Regardless of which type of vitamins you consume, try to get as many of them as you can through whole foods because they're the most *bioavailable* (or most easily absorbed) in that form. Supplements can be a good idea, but look for natural, not synthetic, supplements to avoid chemicals, colorings, and preservatives.

Note: Vitamins are present in whole foods and vegetables in very small amounts, but these small amounts are crucial to good health. They're measured in milligrams (mg; 1/1,000 of a gram), micrograms (mcg; 1/1,000,000 of a gram), or International Units (IU). An IU is the amount of a vitamin that produces a biological effect.

Water-soluble vitamins

You find *water-soluble vitamins* in plants and animals. Your body doesn't store them, so you must consume them in one form or another every day. They include

>> **Vitamin C:** You find this vitamin, which is also called *ascorbic acid,* in citrus fruits and other fresh fruits and vegetables. You should consume a minimum of 45 mg of vitamin C every day to prevent *scurvy,* a vitamin-deficiency disease that results in weakness, rough skin, paleness, and bleeding gums. Your body uses vitamin C to produce *collagen,* a connective tissue that's found throughout your body in skin, bones, muscles, tendons, and blood vessels. Vitamin C helps speed up wound healing and acts as an antioxidant against free radicals that can cause cancer, stroke, and heart disease. It also helps detoxify.

Textbooks of genetics and pediatrics often point out that the human need for vitamin C results from a genetic defect we all share. Check with a doctor skilled and knowledgeable in natural medicine for a recommendation about what amount of vitamin C is best for optimal health for you.

>> **B-Complex vitamins:** This collection of vitamins includes B1, B2, B3, B5, B6, B12, folate, and biotin. You find these vitamins in fish, meat, poultry, fresh vegetables, and whole grains — just the foods you eat on the clean eating plan! Your body uses B-complex vitamins to metabolize carbohydrates, proteins, and fats so that your organs can run properly. These vitamins are particularly important to the health of your brain, heart, liver, and kidneys. They also help form healthy blood cells, minimize the risk of depression, and prevent birth defects. The amount of B vitamins you need varies throughout life.

Your body uses B-complex vitamins quickly when you're ill or under stress, so you need to make sure you get enough of them on a daily basis. Deficiency in vitamin B3 (niacin) causes *pellagra,* which manifests as skin lesions, weakness, confusion, and sensitivity to sunlight. Deficiency in vitamin B1 (thiamine) contributes to *beriberi,* which can cause heart failure.

Water-soluble vitamins are sensitive to light and heat. So look for vitamin containers that are dark colored and store your vitamins in a cool, dark place. Also try to consume uncooked foods that are high in these vitamins.

Fat-soluble vitamins

You find *fat-soluble vitamins* in fruits and vegetables, dairy products, nuts, and meats. Your body can store these vitamins in your fat cells and your liver, and they need fat to carry them to your intestine, where they're absorbed. You can skip a day or two with these vitamins, but for the best health, try to consume some fat-soluble vitamins every day. The fat-soluble vitamins include

>> **Vitamin A:** You find a precursor to this vitamin in brightly colored fruits and vegetables, such as sweet potatoes, cantaloupe, and carrots. But you find actual vitamin A in beef liver, fortified dairy products, cheese, and eggs. Vitamin A helps protect your eyesight and keeps your gastrointestinal tract running smoothly. It also aids in bone and tooth strength and growth, and promotes estrogen production in women and testosterone in men. You need a minimum of 4,000 to 5,000 IU of Vitamin A every day. More than this amount is often useful to reduce the chances of catching a cold or the flu. Check with a physician skilled and knowledgeable in nutritional medicine about what might be good for you.

>> **Vitamin D:** This vitamin is often added to dairy products, and you find it in oily fish and eggs (though the amount in eggs is very small). It's also called the *sunshine vitamin* because your body produces a vitamin D precursor in your skin when it's exposed to sunlight (without sunscreen). Vitamin D helps keep your bones and teeth strong and helps your body absorb calcium and phosphorus, two essential minerals. If you don't get enough vitamin D, you can develop *rickets,* a disease in which your bones become fragile and bend. Research in the last two decades has found that vitamin D also reduces risk of breast, prostate, and colon cancers. Research has also found that higher levels of vitamin D are associated with lower risks of dying of anything (technically called *all-cause mortality*) with the exception of trauma.

The best way to get vitamin D is to get some sun exposure every day. In climates where getting plenty of sun exposure isn't possible, take a supplement every day. For the best health, children need a minimum of 800 to 1,000 IU daily, and adults need a minimum of 2,000 to 3,000 IU daily. Check with a physician skilled and knowledgeable in natural medicine to determine what amount is best for you.

>> **Vitamin E:** You find this vitamin in dark leafy greens and vegetables, nuts, whole grains, butter, eggs, and beef liver. Vitamin E helps protect the other vitamins and fatty acids from oxidation and free radicals. As an antioxidant, it's important to cell health. You need a minimum of 10 to 15 IU of Vitamin E every day, but in many cases, 100 IU or more is best for optimal health. In fact, many physicians skilled in natural and nutritional medicine recommend 300 to 400 IU daily. Talk to your doctor about how much Vitamin E is right for you.

Vitamin E is actually four very similar molecules, termed alpha-, beta-, delta-, and gamma-tocopherols. When together in a supplement (as they are in nature) they're collectively called *mixed tocopherols* and should always be taken together. Research shows that taking alpha-tocopherol alone can actually increase certain health risks.

>> **Vitamin K:** Vitamin K has two natural types: K1 and K2. K2 has several subtypes, the best known at present being MK4 and MK7. You get all the natural types of vitamin K by eating leafy dark-green vegetables, and you find both vitamins K1 and K2 in beef liver. Friendly bacteria in your intestine makes one type of vitamin K2, and you find another form of vitamin K2 in meat and animal protein. Vitamin K is essential to efficient blood clotting and strong bones. Without enough vitamin K, you'll bruise easily and bleed profusely when your skin is cut, and in extreme cases, you can hemorrhage to death. You need a minimum of 80 mcg of vitamin K every day.

The role of minerals

When nutritionists talk about *minerals*, they don't mean chunks of iron or rock salt. They mean the chemical elements, or micronutrients, that are necessary to support a healthy body. Minerals support the biochemical processes of life: metabolism, enzymatic and hormone activity, and cell production.

In this section, we look at which minerals you need to incorporate into your daily diet, what each one does, and what can happen if you don't get enough of them.

Identifying the minerals your body needs

The amount of most minerals you need every day is very small. Even so, getting minerals in proper amounts is essential for good health. And just like with vitamins, clean, whole foods are the best way to get the right amount and proportion of the essential minerals.

The government has established an RDA for 14 essential minerals, which include calcium, phosphorus, and magnesium. Here's what you need to know about these key essential minerals (*mg* stands for milligrams):

>> **Calcium:** You find calcium in dairy products, canned fish with bones, nuts, seeds, and leafy green vegetables. Some processed foods (such as orange juice) are fortified with calcium. You need about 1,000 to 1,300 mg of this mineral every day. Children, nursing mothers, and pregnant women need more. Calcium deficiency can be serious, leading to heart arrhythmia, bones more likely to fracture, and muscle spasms.

>> **Phosphorus:** Phosphorus plays a critical part in life because it's a component of your DNA. You find phosphorus in most foods simply because it's so essential, but dairy products, fish, and meats are especially good sources. This mineral helps build and maintain strong bones and teeth and is essential for a strong metabolism. The molecule your cells use to get energy is called adenosine triphosphate (ATP), and your body uses phosphorus to make it. The RDA for phosphorus ranges from 700 mg for most adults to 1,200 mg for children and teenagers.

WARNING

One troubling source of phosphorus is soft drinks. Phosphoric acid in those sweet beverages can reduce calcium levels in your blood, leading to weakened bones and teeth. So don't get most of your liquid intake from soft drinks!

>> **Magnesium:** You find magnesium in green vegetables (because magnesium is present in chlorophyll, which makes plants green) and in nuts, cocoa, and soybeans. Magnesium plays a part in the production of ATP (the energy molecule we describe in the preceding bullet) and many aspects of metabolism. It also helps keep your bones strong, dilates blood vessels, helps prevent muscle spasms, and has many other functions. You need about 400 mg of magnesium a day.

>> **Potassium and sodium:** These electrolytes are closely linked. In fact, many Americans get too much sodium and not enough potassium because of a diet high in processed foods. Nutritionists think that the main problem with sodium intake isn't that people consume too much; it's that they don't get enough potassium. Eating whole foods is the best way to achieve a good sodium/potassium balance.

Potassium helps the muscles contract and plays a major role in nerve transmission. It also helps maintain the body's pH balance and controls blood pressure. Consuming more potassium can help counteract the effects of too much sodium. You find potassium in fresh vegetables and fruits (particularly in their skins). Especially good sources of potassium include raisins and dates, bananas, sweet and russet potatoes, and white beans.

Sodium also plays a part in muscle contraction and nerve transmission, and it keeps your body's fluid level constant and helps your body absorb nutrients.

Too much sodium can increase the amount of fluid in your body, which puts strain on your heart muscle and blood vessels. Some people are more sensitive to sodium consumption than others.

» **Chloride:** Your body uses this mineral to produce the hydrochloric acid your stomach needs to digest food. Cells also use chloride to obtain energy from the macronutrients you consume. You need about 2,300 mg of chloride daily. Table salts (sodium and potassium chlorides) are the main source of this mineral. Potassium chloride is definitely preferable for those with high blood pressure. Research has shown that potassium chloride can lower blood pressure.

» **Iron:** Iron has two sources: heme and non-heme. Good sources for heme iron include red meats, poultry, and fish. Your body absorbs heme iron more easily than it does non-heme iron, which you find in leafy green vegetables, cocoa, and dried fruits. Non-heme iron is less likely to oxidize, and because it's paired with phytochemicals in plants, the risk of free radicals is even lower. But if you get much of your iron from non-heme sources, you need to get 1.7 times more iron than if you get most of your iron from heme sources. Iron deficiencies can cause anemia, fatigue, and increased risk of infection.

Children, younger men, and menstruating women need about 15 mg of heme iron per day. Older women and men need about 10 mg of heme iron, and pregnant women need about 30 mg of heme iron every day. Your body can store iron, so overdoses of this mineral are possible, especially since iron can oxidize easily and create those nasty free radicals. The tolerable upper limit (UL) for iron is about 40 mg.

» **Zinc:** Zinc is important for prevention of macular degeneration (the gradual loss of vision) and is essential to the production of testosterone and growth hormones. Your body also uses zinc to make enzymes that help it process and digest carbohydrates and alcohol. Low levels of zinc are often responsible for poor wound healing. The RDA for zinc is about 8 to 11 mg per day. Most foods that are high in protein are high in zinc as well: beef, poultry, and seafood. Oysters have the highest zinc content. But you also find this mineral in dairy products, beans, whole grains, and some vegetables, such as potatoes and pumpkins.

» **Chromium:** If you've seen the movie *Erin Brockovich,* you've heard of this mineral in its unhealthy form. There are two types of chromium: chromium 3, or trivalent chromium, and chromium 6, or hexavalent chromium (the bad, unhealthy stuff). Trivalent chromium is the one your body needs, and it's found in many foods. Chromium is used for metabolism of carbs, fat, and protein. It's also critical to the function and action of insulin. Adults need about 25 to 35 micrograms per day; research shows that individuals with type-2 diabetes themselves or in their families may need considerably more. Chromium is found in mushrooms, brewer's yeast, broccoli, whole grains, grapes and grape juice, beef, and garlic.

>> **Copper:** Copper is used to make red blood cells, collagen, elastic tissue, adrenalin, and nerve fibers. This trace mineral regulates blood pressure and heart rhythm and acts as an antioxidant. It's also used in enzyme manufacture and function. The RDA for copper is 2 milligrams per day. Consuming more than 10 mg a day can cause serious side effects, including liver damage, nausea, and muscle pain. Copper is found in fish, legumes, nuts, lentils, soybeans, spinach, and seeds.

>> **Iodine:** Iodine and iodide are both necessary for optimal body function. Iodine's best known use is in the thyroid gland for the synthesis of its many hormones. Low iodine often causes *goiter,* a term for an enlarged thyroid. Our bodies also use iodide to kill germs. Iodine is "preferred" by breast tissue, where it joins with a fat normally present there to actually kill many types of breast cancer cells. Iodine and iodide both help women maintain healthy levels of estriol, an important anticarcinogenic estrogen.

Lack of maternal iodine can lead to diminished mental capacity in infants and children. Low iodine levels can also contribute to diminished mental capacity in children and adults. Although our thyroid glands contain the most iodine, our breasts, ovaries, pituitary glands, salivary glands, and bile made by the liver contain more iodine and iodide than the rest of our bodies. Most adults need a minimum of 120 to 150 micrograms of iodine and iodide per day; pregnant and lactating women need up to 290 micrograms per day. Japan and Iceland — where considerable seaweed and fish are eaten — have the highest iodine intakes and the lowest rates of breast cancer in the world. This mineral is found in powdered kelp, which is available as a mild spice, other seaweed products, fish and other seafood, iodized salt, chard, lima beans, sesame seeds, mushrooms, garlic, and dairy products.

>> **Manganese:** This trace mineral is used to form and create bone and cartilage. It's also a key element in metabolism and helps synthesize amino acids. Manganese is sometimes called the "brain mineral" because it's important for memory and brain function. You need about 3 to 5 milligrams of manganese per day. Good food sources include nuts, seeds, legumes, whole grains, bananas, oranges, and strawberries.

Low levels of manganese can lead to infertility, because our brains need it to stimulate the "releasing hormones" that ultimately lead to adequate progesterone and testosterone synthesis.

>> **Molybdenum:** Molybdenum is key to sulfur metabolism and detoxification. Since all proteins contain sulfur, that makes molybdenum very important in protein metabolism. If you have a bad reaction after eating at a salad bar or drinking certain wines, it's usually due to sulfites used as preservatives. Sometimes taking additional molybdenum can improve your sulfite metabolism enough that the reaction no longer occurs. Molybdenum also helps produce uric acid, a normal component of blood. Adults need a minimum of

45 to 50 micrograms of molybdenum every day. You can find molybdenum in whole grains, nuts, legumes, and dark leafy greens.

>> **Selenium:** Selenium acts as an antioxidant in the body and may help prevent cancer, particularly prostate cancer. Areas in the United States that have higher levels of this mineral in soil have lower cancer rates. It works with vitamin E to help prevent free radical damage to your cells and helps detoxify the body. Adults need about 55 to 60 micrograms of selenium per day. It's found in whole grains, seafood, meats, and nuts, especially Brazil nuts.

Putting clean minerals to work

Like vitamins, minerals assist your body in retrieving energy from macronutrients so that your cells can work, grow, repair themselves, and replace themselves. The minerals in plants, dairy products, and meat all come from the soil. Some nutritionists are concerned that as more and more farmers deplete their soil, the amount of minerals naturally present in these foods also decreases. After all, soil does wear out over time; unless farmers replenish it with decaying plant matter, nutrients disappear from the soil.

Artificial fertilizers, pesticides, and herbicides also take their toll on the soil. Naturally occurring bacteria in the soil convert minerals into the form that plants can use, and those bacteria don't take kindly to poisons such as pesticides. Herbicides, especially fungicides, can negatively affect the mineral content in soils. Some plants have a symbiotic relationship with fungi that helps them pull more minerals and nutrients out of the soil. When farmers use fungicides on their crops, those plants have a reduced mineral content. In fact, studies published by Dr. Linus Pauling have found that the mineral content of fruits and vegetables, from the time frame of 1940 to 1991, has decreased from 20 to 70 percent!

If you're concerned about this trend, consider taking a good multivitamin and mineral supplement, or try to buy organic foods from farms that practice sustainability. Or do both! Sustainable farms practice organic farming techniques and rely on letting fields lie fallow to keep the soil healthy. They also plant *cover crops*, such as clover, which return nutrients to the soil. For more about supporting organic and local farms, see Chapter 10.

Label Issues, Fake Foods, and Clean Eating

In the past few years, a movement has grown, demanding that corporations label the foods they produce with the ingredients that go into them. Consumer activists are concerned about the development of genetically modified organisms (GMOs), trans fats, and the safety of imported foods. Even on the clean eating plan, you'll most likely buy some foods with labels, so you should be informed about these issues.

GMO foods

GMO foods started appearing in the news in the 1980s and 1990s. These foods are made when scientists insert foreign DNA from plants or animals into cells that change the plant or animal's traits. Some GMO foods are bred to be resistant to herbicides and pesticides. Other changes can include increasing the speed with which an animal comes to maturity or reducing the signs of produce spoilage.

In fact, one company just received FDA approval to grow genetically engineered salmon bred to grow faster. Ecologists are concerned that this salmon may escape its breeding grounds and contaminate wild salmon stocks.

Many scientists state that, because we've been eating GMO foods for more than a decade and no serious health effects have been uncovered, GMO foods are safe. But some illnesses take much longer than a decade or two to appear. Testing on GMO foods is controlled by the companies that own the patents on the genes, and no tests have been run longer than three months.

TIP

Most of the corn, soy, canola, and sugar beet crops grown in the United States are genetically engineered. That's just one of the reasons why we tell you to avoid the oils made from these foods, and one more reason why it's important to avoid sugar. Only buy the following foods in their organic form: cornmeal, edamame, tofu, miso, popcorn, and corn tortillas.

One of the problems caused by GMO crops has been the increase in the amount of herbicides farmers use on their crops. Since 1992, the use of glyphosate, the ingredient in the herbicide Roundup, has increased by more than 200 million pounds. This has spurred an epidemic of super weeds that have become resistant to the herbicides, which in turn has forced farmers to apply more and different herbicides. And the cycle continues.

Most consumer advocates believe that any foods that contain GMO crops should be labeled so consumers can choose what they eat. Huge corporations are fighting these labels, and many ballot initiatives requiring these labels have failed.

All you can do is avoid eating corn, soybean, or canola oil, and try to avoid foods with a label, especially highly processed foods. And educate yourself on this issue so you can vote on referendums when they appear on the ballot.

Trans fats

Trans fats appeared on the food scene in the 1950s, and were hailed as an inexpensive and healthy alternative to butter. Unfortunately, all those claims were wrong. Scientists believe that trans fats are the most unhealthy fat you can consume, and may be one of the causes of the skyrocketing heart disease rate in the past 40 years.

These fake fats are made by bubbling hydrogen through polyunsaturated oils. This change makes the oils solid at room temperature. This fake fat raises your LDL cholesterol (the bad stuff) and lowers your HDL cholesterol (the good stuff). And it may literally become part of your cell walls, making them flabby and weaker.

Trans fats was on the generally recognized as a safe (GRAS) list for years. Although foods that contain trans fats must be labeled with them, a sneaky twist let companies claim "0 grams trans fats" on the label as long as each serving had less than 0.5 gram trans fats per serving. But after years of debate, the FDA decided in 2015 to withdraw the approval of trans fats from our food supply. This is good news.

WARNING

Even though producers won't be able to use trans fats by the year 2018, some corporations will be able to petition the FDA to continue to use them. Remember that these corporations can still claim "0 grams trans fats per serving," as long as each serving has less than 0.5 grams. Read labels carefully, and don't buy any foods that have the word *hydrogenated* on the label.

Imported foods

Another labeling issue is called *country of origin labeling.* Your foods — even foods as simple as a steak or an avocado — can be imported into the country. And many foods don't have to be labeled with the country that produced them.

Consumer advocates want to see foods labeled with the country of origin so consumers can make informed choices. Many consumers are worried about foods that come from countries like China, which has had serious food safety issues over the years. The latest news is that the World Court has overruled the U.S. labeling laws, so you won't know where meats such as beef and pork come from.

TIP

To get around this problem, think about buying locally produced foods, including beef, pork, and chicken. You'll avoid this problem altogether and help support local businesses in the process.

Chapter 4

More about Nutrition: Phytochemicals, Water, Fiber, and Probiotics and Prebiotics

A few nutrients are considered "nonessential" even though you must include them in your diet to be healthy. Phytochemicals, water, and fiber are some of these nutrients. You must drink water to live, of course. Fiber is important for digestion and colon health, but your body doesn't absorb or metabolize it. Probiotics are bacteria that live in your gut that are essential to your immune system. Prebiotics are the foods that feed probiotics. And phytochemicals, which are compounds that help protect your body against rapid aging and inflammation, aren't essential for life, but they are essential for good health.

Phytochemicals, probiotics and prebiotics, water, and fiber can make a big difference in your overall health. And the eating clean lifestyle can help you get healthy amounts of water, fiber, probiotics and prebiotics, and phytochemicals into your everyday diet with little effort. These four types of healthy nutrients can have a major benefit on your body but only when you eat them on a regular basis. In this chapter, we discuss the importance of phytochemicals, probiotics and prebiotics, water, and fiber, and we show you how to use the eating clean diet plan to optimize these nutrients.

Natural Body Armor: Introducing the Protective Phytochemicals

Phytochemicals are fairly new to the nutrition scene, having been "discovered" about a hundred years ago. These compounds evolved to protect plant health. Nutritionists have since found that, although they aren't essential nutrients, phytochemicals are necessary for good human health, too. They have become especially important because of the increase in pollution and chemical exposure in today's world that attack cells and bodies, causing cell damage and inflammation that can lead to diseases like cancer and heart disease. Phytochemicals help fight against that cell damage and inflammation. Fortunately for you, thousands of phytochemicals exist in the natural world, and each one plays an important role in maintaining good health.

In this section, we look at why phytochemicals are important to good health, how they help protect you against free radicals and inflammation, and where to find them in the highest concentrations.

What phytochemicals are and what they do

Phytochemicals are natural compounds found in fruits and vegetables that help protect against the many causes of disease. Scientists think that plants developed these compounds to protect themselves against stress and environmental toxins. For instance, the brightly colored skins of many fruits and vegetables protect against the sun's ultraviolet rays.

You won't find phytochemicals in most refined foods. The cooking and processing necessary to produce refined foods destroys many phytochemicals. So why not avoid those products and enjoy whole foods instead? (Head to the later section "Where to find phytochemicals" for more information.)

Phytochemicals have many important roles in your body. They can act as any of the following:

>> **Antioxidants:** Antioxidants are natural chemicals that protect your cells against *free radicals,* which are rogue molecules that can cause damage that leads to diseases like cancer, diabetes, and heart disease. (Check out the later section "Why phytochemicals are important" for a more complete description of free radicals.) Some common antioxidants include carotenoids, flavonoids, polyphenols, anthocyanidins, and allyl sulfides.

>> **Hormone imitators and helpers:** Some phytochemicals can help regulate your body's hormones. For example, isoflavones in soy can imitate the action of female estrogens to help reduce the symptoms of menopause. And a polyphenol in cinnamon can help improve insulin function.

>> **Cholesterol reducers:** Phytosterols reduce the cholesterol counts in your bloodstream and help accelerate your body's natural cholesterol excretion methods.

>> **Collagen producers:** Anthocyanidins help boost collagen production in blood vessels and may help reduce the effects of arthritis.

>> **Immune system stimulators:** Flavonoids and phytoestrogens can help suppress tumor growth, and terpenes block proteins that overstimulate cell growth and reproduction. Other phytochemicals help increase the production and movement of white blood cells that protect your body against infection.

>> **Enzyme stimulators:** Indoles, which are found in cabbage, broccoli, cauliflower, Brussels sprouts, bok choy, and other vegetables, aid enzymes that protect cells against damage by balancing good and bad estrogens in the body. Protease inhibitors and terpenes also boost production of enzymes that inhibit the formation of cancer.

>> **DNA replication interrupters:** This category includes saponins, which are natural detergents found in many plants. These phytochemicals interfere with cell replication, possibly preventing the out-of-control cell growth that's typical in cancer cells, but they don't reduce or interfere with normal cell growth.

>> **Cell binders:** Some phytochemicals go directly to cell walls and bind to them, protecting the cells against pathogens like bacteria and viruses. The proanthocyanidins in cranberries, for instance, can help prevent urinary tract infections by blocking bacteria.

>> **Bacterial, viral, and fungal fighters:** Some phytochemicals destroy the invaders that enter your body through the food, water, and air you take in. For instance, allicin, a compound found in garlic, has antibacterial properties.

Because these powerful chemicals protect your cells, fight bacteria and other intruders (including free radicals), manage hormones, and aid enzymes, it's no wonder that nutritionists have been urging people to eat lots of the fruits and vegetables that provide phytochemicals.

REMEMBER

You can get phytochemicals in pill form, but you benefit more from eating them in their natural form as part of your diet. Here's why:

>> Fruits and vegetables contain phytochemicals in many different forms and combinations that are impossible to replicate in a single pill. And the size of a pill that contained all the antioxidants available in fresh produce would be impossible to swallow!

>> Scientists haven't discovered all the phytochemicals that nature provides, so you can't find them in any available supplement.

>> The way these natural chemicals react in the body is extremely complicated and difficult to test and replicate in a lab, so relying entirely on supplements rather than fruits and vegetables is problematic.

Why phytochemicals are important

As we explain in Chapter 3, essential vitamins and minerals help you prevent specific diseases like scurvy or beriberi. But phytochemicals help protect you against major diseases, like cancer, heart disease, and diabetes, that develop over time due to cell damage. In fact, you can think of phytochemicals as the frontline soldiers in your body's fight against aging and disease. These compounds most likely play a role in health throughout life, even interacting with your genes to affect health.

REMEMBER

Macronutrients keep you alive. Micronutrients, including phytochemicals, keep you healthy by making your cells healthy, protecting your body against inflammation and free radicals, and helping your body repair itself. Phytochemicals are *biologically active*, meaning they perform a role in your body but aren't *nutritive*, or essential to life.

Free radicals are an important part of the discussion regarding phytochemicals. A *free radical* is a rogue atom or molecule that's created by pollution, the aging process, stress, harmful chemicals, radiation, and even by normal metabolism. Free radicals have one or more missing electrons (or one or more too many). This imbalance of electrons makes the molecules very unstable, causing them to attack the cell membranes, DNA, proteins, and fat cells in your body in the attempt to get or give up an electron to become stable. All these attempts to become stable change more and more of the molecules of that cell into free radicals.

This cascading effect can cause damage to your cells and lead to inflammation, which can then result in the following diseases:

>> Alzheimer's disease

>> Cancer

>> Cognitive impairment

>> Depression

>> Diabetes

>> Heart and blood vessel disease

>> Immune problems

Antioxidants give up electrons to free radicals without becoming unstable themselves. As a result, the chain reaction stops the cascading effect and stabilizes the cells in your body. Need we remind you why a diet rich in antioxidants is so important to good health?

We know; all this talk of instability and free radicals sounds a little scary. But don't worry. Eating a diet of whole foods is a great way to achieve good nutrition and possibly sidestep many diseases. If you eat a poor diet and rely on supplements to round out your nutrition, you miss out on many compounds that are essential to good health.

Where to find phytochemicals

Many categories of phytochemicals exist in nature, including phytoestrogens, anthocyanosides, carotenoids, and flavonoids. Each group offers many health benefits, and most fruits and vegetables have different combinations of these compounds. The different phytochemicals are classified in different ways, according to their molecular structure, the ways they protect your body, or the color they create.

The most common and best-understood phytochemicals include the following:

>> **Allyl sulfides:** The vegetables in the onion family, including garlic, leeks, and chives, are good sources of allyl sulfides. These phytochemicals help improve blood circulation, have anti-inflammatory properties, help reduce high blood pressure, and reduce the risk of cancer. They're also antibacterial and act as antioxidants.

>> **Anthocyanidins:** These compounds, which are part of the flavonoid group, create the bright colors in fruits and vegetables like blueberries, grapes, raspberries, radishes, and cabbage. They help strengthen the collagen in your body and act as potent antioxidants.

>> **Beta-glucans:** You find these polysaccharides in oats, barley, and yeast. They can help activate the immune system and may have antitumor and anticarcinogenic properties. Beta-glucans have been used in medicine to help control high cholesterol, cancer, and diabetes.

>> **Carotenoids:** The carotenoid category of phytochemicals overlaps with but can't substitute for vitamin A. Only beta carotene, a precursor to vitamin A, can metabolize into vitamin A. You find beta carotene in orange fruits and vegetables. Other chemicals in the carotenoid category include lycopene, lutein, xanthins, and 600 other pigments that create the yellow, orange, and red color of carrots, bell peppers, tomatoes, apricots, watermelon, and grapefruit. The chemicals in this category can help prevent the hardening of the arteries, preserve mucus membranes, and boost immunity.

>> **Catechins:** You find these phytochemicals in green tea and in smaller amounts in wine, grapes, and chocolate. They may suppress the growth of tumor cells and reduce formation of plaque in arteries. The catechins found in tea are 25 times more potent than vitamin E in antioxidant power.

>> **Flavones:** Found in cereals and in herbs like parsley, these compounds may help protect you against diabetes, different types of cancer, osteoporosis, and atherosclerosis.

>> **Flavonols:** You find these compounds in tomatoes, apples, red onions, cocoa powder, broccoli, kale, berries, tea, and red wine. They help reduce the risk of vascular disease by reducing platelet activity and strengthening blood vessels; they also act as antioxidants. Quercetin is an important flavonol that has anti-inflammatory properties; it may help prevent prostate cancer and can help relieve arthritis pain and asthma symptoms.

>> **Glucosinolates:** You find these bitter and sharp-tasting compounds in brassica vegetables like kohlrabi, Brussels sprouts, cauliflower, and broccoli as well as in mustard, horseradish, and radishes. They act as a natural defense to protect the plant against herbivores. Glucosinolates help block the production of tumors and are potent antioxidants.

>> **Indoles:** You find these compounds in cabbages and other brassica vegetables. They can reduce the risk of cancer by increasing the formation of enzymes that inhibit malignant growth.

>> **Isothiocyanates:** You can get isothiocyanates in brassica vegetables like cabbage, broccoli, cauliflower, kohlrabi, bok choy, and radishes. These powerful compounds are anticarcinogenic, and they seem to be most effective against lung and esophageal cancers.

>> **Phenolic acids:** You can find these chemicals, which include ellagic acid and gallic acid, in whole grains, grapes, citrus fruits, and berries. Phenolic acids help boost your immune system, control inflammation, and improve blood circulation.

>> **Phytoestrogens:** These compounds, which mimic the hormone estrogen, can affect communication between cells, preventing mutations in cells that can develop into cancer. You find them in many whole foods, including nuts, seeds, berries, fruits, grains, and vegetables. Men should avoid eating soy products more than twice a week, because they can cause health issues such as cognitive decline. *Warning:* Be careful about consuming phytoestrogens in supplement form; consuming too much of this phytochemical can stimulate estrogen-dependent tumor growth.

>> **Phytosterols:** Found in whole grains, nuts, legumes, and unrefined vegetable oils, these compounds can help reduce total overall and LDL (or bad) cholesterol levels in the blood. They may also decrease cancer risk.

>> **Polyphenols:** These powerful antioxidants help reduce the bad LDL cholesterol (versus the good HDL type), and they block enzymes that cancer cells need to grow. Some polyphenols include the tannins found in tea and some mushrooms.

>> **Resveratrols:** These polyphenols have anti-inflammatory, antioxidant, anticarcinogenic, and cardiovascular properties. You find them in the skin of red grapes and in red wine.

>> **Saponins:** Found in soybeans, herbs, and peas, these compounds may have potent cholesterol-lowering properties. They also have antimicrobial properties and can stimulate the immune system.

>> **Tannins:** This group of molecules, which you find in tea, grapes, pomegranates, persimmons, red wine, lentils, and beans, has strong anti-inflammatory and antibacterial effects. The puckering feeling you get on your tongue when drinking strong tea or red wine is from tannins.

You can see from this list that phytochemicals are an important part of a healthy diet and that many fruits and vegetables contain a large mix of them. Phytochemicals, which are currently classified as nonessential, may climb to essential status in the future. But for now, get them by eating colorful whole foods in a varied diet. Strive for at least five to nine servings of fruits and vegetables every day, which fit in perfectly with the eating clean lifestyle!

Choose produce that's as deeply colored as possible. For example, if you have a choice between a stalk of light green celery and dark green celery, choose the dark green. It contains more phytochemicals and offers more health benefits.

Protecting Your Health with Fiber

What is *fiber?* It's a complex carbohydrate and the part of fruits, vegetables, nuts, seeds, and whole grains that your body can't absorb or digest. If it doesn't provide any nutrients and your body can't digest it, why is fiber so important? It helps keep your digestive system running smoothly, adds bulk to stools, helps lower cholesterol levels, helps with satiety, and may help prevent against some types of cancer.

Two types of fiber exist: soluble and insoluble. Both are important to good health. The best sources of fiber are the whole foods that are central to the clean eating plan.

In this section, we look at the different types of clean fiber, discuss where to find them, and explain what fiber does for your body as it travels through your gastro-intestinal (GI) tract.

Surveying the different types of clean fiber

The two types of fiber, which perform different functions in your body, are classified by whether or not they dissolve in water. Insoluble fiber doesn't dissolve in water, and soluble fiber does. Fiber is partially fermented by bacteria in your intestines, which helps maintain a good balance of healthy bacteria. It also performs other functions in the trip through your GI tract. Here's the lowdown on what the two types of fiber do:

>> **Insoluble fiber:** This type of fiber helps food and other materials move through your gastrointestinal system. It also makes going to the bathroom a bit easier. In other words, if you eat a lot of clean, fiber-rich, whole foods, you won't have a problem with constipation.

Insoluble fiber helps prevent the development of *diverticulitis* (inflammation of the small pouches in the colon that develop as you age; when these pouches become inflamed, they can harbor bacteria). It also slows the absorption of sugar into your bloodstream and helps control the acidity in your intestines. The bulk provided by insoluble fiber keeps things moving in your intestines, which may help prevent cancer.

You find this type of fiber in the bran of wheat and corn, in seeds and nuts, in other whole-grain products, and in fruit and vegetable skins. Leafy vegetables and fibrous vegetables like green beans are also good sources of insoluble fiber.

» **Soluble fiber:** This type of fiber dissolves in water and forms a gel material. Nutritionists now know that this type of fiber is critical to good health. It can lower blood cholesterol levels and stabilize glucose levels, which may help prevent type-2 diabetes. Soluble fiber binds with bile acids in the intestines, removing them from your body. Your liver then makes more bile acids from the cholesterol in your blood, which reduces overall cholesterol levels. This type of fiber can also reduce inflammation and blood pressure.

Soluble fiber keeps you feeling fuller longer after a meal by slowing down the rate at which your stomach empties so that you don't want to eat again too soon. Good sources of soluble fiber include nuts, barley, fruits, vegetables, oat bran, dried legumes, and psyllium husks.

Bulking up your fiber intake

The average American consumes only about 12 grams of fiber per day. But nutritionists recommend that women eat 20 to 38 grams of fiber per day and that men eat 30 to 38 grams per day. The more calories you consume, the more fiber you should include in your diet. If you eat the recommended five servings of fruits and vegetables and six servings of whole-grain products every day, you can easily meet those fiber requirements.

Getting your fiber from processed foods is okay (check the labels to see how many grams are in a product), but eating whole grains, fruits, vegetables, legumes, nuts, and seeds is the best way to get enough fiber in your diet. In contrast, many processed foods that claim to be enriched with fiber are also high in sugar and trans fats (think those huge bran muffins sold in coffee shops). So depend on whole produce as your main fiber source.

TIP

When you increase your fiber intake be sure to also increase your water intake. Fiber works best when paired with water; water helps it move smoothly and easily through your GI tract.

It's possible to eat too much fiber! So take heed if you're eating whole foods on the eating clean plan and taking fiber supplements. Too much fiber can stop the absorption of minerals because the food speeds through your intestine too quickly. More than 45 to 50 grams of fiber a day is too much.

Chew on this: Connecting fiber and weight loss

Fiber plays an important role in maintaining a healthy weight. Most importantly, you feel more satisfied when you eat high-fiber foods. They add bulk to your stomach so you feel full longer.

Also, high-fiber foods take more time to eat because you have to chew them more before swallowing. (Think about it; you can't just gulp down a couple of apples like you can a handful of chocolate candies.) That extra time spent chewing helps give your stomach time to signal to your brain that you're full. (Head to Chapter 6 for more information on using the eating clean plan — and fiber — for weight loss.)

Just because we say that fiber is a good thing and that it can help you lose weight doesn't mean you should go on a fiber binge to lose 15 pounds in a week. If your diet hasn't been high in fiber and you want to increase your intake, you have to do so slowly. If you add too much fiber to your diet too quickly, your body will rebel. You'll develop gas, bloating, and cramping as the bacteria in your intestines suddenly start to work overtime on the added fiber. So add fiber gradually to allow your system to adjust.

Water: The Essential Nutrient

Water isn't considered an essential nutrient, but you would die without it — and quickly. Your body is made up of about 65 percent water. You can survive for months without food, but you can survive only a few days without water. Every function in your body needs water. You need it for nerves to process signals in your brain; for blood flow; for cell function, repair, and reproduction; for nutrient absorption and waste elimination; for normal metabolism; and for respiration.

Getting enough water

Most nutritionists say that you should consume 8 to 12 glasses of water a day. That sounds like a lot, but if you drink a glass of water with or before each meal, you'll consume six glasses a day on the clean eating plan without even trying.

(The clean eating plan recommends that you eat six times a day. See Chapter 2 for details.) You also get water from the food you eat, especially foods like watermelon, peaches, and berries. Think juicy fruits!

TIP

To make sure you get enough water every day, do the following:

>> Bring a water bottle with you whenever there may not be a clean and easily available source.

>> Drink a glass of water when you wake up and another before you go to sleep.

>> Eat more of the foods, like fruits and vegetables, which can be good sources of water.

Evaluating your tap water

Can you trust that the water that comes out of your kitchen faucet is clean enough to drink? Maybe not. Unfortunately, much of the tap water in the United States has a lot of other things you don't want to consume, including bacteria, lead, chlorine, prescription drugs, and hormones. Overall, tap water is free of infectious microorganisms and thought to be safe to drink. But you still have to consider some important issues.

The nation's wastewater system was designed before many of the chemicals that get into the water were invented and mass-produced. For instance, herbicides, pesticides, and pharmaceutical drugs didn't exist a hundred years ago when the first treatment plants were developed.

WARNING

Tap water can contain chlorine, fluoride, lead, prescription drugs, hormones, and other contaminants that can adversely affect your health. In 2015, doctors in Flint, Michigan, found that the city's water was highly contaminated with lead, which can reduce mental acuity and IQ, especially in children. The outrage after this discovery prompted many investigations into water systems around the country, which revealed that water in some municipal areas runs through aging systems that add lead and other contaminants in your water.

So what can you do to keep yourself and your family safe? You can ask a lab to test your water (including well water), or you can get a water-quality report from the Environmental Protection Agency (EPA). Your water supplier may give you a Consumer Confidence Report every year. For more information, and to find your CCR, visit https://ofmpub.epa.gov/apex/safewater/f?p=136:102. If you're uncomfortable with the results of either test, you can install a water filtration system in your home. Systems range from simple carbon filters to more complex (and more effective) reverse osmosis filters. You also can use a portable filtration system like

Brita. You can buy and drink bottled water as well, but read the following section to get the skinny on it first.

Weighing the pros and cons of bottled water

Is bottled water the solution to the problem of too many contaminants in tap water? Well, yes and no. Many brands of bottled water are simply tap water in a pretty package. However, some bottled water companies do put the water through an extra purification step or two. Some manufacturers strip their bottled water of chlorine before they bottle it, usually using reverse osmosis or distillation methods. And some manufacturers take out the fluoride, too, but many of them add it right back in.

If you can afford a water filtration system, install one in your home. At the very least, buy personal water bottles with a built-in filtration system for your family. After the debacle in Flint, Michigan, it's better to be safe than sorry. Also think about putting the water that you cook with through filters before you use it.

If you think bottled water tastes better than tap water, you're more likely to drink more water in general, so by all means, drink bottled water! However, like everything else, this better taste (and convenience) comes at a price. Bottled water costs up to 500 times as much as tap water. The bottles are made of plastic and are single-use containers. So you have to deal with lugging home lots of bottles and recycling the empty ones. You also have some bigger issues to consider:

>> **Bisphenol A (BPA):** Manufacturers use this chemical to make hard plastics. It's part of the chemical group called *xenoestrogens,* which are endocrine disrupters that interrupt the hormone paths and messages sent throughout your body. This chemical can leach into the water from the plastic bottles, especially when they're stored in high heat.

Water bottles with the recycling number 3 or 7 marked on the bottom may contain BPA. Water bottles with the numbers 1, 2, 4, or 5 don't contain BPA.

>> **Phthalates:** Manufacturers add these chemicals to some plastics to help increase flexibility and reduce shattering. Phthalates are carcinogens and hormone disrupters. They can leach into the water in water bottles, especially if you reuse the bottles, fill them with hot water, or store them in high-temperature conditions.

Water bottles with the number 3 on the bottom contain phthalates.

TIP

Here's what you can do to make sure the bottled water you drink is safe:

>> **Check the recycling number on the bottom of every water bottle.** Never buy water bottles with the number 3 or 7 on them.

>> **Don't reuse bottles intended for single use.** The stress of reusing the bottle can release more BPA and phthalates into the water. Bottles with number 1 are not intended for reuse because that plastic is very porous and can hold on to bacteria you introduce into the bottle when you drink out of it.

>> **Never put hot water into a plastic bottle.** Hot water can degrade the plastic, which then can leach more chemicals into the water. Only use cold or cool water in plastic.

>> **Consider using glass or stainless steel bottles.** You can thoroughly clean these bottles after each use, so you don't have to worry about bacterial contamination. They last a long time, which is more cost-effective and better for the environment.

REMEMBER

Continue to drink water, whether it's from a bottle, glass, or from your (filtered) tap! Don't drink soda pop or sweetened beverages instead. Water is still the best beverage you can drink. If you can afford a good filtration system, the best water choice at present may be well-filtered tap water.

WARNING

If you choose to buy bottled water, be sure to recycle every bottle you use. Although water bottles are recyclable, not everyone recycles them. Water bottles pile up in landfills to the tune of 1.5 million tons every year. Because plastic bottles are light, they easily fly out of garbage trucks and pile up on roadsides, eventually making their way to the ocean. Tons of plastic waste is floating in the earth's oceans, threatening birds and marine life.

Probiotics and Prebiotics: Essential to Your Health

Your gut is teeming with bacteria that are essential to your health. These healthy bacteria compete with harmful bacteria in your intestines for the food you eat. The proportion of the two types of bacteria in most people is about 85 percent "good" bacteria to 15 percent "bad" bacteria.

There are two main kinds of probiotics in food: different species of the genus *Lactobacillus*, found in yogurt and fermented foods, and several species of the genus *Bifidobacteriuim*, also found in dairy products. (There are other probiotics in food, including those from the *Pediococcus, Leuconostoc,* and *Weissella* genera.) These good bacteria help convert carbohydrates into energy sources for your body. They also help your body produce vitamins K and B, make short-chain fatty acids, promote absorption of minerals, detoxify toxins, and aid metabolism.

In this section, we explain the importance of consuming plenty of probiotics and prebiotics for a healthy body. *Probiotics* are live cultures of beneficial bacteria; *prebiotics* are the nondigestible nutrients (in other words, fiber) that feed probiotics.

You and your microbiata

The *microbiata* is the collection of trillions of microorganisms that live in your intestines. The type of bacteria in your gut can affect how you fight off disease, how much you weigh, and how well your body processes nutrients. Your *microbiome* is the collection of genes in those bacteria, which outnumber human genes by 100 to 1.

Scientists are learning more about the microbiata every day. They have recently discovered that bacteria in your gut can affect your daily life. They may even modify your eating behavior! Bad bacteria could generate cravings for foods that they prefer, which includes junk foods and foods that are high in sugar and salt. A higher diversity in gut microbiome could actually help you choose healthier foods and stick to the clean eating plan.

TIP

Scientists are experimenting with fecal microbiata transplants to help people recover from bacterial infections, especially infections of *Clostridium difficile* (or *C. diff.* for short). And studies have shown that transplanting microbiata from obese mice into lean mice made them gain weight. Although these transplants have been conducted in China for thousands of years, this procedure is fairly new in the United States — but it may become more widely available as this technique is studied.

Did you know that 60 percent to 70 percent of your immune system is located in your digestive tract? Probiotics can enhance cellular immune responses by activating macrophages, lymphocytes, and natural killer (NK) cells, which are a type of white blood cell, and influence the level of serotonin, the neurotransmitter that controls your mood. Having good gut bacteria can help protect you against diseases ranging from the common cold to depression to cancer. Good bacteria also compete with pathogens, regulate the inflammatory immune response, and actually produce antibiotics to protect your health.

You need to consume as many kinds of different probiotics as possible for the best diversity of bacteria populating your gut, and enough prebiotics to make sure they have the nutrients they need. Think of probiotics as bees, and prebiotics as the pollen the bees need to do their work.

All about probiotics

You may remember the Dannon yogurt commercial that focused on people from Georgia (or another rustic Eastern European country) who easily lived to be 100 years old. The commercial's claim was that the "friendly bacteria" (also known as *probiotics*) in yogurt can extend your lifespan. Is this claim really true? Maybe!

Your intestines are full of more than 100 trillion microorganisms, both good and bad. These make up your microbiome, which helps you digest food and is part of your immune system. Because your intestines are a critical part of your immune system, you need to keep them healthy. One way to do so is to encourage the growth of healthy kinds of bacteria (that is, probiotics), including those from the *Lactobacillus* and *Bifidobacterium* genera. These bacteria help keep your intestines' pH balance correct, prevent bad bacteria from affecting the intestinal wall, and increase immune system strength.

TIP

When you buy a food for its probiotic benefits, make sure the label says *live and active cultures.* Also look for the specific strain of bacteria that's present in the product. The label should identify each type of bacteria by the genus, species, and strain. For instance, *Lactobacillus acidophilus DDS-1* is the correct term for the bacteria found in most yogurt products.

Several studies have shown that probiotics can help treat intestinal illnesses, including Crohn's disease, irritable bowel syndrome, and ulcerative colitis. They can also help prevent colds and flu, treat diarrhea and yeast infections, reduce the recurrence of bladder infections, and help treat eczema. A healthy microbiome may also control your weight and prevent obesity. Some doctors recommend eating probiotic-rich foods after taking a course of antibiotics to repopulate the good bacteria in your intestines.

You find probiotics in fermented foods, such as yogurt, miso, kefir, sauerkraut, tempeh, and kimchi, as well as in probiotic supplements. Although fermented foods are processed, they're minimally processed, so they still fit into the clean eating plan.

TIP

There is no recommended daily allowance (RDA) for probiotics. But because your intestines are full of trillions of bacteria, it's difficult, if not impossible, to overdose on probiotics. Your body will eliminate what you don't need.

All about prebiotics

After you get the good bacteria in your gut, you need to keep them there and keep them happy! Luckily, the clean eating plan includes lots of healthy foods that contain the prebiotics, or fermentable fiber, that feed the probiotics bacteria. Specifically, the healthy bacteria like to eat carbohydrate molecules called *oligosaccharides*, which you find in many whole foods, including the following:

>> Leafy green vegetables

>> Barley and other whole grains such as oatmeal

>> Legumes

>> Onions and garlic

>> Asparagus

>> Bananas

>> Artichokes

Some probiotic foods even have prebiotic fiber added to them; check the label for details. You can also get fermentable fiber in supplement form.

Unfortunately, the American diet that we're trying to break free from is high in the foods that feed the bad gut bacteria. Eating prebiotics is an important part of eating clean.

WARNING

Be careful when adding prebiotics to your diet because they can cause gas. Your body does not digest these plant fibers, but the bacteria in your gut ferment them, which produces the gas. Fortunately, though, this side effect should subside as your body gets used to friendly bacteria and the food it needs.

Doctors don't yet know exactly how much prebiotic fiber you need every day, but most think that about 4 to 6 grams is right. Almost everyone needs to eat more prebiotic foods for good health. In fact, making this one change, without eating more foods with probiotics, could improve your digestion. In addition, these foods could lower triglycerides, regulate blood sugar, and may reduce cravings. And they're delicious!

Chapter 5

Eat More, Eat Often!

How many times have you looked at the plate of food you allow yourself and wished it contained more? Do you feel deprived when you go "on a diet" and wish you didn't feel so hungry? If you follow the eating clean lifestyle, those days are gone for good. When you eat clean, you get to enjoy many wonderful benefits, including better health and more energy. But best of all, you get to eat more food more often.

The key, of course, is that the types of foods you eat must be nutrient dense. In other words, for each calorie, the food must supply a reasonable amount of vitamins, minerals, fiber, and other nutrients. Empty calories, which are usually found in junk foods and processed foods, just aren't worth the costs to your health and your pocketbook and have no place in the eating clean lifestyle.

In this chapter, we explain how to listen to your body and let it tell you when it's hungry or thirsty and when you just want to eat for emotional reasons. We show you what real hunger cues are and what satiety really means. We also help you discover what you should eat and when you should eat it, how to develop and enjoy mini-meals, and how to work the eating clean lifestyle into your daily routine. We look at ways to enjoy your clean food with natural flavor enhancers. And we examine the Paleo diet, which about one-third of the population should try for better health.

Listening to Your Body

Do you know what being hungry really feels like? Of course, you've felt hunger pangs, especially on days that are so busy you can't find time to eat. But many people have lost the connection between their body's hunger signals and true hunger.

In this section, we look at how your body tells you that you need more food, what forms your body's signals take, and how you can sometimes mistake other emotions or triggers for real hunger. We also explain what satiety means and how to determine when your stomach is really (and comfortably) full.

REMEMBER

The trick to eating clean is knowing how to recognize healthy hunger cues and how to defuse unhealthy cues. When you understand how your stomach and your brain work together and can identify the triggers that prompt overeating and craving, you can do something to stop the cycle of bad food choices.

Decoding hunger cues

Scientist Ivan Pavlov proved that you can prompt hunger in many different ways. Through his experiments, he demonstrated that his dogs would start drooling when they heard a dinner bell. They learned to associate the sound of the bell with food appearing, and their bodies responded. Human beings aren't much different!

Hunger is one of life's biological drives. You have to eat to stay alive, and your body tells you when you need food. But in this modern world, images of food — reminders of everything from chocolate doughnuts to french fries — constantly bombard you. After all, Madison Avenue's efforts to make you crave different kinds of food have been very successful over the years! But with the eating clean lifestyle, you have to figure out what real hunger feels like.

REMEMBER

You can separate hunger into two basic categories. One is the normal hunger that comes when your body needs food to repair and maintain itself. The other is the hunger that occurs when you respond to external cues, such as a picture of food, or internal cues, such as stress or sadness. Within these two hunger categories, you experience several different types of hunger, including

>> **True physiological hunger:** A type of hunger caused by a drop in blood sugar, changes in hormone levels, and an empty stomach and intestine. The brain decodes these signals and sends messages to the rest of your body, making your stomach growl and ache and sometimes causing a headache or feeling of weakness. You must recognize these hunger signals to keep your body properly fueled and healthy.

>> **Psychological hunger:** A type of hunger triggered by thoughts and emotions, like worry, anxiety, or anger, or by the sight or smell of food. Eating junk food, binge eating, and eating out of habit rather than a physical need for nourishment feed this type of hunger.

>> **Appetite:** An interest in or craving for food. Appetite is linked to the physical need for food, but it can override the body's signals that you have eaten enough and can spur you on to eat more than you need — sometimes much more.

Tracking hunger in your household

The biggest challenges to eating well and maintaining a healthy body are understanding and untangling psychological hunger and appetite from physical hunger.

To help you understand the differences between the main hunger types, conduct a little experiment in your household over the next few days. Explain that physical hunger is going to be the standard that prompts eating in your household. Tell your family that they have to pay attention to their own hunger cues. Proposing a hunger rating system, where 1 is "extraordinarily hungry" and 10 is "extraordinarily full," may help. The goal is to stay within the range of about 3 to 7; that is, eat when you feel hunger pangs but aren't uncomfortably hungry and stop when you feel satisfyingly full. Meeting this goal will take some practice, but eventually everyone will become familiar with this natural way to control food intake.

TIP

If you discover that you eat for emotional reasons and have a hard time controlling such impulses, stock your house with healthy foods rather than cupcakes and potato chips. If the tempting, unhealthy foods aren't within easy reach but good snacks like apples with cheese are, your diet will automatically improve.

Ignoring external cues

When everyone in your household understands the difference between physical hunger and psychological cravings, start tackling the external cues that drive you to eat even when you're not really hungry. After all, before you can succeed with the eating clean lifestyle, you must change your bad eating habits.

TIP

To get your body used to eating for health and hunger (rather than for psychological reasons), do the following:

>> **Turn off the television and computer during meal times.** Meal-time distractions turn your attention away from the food in front of you and your body's physical feelings and usually lead to overeating. The goal is to avoid mindless eating, which results when you don't concentrate on your plate.

>> **Slow down meal times.** Take time to talk to your fellow eaters, put down your fork and knife occasionally during a meal, and wait for your stomach to tell your brain it's full. That message takes 20 minutes to travel from your stomach to your brain. And you can eat a lot of food in those last few minutes before the signal arrives!

>> **Understand portion control and proper serving sizes.** Most people are used to the supersized portions restaurants serve. But did you know that a healthy serving of meat is only about the size of a deck of cards and that a serving of ice cream is only ½ cup? Practice measuring food to get used to correct serving sizes until dishing out proper portions becomes second nature to you.

>> **Try to separate emotions from eating.** Stress can prompt overeating or craving unhealthy foods. If you're stressed or angry and want to eat, wait 10 to 15 minutes. If, after that time, you're still hungry — according to physical, not emotional, cues — go ahead and choose something healthy to eat. If you aren't hungry, you know the trigger was emotional or external and not a genuine need for food.

Identifying thirst cues

Water is a basic element of life. In fact, human bodies are about 65 percent water. When your body needs more water, it lets you know through thirst cues. But did you know that people often mistake thirst for hunger?

If your stomach starts rumbling and you want to eat, get a drink of water. Not soda, not coffee or tea — just plain water. Then wait a few minutes. If you were thirsty, not hungry, your craving for food will abate. Drinking water to see whether you're thirsty rather than hungry is especially important if you had something to eat less than three hours ago or if you haven't had any water in the last hour.

Drinking lots of water helps your body do the following:

>> Keep your metabolism at the proper level

>> Decrease food cravings

>> Burn stored fat

>> Maintain muscle tone

>> Increase energy levels

In fact, drinking water or eating a clear soup before a meal is a great way to help fill up your stomach and control hunger pangs. Keeping your body properly hydrated can help you recognize the true feelings of hunger.

Understanding satiety

Satiety (pronounced say-*tie*-uh-tee) is the feeling of satisfaction you have after eating. It doesn't mean that you're full or that you've eaten so much you're uncomfortable. Figuring out what satiety means to you is important to your eating clean lifestyle.

To help you better understand what satiety means, consider the satiety index that Dr. Susanna Holt developed to rank foods according to how satisfying they are to eat, how much of those foods you must eat to feel full, and how soon you feel hunger pangs after eating them.

The index uses an ordinary piece of white bread as the baseline score of 100. Foods that stave off hunger longer receive higher scores, while foods that prompt feelings of hunger more quickly rank lower. Not surprisingly, foods with more fiber, complex carbohydrates, and protein fill your stomach faster, are more satisfying to eat, and keep your blood sugar levels stable longer. Foods high in protein are the best at staving off hunger, while whole grains and fruits and vegetables that are high in fiber are better at helping you feel satisfied longer.

The following foods rank lower on the satiety index:

>> **Candy bar:** Score 70

>> **Doughnut:** Score 68

>> **Potato chips:** Score 91

>> **Cake:** Score 65

The following foods rank higher on the satiety index:

>> **Cheese:** Score 157

>> **Fish:** Score 225

>> **Apples:** Score 197

>> **Baked potato:** Score 322

>> **Oatmeal:** Score 209

The fact that the higher-ranking foods are clean while the lower-ranking foods are highly processed is no surprise. Not only does your eating clean lifestyle improve your health and well-being, but it also helps you feel more satisfied after each meal. Now that's a healthy reward you can build on and learn to enjoy!

The following sections describe two more factors that play a role in satiety — food flavors and stomach processes.

Factoring flavors into the satiety equation

Satiety is more than just a lack of hunger. Your appetite is a complex biological mechanism that engages many parts of the brain. When you eat a meal that contains a lot of different flavors, you activate more appetite centers in your brain. For example, a meal with sweet, salty, sour, and meaty (also called *umami*) flavors turns on many appetite centers in your brain, and you have to eat until all those centers signal that they're satisfied to feel full.

The problem with processed foods is that many of them are high in sugar and salt. As a result, processed foods prompt a lot of appetite centers in your brain, causing you to have to eat more to satisfy them. But you don't really taste all the flavors in processed foods. For example, you know that processed cereals are high in sugar, but did you know that many are also high in salt? The sugar wakes up the sweet appetite center of your brain, and the salt prompts the salty appetite center, urging you to eat more.

This concept plays into what Dr. David Kessler, a former U.S. Federal Drug Administration (FDA) commissioner, calls *hypereating* (an obsessive need to consume processed foods that change brain chemistry). Combinations of sugar, salt, and fat trigger appetite centers in your brain that release feel-good hormones called *endorphins.* In other words, processed foods literally give you feelings of happiness, comfort, and euphoria, very similar to what a drug addict feels after a hit. Food companies understand this fact very well, which is why so many processed foods contain exactly those ingredients in very specific combinations.

REMEMBER

Nobody wants to eat a bland diet. Lucky for you, you don't have to. By eating whole foods, you get the best of both worlds — healthy nutrients and flavor! The key is to choose flavorful, high-volume, and nutritious foods with low density. For example, foods that are high in water and fiber, like grapes or oranges, are more satisfying to eat than fruit juice. Although eating processed foods is often easier because they're usually low volume, eating clean foods is the healthier, more satisfying way to go. Almost anyone can quickly eat an entire package of potato chips, which weighs about 12 ounces, but eating an entire baked potato, which weighs about the same amount, takes more time and is more satisfying and nutritious.

Keeping your stomach busy longer

The rate of *gastric emptying* (how long your stomach takes to process food and empty into the small intestine) also plays a role in satiety. How long your stomach takes to process the food you eat depends on how much fiber, protein, carbohydrates, and fat the food contains. Fruit juices, for example, travel through your stomach quickly because they contain only simple carbs, which break down very quickly; the stomach doesn't have to process any solids.

But a meal full of grains, vegetables, and lean meats takes longer to process. The food stays in your stomach longer, which means you feel more satisfied for a longer period of time. Again, whole foods — the critical part of the eating clean lifestyle — have slower gastric-emptying rates, while highly processed foods have faster gastric-emptying rates.

REMEMBER

Sheer bulk of the food counts, too. In the section "Knowing what (and what not) to eat," we compare the calories and nutrients in a clean meal to those in a processed meal. Not surprisingly, the clean meal has fewer calories and more nutrients, but if you look at the plates of food side by side, you notice something else. The clean plate also has much more volume.

Because you eat with your eyes as well as your mouth, just looking at a plate full of food can help you feel more satisfied. For example, a big salad, full of nuts and vegetables, like mushrooms, avocado, and tomatoes, is more satisfying to eat than a small fried burrito from a fast-food joint.

Getting Started with Good Food Choices

Most Americans suffer from too much choice. Grocery stores are packed full of foods that, unfortunately, aren't very good for you. Although packaged foods taste good and are convenient, the toll they take on your health and your body is very high.

Making good food choices is a basic step toward the eating clean lifestyle. In this section, we look at what the eating clean diet means and what kinds of food you should put in your shopping basket. We compare the calories and nutrition of a typical American fast-food meal with those in a clean meal, and we look at the best times to eat to keep your body properly fueled.

Knowing what (and what not) to eat

Did you know that the average American consumes enough extra calories every seven days to gain more than 50 pounds a year? This alarming statistic corresponds to the explosion of processed food and fast-food availability in modern culture.

The visual and emotional cues you face on a daily basis, along with the chemical makeup of processed foods and your body's natural responses to these cues, make eating a healthy diet very difficult. But you can change course with a little bit of effort, some simple rules, and a better understanding of what your body really needs. Read on to find out what you need to know.

Choosing the right packaged foods (if you must)

You've heard of the food chain that has algae and amoeba at the bottom and lions and tigers at the top, but you may not know about the other food chain — that is, the processed food chain. In this food chain, foods in their natural state, like apples, greens, berries, and whole grains, are at the bottom, and processed foods, like sugary snack cakes and fast-food burgers, are at the top. If you eat low on the food chain, you'll automatically eat a clean diet. So think about food in its natural state before you buy it. A gelatin fruit salad packed in a little plastic cup with chunks of peaches floating in it is very different from a fresh peach picked right off the tree.

In Chapter 13, we offer several plans to help you make the transition from processed foods to clean foods. But if you're still buying foods with a label, use the following rules to help guide your choices:

>> **Read the labels.** If a product like whole-wheat bread contains more than five or seven ingredients, put it back on the shelf. You don't have to stick to a certain ingredient count; just make sure that the number of ingredients is about what you would use if you made the food from scratch.

>> **If you can't pronounce, spell, or understand ingredients on the food label, don't buy that particular product.** Your body doesn't need artificial flavors or chemicals made in the lab. Even chemicals the FDA regards as safe may be problematic in the future.

>> **Avoid foods that have sugars, processed ingredients, or fat as the first or second ingredient on the label.** These foods are made up of empty calories that don't provide much nutrition.

>> **Choose foods that are low on the food chain.** In other words, choose foods that are as close as possible to their natural state. Pick up a head of cabbage rather than a jar of coleslaw. Choose a bag of apples rather than a bottle of sweetened applesauce. If you do so consistently, you'll be well on your way to eating clean.

When you follow these simple rules, you may notice that a lot of the foods you're used to buying are no longer on your grocery list. This switch in what you buy can take some time, but don't stress! You can ease into the process. Becoming aware of what you put in your shopping cart and bring into your house is the first, and most important, step.

Avoiding fast food

As you transition into an eating clean lifestyle, you must begin to consider and choose the foods you eat carefully. Although a fast-food meal is (relatively) inexpensive and quick, a constant diet of such food can have a very expensive and time-consuming effect on your health in the future in terms of medical bills and trips to the doctor.

To help you visualize just how different processed foods and clean foods are, take a look at Tables 5-1 and 5-2, in which we compare a meal comprised of typical American fast foods with one made up of clean, whole foods. If you find yourself sliding back into old habits, just pull out these charts and compare the bottom line. (*Note:* In the tables, *g* stands for gram and *mg* stands for milligram.)

TABLE 5-1   **Fast-Food Meal**

Food	Fat	Carbs	Fiber	Sodium	Protein	Calories
12 ounces of soda	0 g	42 g	0 g	35 mg	0 g	150
1 fast-food cheeseburger	12 g	33 g	2 g	750 mg	15 g	300
1 serving of french fries	19 g	48 g	5 g	270 mg	4 g	380
3 tablespoons of ketchup	0 g	12 g	0 g	500 mg	1 g	45
Total	31 g	135 g	7 g	1,555 mg	20 g	875

The fast-food meal shown in Table 5-1 may be enjoyable to eat, but you'll be hungry soon after eating it, you're not meeting your body's nutritional needs, and you're consuming too much sodium, fat, preservatives, and artificial flavors. The amount of sodium in this one meal is more than half of the daily recommended amount (which is 2,400 mg). The meal also provides almost half of the total calories you should consume in a day (which is 2,000) and is very high in fat.

The fast-food meal is also very low in nutrients. Although the ketchup and tomato on the cheeseburger do provide some vitamin C, you don't get a lot of vitamin D, calcium, or other micronutrients in this meal. In addition, the meal is most likely loaded with hormones from the meat and pesticides from the potatoes, tomato, and lettuce, which were most likely grown on a large factory farm.

The eating clean meal you see in Table 5-2 uses recipes from Part V of this book (the first two come from Chapter 16 and the last one comes from Chapter 18). Feel free to use any clean soup or salad as a substitute.

TABLE 5-2   **Eating Clean Meal**

Food	Fat	Carbs	Fiber	Sodium	Protein	Calories
Chicken Lettuce Wraps	11 g	15 g	3 g	654 mg	23 g	250
Slow Cooker Tomato Barley Soup	1 g	27 g	6 g	512 mg	4 g	126
Frozen Yogurt Bar	1 g	5 g	1 g	12 mg	4 g	39
Total	13 g	47 g	10 g	1,178 mg	31 g	414

REMEMBER

Compare these two charts to look at the fat content, amount of fiber, sodium content, protein content, and total calories. The clean meal has good fats, including monounsaturated fats from olive oil and nuts, less sugar and sodium, and more fiber and protein. Plus, it fills you up, provides you with more nutrients, and keeps you feeling satisfied longer with fewer calories, preservatives, and artificial ingredients. The eating clean diet is one you can live with for life — quite likely a longer, more active, and healthier life, too!

Eating mini meals to combat hunger

Back in the 1980s, the term *grazing* applied to people as well as cows. Scientists thought that eating smaller meals throughout the day (rather than just three large meals) helped keep the body's metabolism going and prevented overeating by keeping blood sugar as stable as possible. When your blood sugar drops, all kinds of nasty things happen: You feel hungry and irritable, your willpower goes out the window, and you reach for any edible substance in sight.

Despite lots of research, scientists haven't found a clear-cut answer about whether eating mini meals offers all those benefits. But if you do eat more often, you may be less tempted to eat processed snack foods, which is one reason why the eating clean diet involves eating five or six smaller meals a day rather than the traditional large breakfast, lunch, and dinner. After all, if you know that you get to eat a turkey sandwich with homemade bread in an hour, that doughnut stand you pass on your coffee break will be much less tempting.

Don't forget the hunger rating system that we describe in the earlier section "Decoding hunger cues." Eating smaller meals at regular intervals throughout the day prevents your hunger from dipping to 1 or 2 on the hunger scale, and eating smaller meals means you almost never reach a 9 or 10 on the fullness scale.

TIP

To get the most out of your mini meals, follow these guidelines:

- » **Make sure each mini meal includes complex carbohydrates, lean proteins, and healthy fats.** You find complex carbs in fruits, vegetables, and whole grains; lean proteins in chicken, fish, lean beef, and pork; and good fats in nuts and nut butters, olive oil, and lean meats.

- » **Always, always eat breakfast.** Eating healthy, filling foods within an hour of waking helps keep your blood sugar from plunging and spiking so that you feel more satisfied the rest of the day.

- » **Make sure the meals stay mini!** Even though you're eating more often, each meal should be smaller. You need to use a little bit of arithmetic to see where this guideline comes from. If you want to consume 2,000 calories a day, each mini meal should be approximately 320 calories. You can allot more calories to each meal and make your snacks a bit smaller, especially when you're just getting started.

- » **Prepare the foods yourself so that you can be sure they don't include any preservatives or additives.** Make your own snack mix or assemble a little wrap sandwich or fruit salad and pack it in an insulated lunch box.

- » **Carry your food with you.** If you work outside the home, make sure to bring your morning snack, lunch, and afternoon snack with you.

- » **Drink lots of water or unsweetened tea throughout the day.** Remember that thirst can masquerade as hunger. Drinking lots of water helps keep your digestive system running smoothly.

- » **Establish fairly regular eating times.** When you eat at about the same time every day, your body uses the calories more efficiently. Because you're not overtaxing or starving your digestive system, you feel stronger.

REMEMBER

Thousands of years ago, when human beings had to scratch and fight for every bite of food, their bodies used hunger to prevent starvation. When you let your body get too hungry or eat too little, it literally goes into starvation mode, which means you burn fewer calories. Your body believes it won't get any more food so it has to protect you! Because your body literally lives in the moment, it can plan only for periods of starvation, not abundance. Eating mini meals every few hours on a regular basis helps your evolutionary survival system relax so that you can relax.

Combining clean eating with your daily routine

Converting your daily routine to the eating clean lifestyle is easier than you think. Sure, you have to spend more time planning, shopping, and preparing meals than you do now, but as with all new skills, you'll get faster as you get more experience.

Especially when you're just getting started, you can eat clean meals with a little help from the grocery store. Whole-grain crackers spread with nut butter or some cheese and a granola bar make for perfectly acceptable mini meals. You don't have to make everything from scratch.

Build your clean eating plan right into your daily routine. Eat breakfast within an hour of waking up. Then schedule a morning snack three hours later. Eat your lunch at the regular time. Then have a piece of fruit during a mid-afternoon break. Eat your dinner at the regular time, and have a snack a few hours later to help you wind down your day and get in the mood for bed.

TIP

You may want to start a journal of your favorite mini meals. Think of the snacks you enjoyed as a child and try to find ways to convert them into clean foods. For example, if you loved eating nacho chips with soda pop, try to make your own crackers with nuts and seeds, and enjoy a few of them with some iced tea sweetened with agave nectar. Before you know it, you'll have a long list of snacks and mini meals that you enjoy eating. Check out the nearby sidebar "Keeping a food journal" for more details.

The Paleo Diet: Essential for Some

The Paleo diet, also called the hunter-gatherer diet, has had a lot of press in recent years. In a nutshell, this diet is designed around the foods our ancient ancestors ate. Before the onset of modern agriculture, people mostly ate foods they killed or found. Their diets consisted of meats, vegetables, nuts, seeds, fish, and some fresh fruits, but only in season. Grains and dairy were never eaten. Notwithstanding the problems of that way of life (such as wild animal attacks and infections), people were generally healthier. They ate as much as they wanted, whenever they were hungry.

REMEMBER

Humans are biologically wired for the hunter-gatherer type of meal. Before the agricultural revolution 10,000 years ago, the foods people ate included wild game, fish, vegetables (leafy and root), nuts, berries, and vegetables. In other words, your ancient ancestors knew nothing of refined carbohydrates, additives, preservatives, too much salt, or trans fats. Sitting around snacking on highly processed foods simply didn't exist; the so-called couch potato had yet to be invented!

Of course, modern humans live longer average lifespans than the cave people did (although some cave people did live into their 80s and 90s — without developing heart disease, high blood pressure, cancer, diabetes, or osteoporosis). But much of that increase in lifespan is the result of the development of antibiotics, which combat infection, and the modern lifestyle, which has significantly reduced human exposure to wild animals and natural accidents.

The development of modern farming, which enabled people to grow huge quantities of wheat, corn, rice, and other cereal grains fairly easily, supported the massive explosion in population and has made modern society possible. But it also changed the human diet to primarily grain-based foods and reduced the amount of work needed to eat.

Defining the Paleo diet

Your ancestors (we're talking cave men and women here, not Grandma who was famous for her coconut cream pie) never knew where their next meal was coming from. They had to work hard to get the food they did eat, and nothing was wasted. Whole foods straight from the animal or plant were the rule.

REMEMBER

The Paleo diet is actually very close to the eating clean diet plan. You avoid processed foods and foods high in sugar and salt, and eat unprocessed, healthy, nutrient-dense foods. But the Paleo diet excludes grains, legumes (including beans), and dairy, because those foods did not exist in ancestral times. These foods stimulate the "favorable" (in prehistoric times, but unfavorable now) mutation that leads to a hyperactive insulin response and triple-fat-gaining. Legumes and beans are also excluded because they contain phytic acid, which binds to nutrients in food so your body can't absorb them, and lectins, which can be toxic to some people.

Triple-fat-gainers (TGFs) are those people who gain triple the amount of fat when they eat the same high-carb and high-sugar foods as those who don't have that response. TFGs have a much more exaggerated insulin response than non-TFG people.

And dairy products are a no-no on the Paleo diet. It's not well known that dairy foods are high on the "insulinemic" index. Dairy products (except clarified butter) evoke an exaggerated insulin response.

But you'll discover that on the Paleo diet, your plate will be very full! As long as you stick to meats, eggs, nuts, seeds, some fruit, fish, and vegetables, you can eat as much as you want until you feel satiated. That is a huge bonus for people who are used to "dieting" by severely restricting food amounts and counting calories.

The following foods are important parts of the Paleo diet:

>> **Lean beef, preferably grass fed:** Choose extra-lean ground beef, lean cuts of steak, or London broil. Grass fed is important because it's anti-inflammatory. Grain-fed beef is pro-inflammatory (and grain is the food given to most cattle since the mid-1800s). *Remember:* Paleolithic cattle and other animals never, ever ate grains!

>> **Lean pork:** The best cuts of pork include the loin and chops. Pork tenderloin is especially good.

>> **White-meat poultry with no skin:** You can enjoy chicken, turkey, and game hens.

>> **Eggs:** These perfect sources of protein are a great addition to the Paleo diet.

>> **Wild game:** If you have a hunter in your family, you can eat elk, goose, buffalo, pheasant, quail, and deer.

>> **Fatty fish:** When you're in the mood for seafood, have a serving of salmon, sardines, perch, herring, cod, halibut, or anchovies. The omega-3 fatty acids in these fish are an important part of any diet.

>> **Brassica vegetables:** Eat plenty of cauliflower, broccoli, kohlrabi, and Brussels sprouts.

>> **Dark-green vegetables:** Eat your fill of asparagus, beet greens, eggplant, spinach, endive, kale, Swiss chard, rutabaga, peppers, and collard greens.

- » **Fresh vegetables:** Focus on eating bell peppers, spinach, celery, carrots, and cucumbers.

- » **Fruits:** Eat berries, cherries, citrus fruits, rhubarb, apples, cantaloupe, peaches, kiwi, cranberries, star fruit, and figs, but eat them in small quantities because they're high in sugars.

- » **Nuts and seeds:** To get your omega-3 fatty acids, eat flaxseed, walnuts, almonds, cashews, hazelnuts, pistachios, pine nuts, pecans, sesame seeds, sunflower seeds, and pumpkin seeds.

In contrast, the following foods have no place whatsoever in the Paleo diet:

- » Dairy products, including milk and cheese

- » Cereal grains, including wheat, corn, amaranth, and buckwheat

- » Russet potatoes and other white potatoes

- » Legumes, like beans, peas, and chickpeas

- » Processed foods (in other words, anything that comes in a box)

- » High-salt foods, including bacon, processed meats, pickled foods, sausages, and commercial sauces and dressings

- » Soft drinks (or any beverages full of empty calories and sweetened with sugar and artificial chemicals)

- » Fruit juices (which are very high in sugar and can easily raise your blood sugar level)

- » Sugary foods

Should you go caveman?

Most people who battle weight gain, have metabolic syndrome (belly fat, high triglycerides, high blood pressure, and high cholesterol), or have type-2 diabetes or a family history of that disease can benefit from the Paleo diet. The number of people with a tendency to those health issues is surprisingly high — about one-third of the population.

If you have osteoarthritis, be aware that recent research reports tell us that you have an 80 percent risk of ultimately developing type-2 diabetes. If you're under 50 when osteoarthritis starts, the chances are even more than 80 percent. If you have osteoarthritis, check with a physician skilled and knowledgeable in natural medicine and ask about the "Kraft pre-diabetes test," which can find pre-diabetes literally decades in advance of the actual onset of type-2 diabetes. If the Kraft pre-diabetes test is positive, for the best of health you should adopt the Paleo diet, too!

Of course, no one diet is best for every single person. But if you've already tried the low-fat route or any other specific diet and haven't had luck losing weight, give the Paleo diet a try. It's healthy and well balanced and may be the key to your weight and health struggle.

TIP

On the first few weeks of the Paleo diet, you may have some issues with digestion. Eating a lot of fiber-rich foods can cause some gastrointestinal distress, such as excess gas. Just stick with the plan and your body will adjust in time.

Just remember that the Paleo diet is a lifestyle change. You can ease into it by eliminating foods from your diet until you're eating only the recommended foods.

On the Paleo diet, if you are TFG, you will experience these changes in your body:

>> Lower blood pressure

>> Improved energy levels

>> Increased insulin sensitivity, lower insulin resistance, and better blood glucose numbers

>> Lower cholesterol and triglyceride numbers

>> Weight loss, sometimes quite considerable!

2

Meeting Your Eating Clean Goals

IN THIS PART . . .

Learn how to meet your eating clean goals, whether you want to lose weight, have more energy, or live longer.

Get information about how to eat clean to prevent diseases.

Motivate yourself to eat clean if you have an illness.

Chapter 6

Eating Clean for a Longer, Healthier, and More Active Life

E veryone wants to live a long life. But life is more than just living a lot of years; it's about the quality of those years. You want to spend your years being active and free from illness and disease so that you can enjoy every second. Although you may have received some bad cards in the genetic lottery, from a tendency to depression to genes that increase your cancer risk, you don't have to stand by and take those cards without a fight. Instead, you can take control of your life and fight for good health.

Eating right is one of the most important ways to help control your health. Years of poor diet can wreak havoc on your body, allowing free radicals, pollutants, and artificial chemicals to attack your cells and organs. But don't panic! No matter how old you are or what you've eaten in the past, choosing an eating clean life-style now can help change the path you've been on and make you healthier.

In this chapter, we look at how eating clean can help you live a longer, healthier, and more active — basically an all-around better — life. Specifically, we look at how to use eating clean to lose weight and fine-tune your body, to increase your energy and strength, and to detoxify your body to get rid of some of the effects of a poor diet, stress, aging, and pollution.

Eating Clean to Live Longer

No matter how much we'd like to, we can't guarantee you a longer life if you eat a good diet. But, all other factors being equal, if you eat healthy foods and forgo processed foods and foods high in trans fats, sugars, and additives, your chance for a longer, healthier life does improve. Yet a longer life isn't the only thing you need to think about. After all, if you live to be 100 but suffer from illness and infirmity the majority of the time, your quality of life will be fairly poor. Whether your life is long or short, the goal is to be as healthy and active as you can for as long as you can.

In this section, we look at how inflammation affects your body and how the foods you choose to eat may slow down this destructive process. We also look at how to boost your immune system, because infectious disease can lead to early death. We finish up by looking at probiotics and prebiotics, which may help keep you healthy.

Reducing inflammation in your body

More and more scientists are discovering that inflammation may be the prime culprit in many chronic and acute diseases. Inflammation affects your body in two ways:

>> **Good inflammation helps treat and heal wounds and injury.** For example, when you cut your finger and the skin around the cut swells and turns red, you're experiencing good inflammation. Your body sends platelets and white blood cells (leukocytes, lymphocytes, and neutrophils) to the injury to stop the bleeding and start the healing process. At the time, all the body's focus is on repairing the damage.

>> **Bad inflammation is low-level and chronic and may be one of the culprits behind some major diseases, including heart disease.** Low-level inflammation isn't as dramatic as the inflammation that occurs after you cut your finger. You won't realize it's happening until a serious acute disease develops. Bad inflammation is partly the result of free radicals that attack your cells. (In case you're wondering, *free radicals* are the byproducts of the natural aging process, pollution, poor diet, stress, allergens, and toxins.)

Chronic (bad) inflammation may cause and certainly exacerbates the following diseases:

- Heart disease
- Atherosclerosis
- Colitis
- High blood pressure
- Arthritis
- Diabetes
- Cancer

So how can you tell if you have chronic inflammation and are at an increased risk of these diseases? Although you can't be 100 percent sure, you can have your doctor run a C-reactive protein test (CRP test). Your body produces CRP in response to inflammation, so higher levels of CRP mean you have more inflammation. A higher CRP level is linked to heart and blood vessel disease.

The good news is that you can minimize chronic inflammation by eating the right kinds of foods. *Phytochemicals* (compounds such as antioxidants that can help prevent disease), vitamins, minerals, and essential fatty acids can all help reduce inflammation by neutralizing free radicals that attack your cells and prompt the inflammatory process. In fact, eating a healthy diet, along with quitting smoking and adding moderate exercise, is one of the best nonpharmaceutical ways to reduce inflammation.

REMEMBER

The best foods to eat to help combat inflammation include

>> **Fatty fish:** Fatty fish is high in omega-3 fatty acids, which are powerful anti-inflammatory compounds.

>> **Olive oil:** This oil, along with walnut oil, helps reduce the risk of heart disease because of its anti-inflammatory properties.

>> **Berries:** Strawberries, raspberries, and blueberries are packed full of phytochemicals, including phenols, flavonoids, and anthocyanins, which protect against free radical damage and oxidation.

>> **Teas:** Green tea contains a polyphenol called EGCG, which stops the expression of a gene that precipitates the inflammatory response.

>> **Orange and yellow produce:** These foods are a good source of beta-cryptoxanthin, a carotenoid that your body converts to vitamin A. When planning your weekly menu, choose more apricots, cantaloupe, mangoes, oranges, peaches, pineapples, carrots, yellow bell peppers, sweet potatoes, and squash.

>> **Spices and herbs:** Add these flavorful ingredients, such as curry powder and ginger, to your cooking to increase the inflammation-fighting properties of whole foods.

Avoid these foods to help reduce inflammation:

>> **Trans fats:** These fake fats are one of the worst substances you can eat. They promote inflammation by blocking enzymes that help stop inflammation. You find trans fats in any food with the word *hydrogenated* on the label. So staying away from foods with labels is the first step. The second step is reading foods with labels to make sure you're avoiding the bad stuff!

>> **Sugar:** When your insulin levels are high because of sugar intake, hormones called *eicosanoids* and the fatty acid arachidonic acid increase. These inflammatory compounds can make inflammation worse. Read labels on foods and avoid those with the terms *sugar, sucrose, fructose, dextrose, syrup, dextrin, corn syrup,* and *lactose,* among others.

>> **Vegetable oils:** Oils made from corn, soybeans, cottonseed, and safflower are high in omega-6 fatty acids, which are inflammatory. In addition, these oils are likely to come from genetically modified (GMO) seeds, which you should avoid on the eating clean plan anyway.

>> **Grain-fed meat:** Meat from grain-fed cows has a higher saturated fat content and many more omega-6 fatty acids than meat from grass-fed cows. Farmers also often feed grain-fed cows hormones and antibiotics because grain isn't their natural food.

>> **Processed meat:** The nitrites and nitrates in processed foods can cause cell damage. The body responds with inflammation to help repair the damage. So avoid processed meats, such as sausages, lunch meats, hot dogs, bologna, ham, and pepperoni.

>> **Food additives:** Additives like MSG, benzoate, and aspartame can trigger inflammation in the body. These compounds can also be toxic and can cause reactions that range from headaches to abdominal pain, breathing troubles, sweating, muscle aches, and mood changes.

>> **Refined grains:** White flour, white rice, and white pasta aren't whole foods. Because the production process removes their bran and germ layers, they have less fiber and a higher glycemic index, which means they raise blood sugar and start the inflammation process.

>> **Allergenic foods:** If you're allergic to a food, it may cause inflammation in your body. See Chapter 14 for more information about dealing with food allergies on the eating clean plan.

Strengthening your immune system

Your immune system is your body's defense against attack. Think of your body as a castle with a moat around it and soldiers poised with arrows positioned at the turrets. The immune system is a complex network of physical barriers (skin, mucous membranes, cell walls, and the entire gastrointestinal tract), cells that attack and kill invaders (white blood cells), organs (thymus and spleen), bone marrow, lymph system, hormones, and antibodies.

A healthy immune system does all of the following to protect your body:

>> Destroys viruses and bacteria that cause disease

>> Stops cell damage that can lead to diseases like cancer and heart disease

>> Fights infection after injuries

When your immune system is weakened or compromised, you're more susceptible to disease. Without a strong immune system, you can't interact with the world. (Remember the movie *The Boy in the Plastic Bubble*? The main character didn't have a functioning immune system, so all bacteria and viruses were a threat to his life and he had to live in a completely sterile environment.)

REMEMBER

Your diet can either strengthen your immune system or make it weaker. For instance, if you eat a lot of processed foods and foods with empty calories or artificial chemicals, your body will likely create free radicals from toxic byproducts; those free radicals will then damage your cells. In contrast, a diet of clean, whole foods can strengthen your immune system by providing phytochemicals, vitamins, and minerals that stop free radical and oxidation damage. By preventing free radical damage through your diet, you reduce the stress on your immune system. Your body also uses the nutrients in whole foods to build T-cells, macrophages, and lymphocytes, which are your immune system's frontline soldiers.

Your immune system's function slows as you age, so supporting it with foods rich in phytochemicals, vitamins, and minerals, which can help protect against free radical damage, is essential. Because appetite can also diminish as you age, you may need to take supplements that contain these important phytochemicals, vitamins, and minerals, even when you consume a healthy diet of whole foods.

Did you know that your intestines are an important part of your immune system? In fact, some doctors estimate that the lining of the intestines contains 60 percent of your body's immune cells. That's where protective gut bacteria live, so eating probiotics and prebiotics to encourage their growth is an important part of your diet. (See Chapter 4 for more information on those nutrients.) So eating a clean diet of whole foods is important to strengthening your immune system and keeping your intestines healthy and functioning at peak capacity.

The best nutrients to focus on for a healthy immune system include

>> **Vitamin C:** This powerful antioxidant is essential for a strong immune system. It supports T-cell function and stimulates the immune system by promoting white blood cell function. It also increases production of *interferon,* the antibody that protects cells from viruses. This vitamin is present in citrus foods, bell peppers, dark leafy greens, and berries.

>> **Vitamin E:** People with vitamin E deficiencies are more susceptible to disease-causing germs. You can get the recommended daily amount of vitamin E (about 10 mg) in a handful of almonds or other nuts, avocados, and wheat germ, but if you have a weakened immune system, you may need to take a daily supplement of 400 mg. Check with your doctor for more details. Just make sure your supplement consists of mixed tocopherols, because alpha-tocopherol alone can put your vitamin E ratio out of balance and can actually cause problems.

>> **Vitamin D:** Your body uses the sunshine vitamin to make germ-killing proteins. Getting enough vitamin D from foods is difficult, so unless you live in a tropical area and get lots of sunshine, you need to take a supplement. Check with a physician skilled in natural and nutritional medicine to help determine what amount is right for you.

>> **B-complex vitamins:** B vitamins help promote antibodies and T-cells, which are the immune system's first line of defense. Vitamin B6 supports blood lymphocytes, and folate increases T-cell distribution and immune cell activity. Foods high in B vitamins include fortified cereals, nuts, lentils, eggs, chicken, and dark green leafy vegetables.

>> **Carotenoids:** Beta carotene, the precursor to vitamin A, and other carotenoids help increase the activity of immune compounds that kill cancer cells. They can also protect cell membrane fats from oxidation, which damages them. Find this nutrient in green leafy vegetables, carrots, sweet potatoes, squash, and cantaloupe.

>> **Zinc:** This mineral is an *immunostimulant,* which means it promotes T-cell function. You may have noticed the proliferation of zinc lozenges sold to reduce the length and severity of colds; now you know why! Foods high in zinc include lean beef, wheat germ, chickpeas, and nuts.

>> **Selenium:** Trace minerals like selenium help build your immune system and keep it functioning efficiently. Your body uses selenium to help white blood cells clear viruses and bacteria from your body. Get this nutrient in fish, Brazil nuts, dried beans, mushrooms, chia seeds, and brown rice.

>> **Magnesium:** This mineral helps regulate the immune system and reduces the risk of infection. By regulating the immune system, it helps reduce the risk of *autoimmune diseases,* which are diseases caused by an overactive immune

system. (See Chapters 7 and 8 for details on preventing and managing these diseases with the eating clean plan.) Magnesium is found in dark leafy greens, nuts and seeds, and fish.

>> **Omega-3 fatty acids:** These essential fatty acids help promote strong cell membranes and membranes in your gastrointestinal tract. Omega-3 fatty acids can also boost the immune system and help slow down the aging process. Find them in fatty fish and eggs.

Eating Clean to Lose Weight

Everybody seems to want to lose weight these days. And because 60 percent of the American population is overweight and obese, we suppose that makes sense! But while fad diets, crash diets, and weird diets (bananas and oat bran, anyone?) can help you lose weight, they can also damage your health.

The clean eating plan is really the best diet for weight loss, simply because it's easy to follow and maintain. You can be on this diet for a lifetime, you don't have to count calories, carbs, or fat grams, and you certainly don't have to suffer from feelings of deprivation. Just eat whole, unprocessed foods, including lean meats (grass-fed only, if possible), fish, vegetables, whole grains, and fruits, and then watch the weight come off.

In this section, we look at specific tips for losing weight on the eating clean plan. We look at the calories consumed on the typical American fast-food diet compared to a diet of clean, whole foods. We finish up by discussing the importance of willpower and describing some other key behavior changes that can help you keep the weight off for good.

THE SAFEST FISH

Everyone has heard a lot about the mercury content of fish, and unfortunately, the hype is true. Although fatty fish is a fabulous source of omega-3 fatty acids, the large fish, which eat smaller fish (think of those Russian nesting dolls), can consume too much mercury, and that mercury concentrates in their fat. So avoid large fish like tuna, swordfish, shark, red snapper, moonfish, orange roughy, king mackerel, and tilefish. Stick with smaller fatty fish like wild salmon, mackerel, sardines, herring, and flounder. These fish have a much lower level of mercury.

Being aware of your calorie consumption

One of the nicest things about the clean eating plan is how much food you get to eat. If you've ever been on a diet that severely restricts calories, you know how easily you can get off track. Not only are whole, unprocessed foods good for you health-wise, but they're also high in fiber and water, which helps you feel full and reduces the number of calories you get in each bite.

To see just how much food you get to eat on the eating clean plan, compare a typical "diet plate" to a plate of clean foods. On the typical diet plate, you may have a 4-ounce piece of fish, a few pieces of broccoli with nonfat cheese melted on top, a piece of low-carb bread with diet margarine, and a fruit cup. A plate of clean foods, on the other hand, may contain a grass-fed steak, lots of sautéed veggies seasoned with fresh herbs, and a big spinach salad with strawberries and walnuts — all for about the same number of calories. Which one would you rather eat?

The typical American fast-food meal contains at least 1,000 calories, or more than half of your quota for the entire day. In fact, some meals contain enough calories, fat grams, and sodium to meet your quota for several days! One hamburger at a popular fast-food chain contains 1,300 calories, 3,150 mg of sodium, and 38 grams of saturated fat. On the other hand, a satisfying clean meal can contain about 500 calories, the right amount of healthy fat and little sodium, and a good one-third of your daily requirement of vitamins, minerals, fiber, and phytochemicals.

Strengthening your willpower

When you think about eating and plan what you want to eat, three parts of your brain are literally at war. The part that seeks pleasure and the part that's afraid you'll starve if you don't eat right now are battling the part of your brain responsible for restraint. The first two parts reside in an older, more primitive part of your brain called the *basil ganglia* and are stronger than the self-restraint part (the prefrontal cortex), which resides in a newer part of the brain that survival instincts can easily overrule.

Is this internal battle the reason why 95 percent of all dieters eventually regain any weight they lose? Yes! Is all hope lost? No! Now that you know that your brain is suffering from an internal fight for control, you can use some basic techniques to fight the primitive urges and give in to your self-restraint.

Willpower, another word for self-restraint, is like a muscle. You have to use it and exercise it to make it stronger. But also like a muscle, willpower can collapse under some conditions. When it does, you must coax it into a stronger presence in your brain. Because successful weight loss has so many different components (eating less, choosing the right foods, not eating under stress, and adding exercise, just to name a few), your willpower can easily be overwhelmed. Imagine if you tried to run a marathon without training for it. You'd collapse! The same thing happens to your willpower when you make too many changes at once.

Unfortunately, most people who are overweight have heard criticisms that they have no willpower. Not surprisingly, the people doing the criticizing have usually never had a weight problem, not to mention that such criticisms are downright wrong. Everyone has a limited amount of willpower; you just have to use it where it counts. In other words, don't try to do too much too soon.

REMEMBER

Losing weight should take a long time. After all, you didn't pile those pounds on in a month or two. Safe weight loss consists of about 1 to 2 pounds a week. Any more than that and you're pushing your body too hard and you'll be losing muscle and water weight, not fat. Weight loss programs that promise 10 pounds per week are not only untruthful but can also threaten your health.

Developing good habits

Losing weight is all about developing good habits. To lose weight successfully on the clean eating plan, make a habit of doing the following:

>> Avoid processed foods and eliminate fast foods from your diet.

>> Add healthy whole foods to your menu. Focus on foods in their natural state and eat lower on the food chain.

>> Eat when you're hungry and stop when you're full. (This advice sounds simple, but not everyone follows it without deliberately thinking about it.) One way to accomplish this is to eat slowly, without distractions — don't watch TV or read while eating. Pay attention to how your body feels and learn to recognize the true signs of hunger and satisfaction.

>> Concentrate on eating the type of foods that are best for your body. You may want to follow the Paleo diet plan if you have a family history of diabetes. Or you may want to try out the Mediterranean diet, with its emphasis on produce, fish, and olive oil. You'll know you're eating the right foods when your weight stabilizes, you feel wonderful, and your skin glows. Whichever diet you choose, just make sure it's clean.

>> Add exercise to build muscle, boost your mood, and enhance weight loss.

Don't try to adopt all these habits at one time. Instead, try to make one change every couple of weeks, keeping in mind that each change takes at least three weeks to become a habit. Limiting yourself to one change per every couple of weeks gives your body time to get used to your new lifestyle and gives your brain positive feedback as you accomplish each change. Build on each healthy diet change with positive affirmations. As you get into a habit of eating healthy foods, you literally train your basil ganglia into new patterns and you may be surprised to discover that you automatically reach for the fruit salad and roasted chicken rather than the fudge brownie and french fries.

TIP

Here's a psychological trick you can use on the clean eating plan to help you create good habits and strengthen your willpower. Most people try to get rid of bad habits by banishing them from their lives. Although throwing away all the junk food in your house is a good first step in the clean eating plan, doing so creates a big hole in your psyche (and pantry) that you need to fill with something else. Think about weeding a garden: If you don't plant something else where the weeds used to thrive, more weeds will move right in. So bolster your willpower and your eating clean plan by adding satisfying and healthy snack foods in place of the junk you get rid of. Add clean foods to crowd out the unhealthy foods you're used to eating. Fill your fridge with healthy, ready-to-eat snacks. Keep health-promoting snacks made with whole foods with you at all times, and make sure that you never get so hungry you'll fall on anything edible. (Turn to Chapter 9 for tips on how to stock your kitchen to fit your new eating clean lifestyle.)

As you begin any new diet plan or lifestyle, be sure to build failure right into that plan. Accept the fact that you will fail. Maybe you'll eat a doughnut, maybe you'll snack on some french fries, or maybe you'll eat some potato chips. However you fail, remember that one important difference between the eating clean lifestyle and all other diet plans is that you don't have to adhere 100 percent to its precepts. When you snarf down that brownie, enjoy it, accept it, and start over again at the next meal.

REMEMBER

Junk food and processed food is addictive. In fact, sugar, fat, salt, and additives can be as addictive as heroin. You need to treat yourself gently, add good habits to crowd out the old, reward yourself for accomplishments, and stop beating yourself up when you fall off the plan. (See Chapter 2 for more on how to deal with backsliding and lapses on the eating clean plan.)

Eating Clean for Energy

Just about everyone we know wants more energy. After all, no one wants to drag through life, feeling tired and worn out and having to make a major effort to get off the couch. Fortunately, you can control your energy levels, at least in part, by what you eat and what you don't eat — another reason why the eating clean plan is so good for you!

In this section, we look at clean foods that help increase your energy level. Because blood sugar levels directly affect your energy level, we point out foods that give you a boost of energy without the sugar rush and inevitable crash that follows. We also take a look at clean foods that promote better thyroid health because your thyroid is a critical part of living an energetic life.

Jumping off the sugar roller coaster

Everyone has experienced the sugar roller coaster. You know what we're talking about: Your energy lags in mid-afternoon, so you pick out a candy bar from the vending machine and gobble it down. Instant energy! You feel revved up and ready to go. But an hour later, you're more exhausted and limp than you were before your little sugar infusion. What's going on?

You're taking a ride on the classic sugar roller coaster. When you eat sugary foods, your blood sugar spikes, prompting insulin to enter the bloodstream to help process all that sugar. Insulin quickly lowers the blood sugar level and prompts hunger pangs, making you want to eat even more sugar.

Instead of eating sugary snacks to boost energy, many people turn to caffeinated drinks. These drinks affect blood sugar levels in ways that are similar to sugary foods. Plus, they're addictive. Whether you try to boost your energy via sugary snacks or caffeinated beverages, you put undue stress on your body, especially your pancreas, liver, and adrenal glands. That undue stress can result in fatigue.

The best way to get off the sickening sugar roller coaster is to adopt the clean eating plan by doing the following:

>> Eliminate or reduce your intake of processed foods.

>> Focus on eating healthy, whole, natural foods.

>> Eat small meals throughout the day.

>> Eat regular meals and snacks.

>> Combine protein, carbs, and fat at every meal and snack.

>> Always have healthy snacks with you.

>> Never let yourself get so hungry that you'll eat anything within reach.

If you want to boost your energy, incorporate the following foods into your daily menu:

>> **Nuts and seeds:** These foods are high in fiber, zinc, protein, and magnesium, which are all essential for converting food into energy. They also help you feel satisfied longer, and their good fats chase away hunger.

>> **Lean meats:** The healthy fats and protein in meats help boost your energy and balance your blood sugar levels. Protein contains tyrosine, which is essential for the production of dopamine, which helps you feel alert. If you choose to eat carbohydrates, pair them with meats or other protein sources to slow down your digestion and boost your energy level for a longer period of time.

>> **Fruits:** Whole fruits (not fruit juices) can provide a burst of energy because of their sugar content. Pair them with nuts or cheese to help slow down digestion and to satisfy your hunger pangs.

>> **Vegetables:** Concentrate on whole vegetables like broccoli, bell peppers, and mushrooms; they have plenty of fiber, which slows down digestion for a steady supply of energy, stabilizes blood sugar, and helps you feel satisfied longer. You may also add some sea vegetables to your diet to help improve your iodine intake; seaweed, nori, and kelp are delicious and very nutritious.

>> **Leafy dark greens:** These foods provide fiber, which slows down the digestion process so that your blood sugar stays level. Plus, dark greens are rich in phytochemicals, which help make your cells stronger, giving you more energy.

>> **Water:** Water is an essential part of the clean diet plan. Dehydration is an energy-zapper, and it slows down your metabolism. For more information about the importance of water, see Chapter 4.

Improving your metabolism by keeping your thyroid healthy

Your thyroid is a gland located at the base of your neck. As part of the endocrine system, your thyroid controls your energy use, metabolism, sleep cycles, and weight gain and loss. Because the foods you eat (and the nutrients in them or lack thereof) greatly affect your thyroid, you must eat well to keep your thyroid healthy. Not surprisingly, you can get all the nutrients your thyroid needs through the whole foods on the eating clean plan.

ENERGIZING YOUR LIFE WITH SUPPLEMENTS

You can take several different supplements to help potentially help give you more energy. Here are just a few:

- **Coenzyme Q10:** Helps supply energy to your body

- **L-carnitine:** Helps your body turn fat into energy and is tied to improved brain function in elderly people

- **Nicotinamide adenine dinucleotide (NADH):** Helps convert carbs, protein, and fat into energy

- **Kelp powder and seaweed:** The iodide in kelp powder and seaweed actually does boost function of the thyroid gland. As a bonus, the iodine in kelp lowers breast cancer risk. It's very difficult to overdose on kelp powder, but much easier to overdose on iodine and iodide as liquid or tablets.

- **Multivitamin with the complete B-complex vitamin, iron, and vitamins A, D, E, and K:** Can help improve your energy levels

Feeling lethargic, weak, and sluggish are all signs that your thyroid isn't functioning well. For example, if you have a low-functioning thyroid, also called *hypothyroidism*, you may experience feelings of exhaustion. If you have an overly active thyroid, or *hyperthyroidism*, you may suffer from insomnia, which leads directly to lethargy. So whether you suffer from hypothyroidism or hyperthyroidism, low energy is an issue.

Of course, you should talk to a doctor knowledgeable in nutritional medicine and get tested for thyroid disease if you suspect you have it. But you can help improve your thyroid function, increase your energy level, and feel better by taking the following diet-related actions:

>> **Always eat breakfast.** A healthy, nutritious breakfast is important for everyone, but it's especially crucial for those who suffer from thyroid disease. People who eat breakfast have better metabolism, more energy all day, and weigh less. And because one of the effects of thyroid disease is weight gain, it's important to eat a healthy breakfast.

>> **Follow the clean eating plan and eliminate (or reduce) processed foods, refined carbohydrates, and sugar from your diet.** These products wreak havoc on your blood sugar levels and put more stress on your thyroid.

>> **Eat more often throughout the day.** Doing so keeps your blood sugar levels stable and puts less stress on your thyroid. (Plus, eating more often is one of the keys to the eating clean plan.)

>> **Eat smaller meals as you move through the day.** Again, doing so helps stabilize your blood sugar levels and puts less stress on your thyroid.

>> **Don't let yourself get too hungry.** Low blood sugar prompts hunger and can make you reach for anything edible. Check out Chapter 5 for more on hunger cues.

>> **Concentrate on the B-complex vitamins.** These vitamins are essential for converting fuel into energy. Foods high in the B vitamins include beef, turkey, Brazil nuts, avocados, potatoes, bananas, and legumes.

>> **Get enough iodine and iodide.** *Iodine* is a rare element, but when it combines with other minerals, like potassium, it's called *iodide.* This trace element is central to thyroid function. The hormones your thyroid creates are the only ones that use iodine. Good food sources for iodide and iodine include seafood, iodized sea salt, eggs, mushrooms, spinach, sesame seeds, and garlic.

>> **Eat seaweed.** Although seaweed isn't part of a traditional American diet, many people around the world use various forms of seafood in their everyday cooking. (Think sushi at the Japanese restaurant.) Cultures that use the most seaweed generally have healthier thyroid function and, as a bonus, less breast cancer. Nori (dried, pressed seaweed) is available at a few stores, and powdered kelp is available in all natural food stores for use as a very mildly

salty spice. Sprinkle some kelp powder into your food. It's relatively bland in taste, unlike other types of seaweed. Using any of these products as part of a clean diet plan can help keep your family's thyroid glands healthier.

>> **Consume foods with vitamin D.** This vitamin is now considered a co-hormone, because it's essential to a properly functioning thyroid. Without enough vitamin D, your cells don't absorb thyroid hormones. You find the so-called sunshine vitamin in mushrooms, mackerel, herring, sardines (especially in the bones of those small fish), and eggs. Consider taking a supplement (make sure it's vitamin D3) if you don't live in a tropical climate.

>> **Focus on selenium.** This mineral helps regulate thyroid function and active thyroid hormone synthesis. It also helps your body regulate and recycle iodine. Brazil nuts are the very best source of selenium. Soybeans, sunflower seeds, mushrooms, and beef also contain more selenium than other foods.

>> **Get enough zinc, iron, and copper.** These essential minerals help regulate thyroid hormone production. Zinc and copper occur in the highest concentration in oysters and shellfish, next in beef and other animal proteins, and then in sunflower seeds, pumpkin seeds, lentils, and dark chocolate.

Eating Clean to Detoxify Your Body

The detox craze hit its peak a few years ago. The philosophy behind this trend started with the treatment of alcoholics and drug addicts: Because the liver metabolizes alcohol and drugs, many people think that the organ can become overstressed and weakened when a person consumes too much of either product. Thus, you need to detoxify it. Similarly, the detox diet seeks to rid your body of toxins and other chemicals you consume through processed food and pollutants that can harm your liver and other organs.

In this section, we look at how to tweak your clean eating plan to detoxify your liver. We discuss the foods and herbs to add to your diet for detoxification and look at some foods to avoid.

Understanding clean detoxification

By definition, a *detox diet* does the following:

>> Reduces or eliminates processed foods and the chemicals they contain

>> Emphasizes clean and nutritious foods

>> Focuses on increasing fiber and water intake

Sounds similar to the eating clean plan, right? In fact, the benefits of a detox diet are very similar to those of the eating clean plan: better digestion, clearer skin, more energy, and sharper concentration skills. (See Chapter 19 for more about the benefits of the eating clean plan.)

The aim of detoxification is to make toxins water-soluble so that your body can excrete them. Your liver performs this function in a process called *biotransformation*, which takes place in two phases. In the first phase (cleverly called phase I), the liver activates the toxins so that enzymes can recognize them and neutralize them. In the second phase (you guessed it — phase II), the liver pairs water-soluble molecules with the activated toxins and excretes them through urine or bile.

Toxins need to go through phase I to phase II as quickly as possible, because they can be carcinogenic in the first phase. This quick transition is where the foods you eat (and avoid) and the herbs and supplements you add to your diet come into play. The nutrients in certain clean, whole foods, herbs, and supplements can increase the production of your liver's key enzymes so that your liver can process toxins and eliminate them as quickly as possible.

Most people follow detox diets only once or twice a year. However, if you follow the eating clean plan, you may not need a detox diet, because your everyday diet is so healthy and toxin-free! But if you do choose to up the ante occasionally for detoxification, you need to know which foods to avoid and which foods to include in your diet.

REMEMBER

Unlike the eating clean diet, the detox diet requires you to avoid the following foods, which can be hard on the body, especially for people who are sensitive to them:

>> **Dairy products:** Dairy products can cause irritation and inflammation in the stomach and intestines, especially in people who are lactose intolerant.

>> **Wheat products and any food containing gluten (including rye, barley, and oats):** The gluten in wheat and other products can interfere with nutrient absorption in the intestines.

>> **Sugar:** Sugar is just another name for empty calories, and the foods high in sugar are usually high in saturated fat, additives, preservatives, and other chemicals, as well. Plus, sugar can cause inflammation and is addictive.

>> **Yeast:** A certain type of yeast called *Candida albicans* can be problematic if it overproliferates in the body, because it can trigger autoimmune diseases and yeast infections. This is not the same type as brewer's or baker's yeast.

>> **Chocolate:** While dark chocolate is good for you (in moderation), on a detox diet you want to eliminate sugar, so you must eliminate chocolate. Chocolate also contains caffeine, another no-no on the detox diet.

Because the point of detoxification is to support the liver, you need to emphasize certain liver-healthy nutrients as part of a detox diet. When you want to tweak your eating clean plan for detoxification, be sure to include these foods:

>> **Fresh fruits and veggies:** Organic and unprocessed fruits and veggies provide the cornerstone of a detox diet because they're free of toxins and contain large amounts of vitamins, fiber, and antioxidants.

>> **Beets:** These root vegetables contain the amino acid betaine, which can help heal the liver and improve production of bile acids.

>> **Cruciferous vegetables:** Broccoli, cauliflower, watercress, Brussels sprouts, kohlrabi, cabbage, and kale help support the liver. These foods are very rich in antioxidants, fiber, and phytochemicals like glucosinolates, which help liver enzymes eliminate toxins.

>> **Onions and garlic:** In addition to being delicious, these veggies are rich in allyl sulfides and other sulfur compounds that help enzymes in the liver eliminate toxins and can help eliminate heavy metals from cells.

In the detox variation of the eating clean plan, try to rely on natural, unprocessed, whole foods rather than medical foods or supplements. However, keep in mind that supplements (especially for those important nutrients, such as vitamin C, vitamin D, and calcium with magnesium) are a good idea for many people just to ensure that they meet their special nutritional needs.

Taking herbs and spices for detoxification

Cooking with herbs is an important part of the clean eating plan. These fragrant additions to your food can help reduce your dependence on salt, add important phytonutrients to your diet, and make healthy food taste wonderful.

Fortunately, herbs and spices are key to a detoxification plan, too. Just make sure the herbs and spices you incorporate into your meals are fresh, not dried. Most spices last only about six months in the average kitchen; then they lose their potency (and flavor!).

Certain herbs play an important role in liver function and health. Try to include these herbs in the recipes you make:

>> **Peppermint:** This herb is a tonic and digestive stimulant for women. Try sprinkling chopped peppermint leaves on chicken dishes or adding them to green salads. But spearmint or spearmint tea should not be given to men, since it reduces testosterone levels, which can increase his risk of cardiovascular disease, osteoporosis, and Alzheimer's disease. Men should stick with regular green or black tea varieties.

>> **Parsley:** Parsley is rich in phytochemicals, vitamin C, and chlorophyll, which can act as a cleansing agent.

>> **Garlic:** Garlic has many healthy compounds that support detoxification and increase phase II enzyme activity in the liver. Although some of these compounds have been isolated and sold in pill form, many scientists think that garlic is more helpful when you consume it in its natural form.

>> **Turmeric:** The all-important phytochemical curcumin, which you find in large quantities in turmeric, is essential for detoxification. The curcumin in turmeric increases the phase II enzymes in the liver, which make toxins easier to remove from the body. And the curcumin fraction of turmeric can significantly lower the risk of developing Alzheimer's disease.

>> **Rosemary and sage:** These herbs contain carnosol, a phytochemical that helps increase phase II enzymes.

>> **Green tea:** Compounds in green tea increase both phase I and phase II enzyme activity.

Add peppermint to your green tea if you're female. Chop parsley and put it in everything from soups to meatloaf. Include curry powder in stir-fries and casseroles. You get the idea!

Whether you choose to detox occasionally by concentrating on these foods and eliminating others or you think the eating clean plan is enough, be sure to get a good mix of foods in your diet. Not only do new foods make mealtime interesting, but they can also add a new mix of vitamins, minerals, and phytochemicals to your diet.

Recovering after a sugar binge

If you've eaten a lot of sugar — whether it's because of Valentine's Day, Halloween, Christmas, or because your neighbor made her famous caramel fudge brownies — there are things you can do to feel better and get back on the clean eating plan.

After a sugar binge, you won't feel very good. Your insulin levels are bouncing around and you may even feel slightly nauseated. Here's what you can do to make yourself feel better physically:

>> Drink lots of water to help your kidneys function and process the sugar out of your body.

>> Consider some mild exercise to help your body use the sugar instead of storing it.

>> Eat a snack high in protein, such as some nuts, to help your body recover and to slow digestion. Don't skip a meal — you want to get your blood sugar back in balance.

>> Plan your meals for the next day, including foods high in protein and low in carbs, with healthy fats.

The next step is to forgive yourself. Don't beat yourself up over this misstep. Something happened to make those sweets look tempting. Was it upsetting news? A bad day on the job? Or did you just feel like binging?

USING SUPPLEMENTS TO ENCOURAGE DETOXIFICATION

Some supplements that can help detoxify your liver include

- **Schisandra chinensis:** This medical plant protects liver cells from toxin damage and increases enzyme activity in phase I and phase II.

- **Milk thistle:** This plant increases the liver's production of glutathione, which aids in phase II enzyme production.

- **Citrus oils:** These ingredients contain limonene, which can help increase levels of essential liver enzymes that help detoxify carcinogens, and vitamin C, a powerful antioxidant, which can help your liver remove free radicals.

- **Probiotics and prebiotics:** These bacteria and bacterial growth supporters help repopulate your intestine with "good" bacteria, which can relieve strain on your liver. (See the section "Getting your probiotics and prebiotics" for more details.)

- **Vitamin C:** Vitamin C is a vital part of the detoxification process. When an animal's liver detoxifies anything at all — a poison, a carcinogen, a patient medication, a chemical — it immediately makes more vitamin C (ascorbic acid). Under the same circumstances, your liver tries to make more ascorbic acid, too, but humans are missing the last of the four enzymes that animals' livers use to make vitamin C from glucose.

  Because many people barely get enough ascorbic acid in their diets to prevent scurvy (a serious and sometimes deadly disease caused by an ascorbic acid deficiency) and not nearly enough for optimum health, most physicians skilled in natural and nutritional medicine recommend a daily vitamin C supplement.

REMEMBER

The aim of eating clean is to improve your life. If you enjoyed the treat, forgive yourself and move on. And the next time you see something tempting, stop and think: Do you really want that slice of cheesecake, or are you trying to fill a hole in your life or solve a problem with food? If everything is okay and the sugary treat looks tempting, think about having one bite, enjoying it completely, and then moving on with your healthy life. Don't give up on your clean eating plan or fall off the wagon. This is just a small misstep in your lifelong plan of eating clean.

Chapter 7

Eating Clean to Prevent Disease

No one wants to get sick. Yet every day thousands of people develop serious diseases that need invasive and expensive medical treatments. Although genetics plays a part in some disease development, what you eat and how you live your life are very significant factors in whether you stay healthy or get sick.

Just eliminating processed and refined foods from your diet is a great first step toward disease prevention. After you wean yourself off of these chemical-laden foods, you can fine-tune your eating plan to take disease prevention to the next level.

In this chapter, we look at specific ways to modify the basic eating clean plan to help prevent certain diseases. We discuss what you should eat to help prevent heart disease and reduce cancer risk, how you can plan your diet to reduce cholesterol levels and prevent diabetes, and how you can eat clean to prevent autoimmune diseases.

As you read this chapter, notice that we mention the same substances over and over again as tools in fighting many diseases. The beauty of the eating clean plan is that the wholesome clean foods you eat on the plan can play many roles in keeping you as healthy as possible.

Eating Clean to Help Prevent Heart Disease

Heart disease is the number-one killer of men and women in the United States. Yet many of these deaths could be prevented with proper nutrition — starting with a clean diet — as well as exercise and a few lifestyle changes.

In this section, we look at the foods to eat (and the foods to avoid) to keep your heart and circulatory system healthy. Because most of the foods on the do-not-eat list include processed foods and those high in saturated and trans fats, sugar, and artificial ingredients, the clean eating plan can automatically get you on the right track.

TIP

Add exercise to your clean eating plan for heart health. It helps reduce stress, helps you lose weight, and strengthens all the muscles in your body — including your heart!

Getting some variety in your diet (with lots of fruits and vegetables)

As you work toward heart disease prevention, you can follow one of several special diets, including the Dietary Approaches to Stop Hypertension (often called the DASH diet), whose main purpose is to reduce the number of foods you eat that are high in saturated and trans fats, cholesterol, and salt. But the eating clean plan automatically reduces your fat, cholesterol, and salt consumption (and offers many other health benefits) by focusing on fresh, whole foods.

Really strive to consume five to ten servings of fresh vegetables and fruits every single day. Not many Americans eat this much produce, and their health is poorer as a result. After all, fresh fruits and veggies contain the phytochemicals and vitamins and minerals that can help reduce blood cholesterol levels, strengthen the circulatory system, prevent cellular damage, reduce blood clots, prevent hardening of the arteries and plaque buildup, and increase blood flow.

Focus on getting plenty of the following phytochemicals for heart health:

>> **Antioxidants:** These chemicals, found in colorful fruits and vegetables, prevent damage to your heart and blood vessels from free radicals. They also help keep cholesterol from oxidizing and sticking to artery walls. Although single supplements of these phytochemicals are useful, they're not as effective as whole foods, which offer many additional benefits.

>> **Phytosterols:** You can reduce cholesterol counts in your bloodstream with these phytochemicals, which speed up your body's cholesterol excretion. Find them in whole grains, legumes, and nuts.

>> **Flavonols:** These compounds, which you find in tomatoes, apples, broccoli, and tea, can strengthen blood vessels and reduce the blood-clotting activity of platelets. Strong blood vessels are key to fighting heart disease.

>> **Polyphenols:** Reduce the LDL, or bad, cholesterol in your blood by eating foods rich in these compounds. Polyphenol-rich foods include whole vegetables, fruits, whole grains, and legumes. The polyphenols in olive oil may actually modify atherosclerosis-related genes (the genes that can cause a thickening of artery walls).

>> **Catechins:** Eating a diet rich in catechins, which you find in wine, grapes, and dark chocolate, can help reduce plaque formation in your arteries. (Plaque formation can lead to coronary artery disease and heart attacks.)

>> **Allyl sulfides:** Found in garlic, leeks, and chives, these compounds can help improve blood circulation, reducing the risk of plaque and blood clots. Allyl sulfides also help keep triglycerides from clotting, which reduces the risk of heart attack.

>> **Carotenoids:** These compounds can help prevent hardening of the arteries, which is a major risk factor in the development of heart disease. Find carotenoids in all orange, yellow, and red fruits and vegetables.

To maximize your intake of phytochemicals and whole foods, try new fruits and vegetables on a regular basis. Add a new food to your diet every week, visit a farmers' market and ask questions about unusual produce, and look through the produce aisle of your supermarket for interesting fruits and vegetables. Adding more fruits and veggies keeps your diet more varied, making you less likely to turn toward processed, unhealthy foods.

Focus on consuming foods that contain these vitamins and minerals for heart health:

>> **Vitamin E:** This vitamin is a powerful antioxidant that helps reduce inflammation. In vitro studies found that LDL cholesterol doesn't oxidize in the presence of vitamin E, which could prevent the first step in atherosclerosis. This vitamin also helps prevent blood cells from aggregating. Eat foods high in this vitamin instead of relying on supplements. Foods high in vitamin E include nuts, tomatoes, spinach, fortified cereals, dark leafy greens, sunflower seeds, peanut butter, and avocados.

>> **Coenzyme Q10 (CoQ10):** You find this vitamin-like antioxidant in many foods, including liver, beef, sardines, and peanuts, as well as in your heart muscle

where it helps increase your cells' energy capabilities (which is important given how much energy your heart uses!). Your body synthesizes CoQ10, but synthesis decreases with age. You may want to consider a CoQ10 supplement, especially if you're taking statins or other heart medications and if you're past age 55. By then the body's internal CoQ10 synthesis has almost always declined.

>> **Vitamin C:** Most studies have found that vitamin C intake is critical to heart health. This vitamin helps maintain cell strength and tissue integrity, which are particularly important to the heart muscle and artery walls. Good food sources for vitamin C include all citrus fruits, red bell peppers, broccoli, cantaloupe, tomatoes, strawberries, and other brightly colored fruits and vegetables.

>> **Vitamin D:** Cardiologists are recommending more vitamin D for their patients. Vitamin D can help control inflammation and blood glucose levels and regulate blood pressure. Despite the importance of vitamin D, deficiency of this vitamin is quite common in the United States. Get some sunshine on bare (no sunscreen) skin every day if possible. However, if you live to the north of a line drawn roughly from Los Angeles to South Carolina, the vitamin D-producing rays of the sun don't reach the earth's surface between late October and early April, so getting sunshine on your bare skin during those months doesn't help your vitamin D levels at all! So take a supplement and look for these vitamin D-rich foods: cod liver oil, salmon, tuna fish, fortified cow's milk, eggs, liver, and cheese.

>> **Vitamin B complex:** Vitamins B6, B12, and folate can reduce homocysteine levels in the blood. Too much homocysteine in your blood may increase your risk for cardiovascular disease. The active forms of vitamin B6 can also help reduce inflammation in the body. Get these vitamins from vegetables and fruits, whole grains, legumes, fortified cereals, and in lesser amounts from lean fish, poultry, and dairy products.

>> **Calcium:** When paired with magnesium, this mineral helps control blood pressure. Like with other nutrients, try to get calcium from food first. Good calcium sources include yogurt, blackstrap molasses, white beans, cheese, broccoli, quinoa, and sesame seeds. But you'll probably need calcium/magnesium supplements when you pass age 40.

WARNING

Some studies have shown that taking calcium supplements without magnesium may increase the risk of a heart attack, so if you take a calcium supplement, make sure it contains magnesium, too.

>> **Magnesium:** This mineral helps regulate heart rhythm and stops the spasming of coronary arteries and muscles all over the body. It's the major mineral involved in your body's synthesis of ATP, the number-one energy molecule. Magnesium also controls high blood pressure. Get magnesium from leafy dark-green vegetables, whole grains, and nuts. Try to eat the greens raw for the most absorption.

>> **Potassium:** Along with magnesium, potassium helps balance the effects of sodium on your heart. This electrolyte relaxes artery walls, helping to reduce blood pressure. Higher potassium intake is associated with lower risk of stroke. Getting potassium from whole foods is the best way to achieve a good sodium/potassium balance. Foods rich in potassium include potatoes, bananas, apricots, avocados, beets, spinach, and tomatoes. For people with high blood pressure, many doctors recommend replacing sodium chloride salt with potassium chloride salt, which is available in grocery stores and natural food stores.

>> **Selenium:** This antioxidant helps prevent inflammation and reduces the levels of homocysteine in the blood. Selenium also reduces the risk of prostate cancer. Selenium deficiency leads to Keshan disease, which is a form of cardiomyopathy (severe heart muscle weakness). Plant foods are a great source of selenium, but the best source is the Brazil nut. Other good sources of selenium include fatty fish, asparagus, garlic, spinach and other leafy greens, wheat germ, eggs, oats, tofu, brown rice, and cashew nuts.

So how do you make sure you get enough of all these heart-healthy phytochemicals, vitamins, and minerals? Eat a diet that's rich in the following clean, whole foods:

>> **Vegetables:** Choose colorful vegetables to make a rainbow on your plate. Consuming a variety of vegetables is the best way to get enough phytochemicals, vitamins, and minerals.

>> **Whole grains:** Fiber from these foods is important for regulating cholesterol in your body. Soluble fiber helps remove cholesterol from your GI tract. Whole grains are also an important source of B vitamins.

>> **Fruits:** Fresh fruit is an excellent source of phytochemicals, fiber, and essential vitamins. Stick with whole fruits and avoid fruit juices if you or someone in your family has a history of obesity, diabetes, or heart disease. Remember that eating whole fruits ensures that you get nutrients that scientists don't even know about yet. Plus, whole fruits satisfy your hunger pangs.

>> **Oily fish:** Make wild salmon, sardines, and herring a part of your weekly diet plan. In fact, strive to eat them twice a week! These fish are high in omega-3 fatty acids, which help lower triglyceride levels in your blood. They're also high in protein and are satisfying to eat.

>> **Nuts:** People who regularly eat nuts have lower levels of LDL cholesterol. These foods improve the lining of your arteries and reduce the development of blood clots. The monounsaturated fats, fiber, vitamin E, plant sterols, and l-arginine that you find in nearly all nuts make them an excellent heart-healthy food. Add walnuts, almonds, hazelnuts, macadamia nuts, pecans, and pistachios to your diet.

» **Seeds:** Sunflower seeds, sesame seeds, and pumpkin seeds are good sources of zinc, protein, vitamin E, and magnesium. Try to eat unroasted seeds, since heat reduces the antioxidant levels in these foods and oxidizes much of the essential fatty acid content. Flaxseed is okay in small quantities, but large quantities may increase the risk of prostate cancer.

» **Legumes:** All legumes are whole foods and good for your heart. Look for canned varieties with no added salt and packed in BPA-free cans or cook dried legumes. The fiber in legumes helps reduce cholesterol levels, and the saponin in many legumes helps reduce inflammation, which is a cause of atherosclerosis.

SUPPLEMENTS FOR HEART HEALTH

Before you add any supplements (even those recommended for heart health) to your diet, be sure to talk to your doctor. But remember that many physicians know much more about patent medicines, or pharmaceuticals, than vitamins and minerals, so you may want to check with a physician who specializes in natural medicine.

Consider taking the following heart-healthy supplements:

- **Fish oil:** Its omega-3 fatty acids reduce inflammation throughout the body, inhibit abnormal blood clotting, and lower triglycerides.

- **Plant sterols:** They help lower LDL cholesterol levels.

- **Niacin:** Niacin, particularly the slow-release form, lowers cholesterol and improves HDL levels. Recent studies have shown that it can also reduce abnormal arterial thickness.

- **Green tea extract:** It decreases LDL levels.

- **CoQ10:** This antioxidant helps increase your cells' energy capabilities. Consider taking a CoQ10 supplement especially if you're taking statin drugs and are over age 55.

- **Red yeast rice:** It lowers total cholesterol, LDL cholesterol, and triglyceride levels.

- **Magnesium:** This mineral dilates blood vessels, helps lower blood pressure, helps with the production of ATP, and helps maintain normal heart rhythm.

- **Herbs and extracts like yarrow, holy basil, and artichoke leaf extract:** These ingredients can help reduce cholesterol and triglyceride levels.

After you decide which supplements you want to take, be sure to buy the supplements from a highly reputable source. But remember that food comes first. A healthy diet based on the eating clean plan is your most important tool in the fight against heart disease.

TIP

Even when you're eating heart-healthy foods like the ones we mention in the preceding list, you must remember to control portion sizes. When asked to self-regulate food portions, most Americans eat way too much of any product. A healthy serving of whole-grain pasta is only ½ cup, while a serving of lean meat is only 3 ounces, about the size of a deck of cards. Making portion control a big part of your eating clean plan is a great way to improve heart health.

Avoiding the bad foods

If you want to eat a heart-healthy diet, try to avoid the following foods. (The best way to do so is to follow the eating clean plan because it automatically eliminates processed foods, foods with artificial ingredients, foods high in trans fats, and foods that provide empty calories.)

>> **High-sodium foods:** Some authorities say that most adults should consume less than 2,400 milligrams of sodium per day, but most Americans consume at least 3,400 milligrams per day. This electrolyte, especially when coupled with poor potassium consumption, can increase blood pressure and increase the risk of heart attack.

Most processed foods contain sodium in large quantities. So reducing your intake of processed foods on the eating clean diet plan automatically helps you reduce your sodium intake. Use spices and herbs rather than salt to enhance your food's flavor and get used to a less salty taste in your foods.

>> **Trans fats:** Trans fats have been linked to some serious health problems. Very few trans fats occur in nature; manufacturers create them by hydrogenating polyunsaturated fats to make them solid at room temperature. Trans fats actually become part of the structure of your cells, making them weaker and more prone to errors. The Nurses' Health Study found that women who eat foods with trans fats are more than three times as likely to develop heart disease as those who avoid them.

Avoid processed foods, especially bakery foods, crackers, cookies, and snack foods. Although you can read food labels to find trans fat amounts, manufacturers are allowed to claim "0 grams of trans fats" as long as the product has less than 0.5 gram of trans fat per serving. So if you eat five servings of that product, you've consumed up to 2.5 grams of trans fat, and there is no safe intake threshold for this fake fat.

>> **Processed meats:** Consuming processed meats increases the risk of heart disease. Salt and preservatives, like sodium nitrate, in these foods can increase blood pressure and may promote atherosclerosis. For this reason, many scientists believe that the salt and preservatives, not the saturated fat, actually make processed meats a health risk. Sodium nitrate and nitrite react

with compounds in meat to form nitrosamines, which are carcinogenic. So if you do eat processed meats, consider consuming a food high in vitamin C at the same time to help stop the formation of nitrosamines.

>> **Fast food:** Everyone knows that a steady diet of fast-food burgers and french fries isn't good for you. But why are these foods so bad? They contain many preservatives, additives, and artificial ingredients. Fast food is high in fat, sugar, and trans fats and low in healthy ingredients like whole grains, fruits, and vegetables. Plus, these foods are high in advanced glycation end products (AGEs), which form when you cook fatty food at a high heat. AGEs irritate cells and can lead to heart disease, diabetes, Alzheimer's disease, and stroke. Canadian scientists have found that fast food may cause 35 percent of all the heart disease in the world.

>> **Foods high in sugar:** The average sugar consumption in America is 150 pounds per person per year! Studies have linked a high intake of sugar to increased coronary heart disease. Sugar can cause changes in lipoproteins. These changes reduce HDL cholesterol (the good stuff) in your blood, and a diet high in sugar increases blood triglyceride levels. For one-third of Americans, high sugar consumption can lead to high blood pressure, high cholesterol, and ultimately type-2 diabetes. For men over 40 with this tendency, high sugar intake also lowers testosterone levels while raising estrogen levels.

Diets high in sugar are usually deficient in many nutrients because many foods that are high in sugar lack nutritional value but provide lots of empty calories. So try to reduce your sugar consumption and satisfy your sweet tooth naturally through fresh fruits.

TIP

If you can't eliminate these foods completely from your diet, try to limit them as much as possible. Remember that you can have a treat every now and then. But if you choose to have one of these foods as a treat, have only a small amount and don't go on a binge.

Adding clean monounsaturated fats to your diet

Monounsaturated fats are one type of fat that's actually good for your heart. In fact, when you use them to replace trans fats and saturated fats, monounsaturated fats, especially from food sources like nuts and vegetables, can lower your risk of heart disease. You find these fats in foods that are high in vitamin E, an important antioxidant. Studies have found that monounsaturated fats may actually remove plaque from your arteries and may reduce LDL cholesterol levels in your blood. As a bonus, they increase HDL cholesterol levels at the same time!

REMEMBER

Look for monounsaturated fats in avocados, peanut butter and other nut butters, whole nuts, and seeds. Olive and macadamia nut oils are highest in monounsaturated fats, so use these oils for cooking. But beware of oils made from genetically modified (GMO) foods. Canola oil, which is also high in monounsaturated fats, usually comes from GMO corn, the long-term effects of which are unknown at this time.

Note: Overall, your fat intake shouldn't total more than 35 percent of the calories you consume during the day. On the eating clean plan, when you focus on whole produce, whole grains, and unprocessed foods, you shouldn't have trouble sticking to that number.

If you're on a diet intended to reduce cholesterol levels (if your doctor has told you to reduce cholesterol intake), you can make that diet even better for you by adding monounsaturated fats. (Remember that in those who are genetically predisposed to type-2 diabetes, the Paleo diet reduces cholesterol levels. The Paleo diet does *not* do this for those not genetically predisposed to type-2 diabetes.) Many nutritionists recommend the Mediterranean diet, which is high in monounsaturated fats, for people trying to reduce cholesterol levels. This diet incorporates the eating patterns of people who live around the Mediterranean Sea. If you have high cholesterol, before choosing either Paleo or the Mediterranean diet, check with a doctor skilled and knowledgeable in natural medicine to have the Kraft pre-diabetes test done.

WHAT ABOUT THE PALEO DIET?

The Paleolithic (Paleo) diet, which is based on the diet your ancestors ate as hunters and gatherers, can be a powerful tool against heart disease. This plan works because the animal protein in the Paleo diet comes from free-range and wild animals and fish. These animals have much higher concentrations of omega-3 fatty acids and much lower overall fat content than commercial meats raised on grain. Because grain is an unnatural source of food for these animals, their meat is much higher in pro-inflammatory omega-6 fatty acids and has a higher overall saturated fat content. Talk to a doctor skilled in nutritional medicine if you want to try this diet to help prevent heart disease. Also check out Chapter 6 for more details on the Paleo diet in general.

UNDERSTANDING THE OMEGA-3: OMEGA-6 RATIO

When you're eating to prevent heart disease, you need to make sure you find the right balance of omega-3 and omega-6 fatty acids in your diet. You have to eat these essential nutrients because your body can't make them on its own. But you need to be aware of how many of each kind you eat. Estimates of the ideal ratio range from 1:1 to 1:4 (omega-3:omega-6). But the typical American diet has a ratio of between 1:10 and 1:20!

Why is the 1:1 or 1:4 ratio so important? Generally speaking, omega-3 fatty acids are anti-inflammatory, which means they reduce inflammation throughout the body. Omega-6 fatty acids are almost exclusively pro-inflammatory, which means they contribute to inflammation in the body. Although inflammation is a very necessary step in healing, if you allow it to go on and on because of inadequate omega-3 fatty acid intake, your body can suffer tissue damage and disease.

In fact, many experts now believe that chronic inflammation is, in large part, the cause of atherosclerosis. The natural imbalance of omega-6 to omega-3 fatty acids is largely responsible for the consumption of so many anti-inflammatory medications.

Omega-3 fatty acids are very good for your heart. They help prevent platelets from clotting and sticking to artery walls, which helps reduce abnormal blood clotting and plaque. Good sources of omega-3 fatty acids include seafood, especially fatty fish like salmon and sardines, free-range beef, bison, and other animals, omega-3-enriched eggs, walnuts, and flaxseed. Increasing the intake of these fatty acids reduces the risk of chronic heart disease.

You find omega-6 fatty acids in avocados, whole grains, and nearly all nuts and seeds. (Remember, though, that roasting nuts and seeds oxidizes much of their essential fatty acid content. You may want to consider eliminating roasting these ingredients if a recipe calls for it.) Many processed and refined foods, like snack foods, cake mixes, and junk food, are made with omega-6-containing plant oils, especially corn oil, safflower oil, sunflower oil, and peanut oil. Because many Americans eat so many of these foods and fewer foods high in omega-3 fatty acids, the ratio of omega-6 to omega-3 has swung in the wrong direction.

Scientists are divided as to whether or not omega-6 fatty acids are actually bad for your heart. But they do agree on one point: People should consume more omega-3 fatty acids, especially from sources recommended by the eating clean diet plan.

In many ways, the Mediterranean diet and the eating clean diet are one and the same. They both involve

>> Eating lots of fresh, whole produce, including brightly colored fruits and vegetables

>> Eating oily fish at least three times a week

>> Adding lots of olive oil to recipes and using it for cooking and baking

>> Eating nuts as snacks

>> Consuming lots of legumes and whole grains

>> Eating lean produce in moderate amounts

One difference between the Mediterranean diet and the eating clean plan is that the Mediterranean diet calls for consuming a glass of red wine every day. While you can certainly drink wine on the eating clean plan, if you don't consume alcohol normally, don't start just for the purported health benefits.

Eating Clean to Lower Blood Pressure

Hypertension (high blood pressure) is a silent killer in this country. As many as 80,000,000 Americans have high blood pressure, which can lead to heart attacks, kidney failure, and stroke. Fortunately, the clean eating program can help get that blood pressure under control.

If your doctor says you have high blood pressure, take the medications prescribed, and think about changing your diet. The diet recommended by the American Heart Association is the DASH diet. (*DASH* is short for *dietary approaches to stop hypertension.*)

Fortunately, this diet encourages you to eat a variety of foods rich in potassium, calcium, and magnesium that can help lower blood pressure. It's really the clean eating plan! Eat whole foods; avoid packaged, processed, and fast foods; and reduce sodium.

And you can include the following foods in your diet that are high in potassium, calcium, and magnesium:

>> Bananas for potassium

>> Red and white beans for potassium and magnesium

>> Lowfat yogurt for calcium and magnesium

>> Peaches and nectarines for potassium and magnesium

>> Kale for calcium, magnesium, and potassium

REMEMBER

Eating whole and unprocessed foods will automatically lower your sodium intake. Most of the sodium in our diets comes from processed foods. Always read labels on any products you buy and look for the sodium content. People with hypertension should consume no more than 1,500 mg of sodium every day.

There's one other very simple thing to do with your diet that helps lower blood pressure and keep it lowered: Change to potassium chloride salt, available in most supermarkets and natural food stores. In his book *The High Blood Pressure Solution*, Dr. Richard Moore describes in easy-to-understand language that discarding sodium chloride salt and using only potassium chloride salt — as much as your taste buds will allow — can significantly lower blood pressure.

The other option is a salt that can do as well as or better than potassium chloride salt — potassium-magnesium salt — which also contains very small amounts of lysine, silicon, zinc, copper, selenium, and iodide. This is the same salt that was responsible for a significant part of the 30-year (1976–2006) "Medical Miracle" in Finland. In this nationwide effort, all sodium chloride salt was replaced nationwide with potassium-magnesium salt and they worked to reduce saturated fat and increase unsaturated fat consumption.

What was the result? According to the 2006 report on this 30-year nationwide effort: a 75 percent to 80 percent decrease in both stroke and coronary heart disease mortality. There was also an increase in life expectancy of both male and female Finns of six to seven years. A prior report noted that only 10 percent to 15 percent of this improvement could be attributed in any way to pharmaceuticals.

The potassium-magnesium salt used in this 30-year nationwide research project in Finland has been duplicated in the United States. Unfortunately, as this is written it's available only in a few natural food stores and the Tahoma Clinic Dispensary (www.tahomadispensary.com).

Eating Clean to Reduce Cholesterol

Cholesterol is a waxy substance found in all cell membranes and in all animals. Despite its bad rap, it performs several useful functions:

>> It makes membranes permeable so that cells can absorb nutrients.

>> It transports nutrients.

>> It helps your body absorb fat-soluble vitamins when your liver converts it into bile salts.

Your body synthesizes much more cholesterol in a day than you could ever eat. But because your body's system self-compensates, the more cholesterol you eat, the less your body synthesizes.

So why has cholesterol turned into such a boogeyman? This section answers that question and offers a few ways to help you reduce your overall cholesterol count, increase your HDL cholesterol, and reduce your LDL cholesterol with the clean eating diet plan. Reducing cholesterol is more than just reducing the number below 200. It's also about preventing the oxidation of LDL cholesterol, which is why antioxidants are so important.

REMEMBER

A high blood cholesterol level is a marker that something may be wrong with your circulatory system and that you may have chronic inflammation. But your HDL/LDL ratio is more important because high LDL cholesterol indicates a more significant risk for heart disease than total cholesterol numbers. Phytochemicals and vitamins in whole foods can help you improve your cholesterol counts and, we hope, your overall health.

A high cholesterol reading can also indicate that you've inherited that "hyper" insulin response to dietary carbohydrates, In that case, following the Paleo diet, which reduces that insulin signal, is very likely to reduce both your cholesterol and triglycerides. Check with a physician skilled and knowledgeable in natural medicine to see if this is the case for you.

Inflammation and your arteries

Inflammation can be a good thing. Sending white blood cells and other compounds to a point of injury is how your body heals itself. But chronic inflammation, which occurs when the body doesn't face any acute, direct threat, injures arteries and other tissues and is the starting point for the calamitous process of atherosclerosis.

Many scientists now believe that inflammation may also be a primary cause of high cholesterol levels. When LDL cholesterol (the bad stuff) collects in your arteries, plaque forms. Plaque deposits can then become inflamed and attract even more cholesterol. When those deposits become too big, they can block arteries, causing a heart attack — or break off and become a clot, which can also cause a heart attack or stroke.

The key factors that lead to chronic inflammation in the body include

>> **Ordinary aging:** As you age, free radicals in your body become more numerous, your cells' structures get weaker as the oxidized compounds damage them, and chronic inflammation begins. This chain of events spurs on more aging, and a vicious cycle ensues.

>> **Poor diet:** A diet low in whole foods and high in processed foods can increase inflammation. Sugar, excess sodium, and additives can aggravate cells, and a diet low in phytochemicals, vitamins, and minerals hinders your body's natural healing process. A person can be overweight and still be quite malnourished.

>> **Trans fats:** These fake fats, which become part of your cell walls, are a primary cause of inflammation in the modern diet. While many manufacturers are eliminating these fats from their products, trans fats remain too prevalent in the American diet. These fats increase LDL cholesterol and reduce HDL cholesterol, and they damage the cells lining your blood vessels.

>> **Obesity:** Fat cells promote inflammation, but inflammation may be a cause of obesity — what a vicious cycle! Fat cells make macrophages (a type of immunity cell) and other chemicals like resistin that are inflammatory. These chemicals leave the fat cells and enter the bloodstream.

>> **Pollution:** Long-term exposure to air pollution causes inflammation in the body. Chemical pollution enters your lungs and generates those nasty free radicals, which cause injury and inflammation in the body.

>> **Stress:** Stress causes your body to enter the fight-or-flight response. Adrenaline enters the bloodstream, preparing the body for a quick reaction to a threat. But in the modern world, people don't face life-threatening situations every day, so this response actually has a negative effect on your body. It can keep your blood pressure high, damaging blood vessels, making them rough, and creating the perfect spot for plaque to develop. Adrenaline itself can also promote inflammation.

Another key factor directly related to inflammation in the very areas where the most cholesterol plaque forms is the thickness of blood. Two research studies have found that blood donation (which reduces blood thickness) reduces heart attack risk in men and postmenopausal women by 45 percent to 88 percent. This does not apply to premenopausal women, who have blood loss every month during their periods. For more about this approach to blood vessel inflammation reduction, see *The Blood Thinner Cure*, by cardiologist Dr. Kenneth Kensey.

REMEMBER

Fortunately, the eating clean plan can help you counteract many of the inflammation factors we describe in the preceding list. (In fact, studies have shown that eating a diet very high in plant foods can be as effective in lowering cholesterol as prescription drugs.) For instance, eating whole foods provides lots of phytochemicals and nutrients, which your body needs to fight free radicals, and can help you lose weight. In addition, avoiding processed foods as part of the eating clean plan reduces the number of trans fats, additives, and preservatives you eat, which reduces free radical activity in your cells. And the whole foods you eat help fight inflammation caused by aging, pollution, and stress.

Specifically, eat foods that directly combat inflammation, such as fatty fish, fruits (especially tart cherries), vegetables, essential fatty acids (especially omega-3 fatty acids), and nuts and seeds. Spices, supplements, and herbs that fight inflammation include cinnamon, ginger, turmeric, vitamins C and E, biotin, the entire B complex, ginkgo, magnesium, *Boswellia*, and oregano and basil, which are two powerful antioxidants.

How sugar, fats, and simple carbs raise cholesterol levels

Diets high in sugar, certain fats, and simple carbohydrates can raise cholesterol levels, especially the bad type, LDL cholesterol. These ingredients are common in the typical American diet and are prevalent in processed and refined foods. The eating clean plan minimizes (or maybe even eliminates) these foods from your diet.

Sugar and cholesterol

A 2010 study published in the *Journal of the American Medical Association* found that people who ate one-quarter of their daily calories in the form of sugar were three times more likely to have low levels of HDL cholesterol. This group also had high levels of triglycerides, another type of fat found in the blood.

Foods high in sugar are damaging to the body in and of themselves, and they usually have very little nutritional value. The empty calories in high-sugar foods cause obesity (another risk factor for inflammation), high LDL cholesterol levels, and heart disease.

Sugar suppresses the immune system, causes hormonal imbalance, and increases the risk of high blood pressure. In addition, some scientists believe that sugar molecules can actually damage cell walls and the interior walls of arteries, leading to inflammation that attracts cholesterol and eventually creating plaque and disease.

"Sugar risk" is significantly greater if you have inherited the "hyper" insulin response that precedes type-2 diabetes. Check with a physician skilled and knowledgeable in natural medicine to determine if you have this extra risk from sugar consumption.

Fats and cholesterol

Certain types of fats raise cholesterol levels in your blood. Trans fats increase LDL cholesterol, which creates plaque, and reduce HDL cholesterol, which actually removes cholesterol from arteries. Polyunsaturated fats can reduce LDL cholesterol in some people but not all; they also can reduce HDL cholesterol levels. Saturated fat can raise LDL levels, but it can also protect against stroke.

On the eating clean diet, you avoid the harmful trans fats and polyunsaturated fats made from genetically modified (GMO) vegetables. Polyunsaturated fats are reactive and can oxidize and become rancid easily; as a result, these fats lead directly to inflammation when you consume them.

However, some naturally occurring polyunsaturated fatty acids such as omega-3 fatty acids are good for you. To reduce potential oxidative damage from otherwise beneficial polyunsaturated fatty acids, eat foods high in vitamin E such as Swiss chard, spinach, turnip greens, kale, hazelnuts, almonds, and seeds, and perhaps take a mixed tocopherol vitamin E supplement.

Monounsaturated fats are a much better choice whether you're on the eating clean plan or not, and saturated fats aren't as bad for you as you may have been told. In fact, people who have type-2 diabetes or have a family history of it do better on high-fat, low-carb diets. For these people, carbohydrates wreak havoc on the insulin system, causing elevated total cholesterol and LDL cholesterol while lowering HDL cholesterol and raising blood pressure and the presence of serum uric acid. Put together, the results of high-sugar, high-carb diets are called *metabolic syndrome* and, if not reversed, will proceed to type-2 diabetes. (See the later section "Eating Clean to Prevent Diabetes" for more details.)

Talk to a doctor knowledgeable in nutritional medicine if your family has a history of inflammation-caused diseases or type-2 diabetes. Eat a clean diet for a month or two and get your blood cholesterol, C-reactive protein, and HDL/LDL levels checked. Keep working with your doctor until you find a diet that works for you — whether it's low fat/high carb or high protein/low carb. Because every *body* is different, everybody's reaction to fats is different, too.

Simple carbs and cholesterol

Simple carbohydrates include sugar, honey, molasses, white flour, white pasta, and processed foods. Many of the foods that contain these ingredients are high in calories and low in nutrients; as a result, consuming them causes inflammation and adds pounds.

Scientists developed the glycemic index to categorize foods by how much and how fast they make your blood sugar content rise. Foods with a high glycemic index number have a strong effect on blood sugar and can lower HDL cholesterol. And consider the *insulinemic index* (exaggerated insulin response) that is produced in those predisposed to type-2 diabetes in response to many foods, including dairy products, breakfast cereals, and bakery products that are high in refined carbohydrates. Read more about this in Chapter 5.

TIP

If you have a sweet tooth and choose to eat simple carbs, pick foods like fruits and products made with whole grains. These foods have a mitigating effect on blood sugar increases because they contain fiber and other vitamins and minerals that take longer to digest.

The role of folate, lutein, resveratrol, and other nutrients

Certain nutrients reduce LDL cholesterol levels and increase HDL cholesterol levels. If you have high cholesterol levels and a poor LDL/HDL cholesterol ratio, concentrate on foods that contain these nutrients:

>> **Folate:** This vitamin may reduce levels of LDL cholesterol. A 2010 study in *Nutrition Journal* found that people with higher levels of folate in their blood have lower LDL levels. Getting folate from foods is better than getting it from supplements. Find it in leafy green vegetables, legumes, fruits like bananas and melons, organ meats, and vegetables like mushrooms, broccoli, and tomatoes.

>> **Niacin:** One of the two forms of vitamin B3, niacin lowers total cholesterol and raises HDL levels by at least 15 percent when taken at the right doses. Short-acting niacin supplements can cause side effects like upset stomach and flushing of the skin, so more people are switching to timed-release or extended-release forms of this supplement. Although getting niacin from food sources is the best way to go, getting enough to significantly affect cholesterol levels can be difficult. You find it in dairy products, whole grains, fish, and nuts.

>> **Lutein:** This antioxidant helps neutralize free radicals in your body, preventing the oxidation of LDL cholesterol. It can also help reduce the formation of LDL particles, resulting in fewer deposits of plaque in your arteries. Foods rich in lutein include spinach and other leafy dark greens, zucchini, Brussels sprouts, corn, and peas. Lutein is sensitive to heat, so try to eat these foods raw or lightly cooked.

>> **Resveratrol:** This phytochemical helps reduce the oxidation of LDL cholesterol and decrease platelet stickiness, which, in turn, could help prevent plaque formation. You can find this compound in red grapes, grape juice, red wine, peanuts, and some dark-colored berries.

>> **Chromium and magnesium:** Both of these minerals raise HDL cholesterol levels. Magnesium-rich foods include leafy dark-green vegetables, whole grains, and nuts. Foods high in chromium include mushrooms and brewer's yeast.

>> **Vitamin D:** This vitamin comes in two forms: Plants synthesize vitamin D2, and your skin synthesizes the precursor D3 when you bask in the sun. Vitamin D2 reduces overall cholesterol levels, LDL cholesterol, and triglycerides. Vitamin D3 helps build up HDL cholesterol. So get some exposure to sunshine every day if you can, and consume vitamin D-rich foods, including fortified foods like orange juice and milk. Supplementation is usually necessary for optimum health, because you likely can't get enough sunshine to produce optimal levels of this vitamin — unless, of course, you live in the tropics.

REMEMBER

Eating lots of fruits and vegetables on the clean eating plan is the perfect way to get plenty of these nutrients in the proper ratios and doses. As a bonus, eating clean automatically helps you reduce consumption of the foods that raise cholesterol, while increasing your consumption of the foods that reduce it and promoting good cholesterol levels.

Eating Clean to Help Reduce Cancer Risk

For many people, cancer is the scariest disease out there. Modern treatments are very difficult and hard on the body, and a cancer diagnosis carries with it a lot of uncertainty. Luckily, you can take action and eat more of certain foods to help reduce your cancer risk.

In this section, we look at some of the diet-related causes of cancer. (Did you know that scientists estimate that at least one-third of all cancer deaths are directly related to a poor diet and sedentary lifestyle?) Then we look at how certain phytochemicals, vitamins, and minerals can help reduce cell damage that can lead to cancer. Finally, we help you stock your cancer-fighting arsenal with lots of clean foods that taste great.

REMEMBER

The substances we describe in this section are not treatments for cancer or a guarantee against the disease's development. The eating clean diet focuses on healthy foods that can only help minimize (not eliminate) your risk of developing cancer and other diseases.

Looking at what causes cancer

Unfortunately, cancer has many causes. Smoking is the biggest single preventable cause of cancer. But poor diet, chemical pollution, lifestyle, genetic predisposition, and even viruses also cause the disease. The one bright side is that you can minimize all these causes with a good diet and a healthy lifestyle.

Cancer is the end result of cells that grow uncontrollably and don't have normal life cycles. Healthy cells die after a certain amount of time, and new cells replace them. With cancer, abnormal cells start to grow out of control and form one or more tumors. Those abnormal cells can spread throughout the body, eventually causing death.

REMEMBER

Phytochemicals, vitamins, and minerals (which are all a big part of the eating clean lifestyle) help give your cells a fighting chance at staying healthy. These compounds deflect substances like free radicals, which can cause cell changes, and help your damaged cells heal. Studies have found that phytochemicals may act on cancer cells at any stage of development, from the initiation stage to precancerous cells to the promotion stage and full-blown tumors. The foods on the clean eating plan are also high in fiber, which is an essential component in the cancer fight because it moves contaminants through your digestive system quickly.

The foods that may increase your risk of developing cancer include processed foods, especially processed meats and very salty pickled foods. How you cook your food can also increase your cancer risk. Smoked and grilled foods contain polycyclic aromatic hydrocarbons (PAHs), which are carcinogenic. Frying and roasting at very high temperatures can produce heterocyclic amines and acrylamide, more chemicals that are carcinogenic. So for better health, reduce your consumption of foods prepared in these ways (see Chapter 11 for more details).

As part of your cancer prevention, try to maintain a normal weight. Gaining weight is easy to do when you're eating processed, refined, and other unhealthy foods (not to mention that these foods are low in cancer-fighting nutrients). But fat cells can actually keep damaged cells in your body and may interfere with *apoptosis*, or normal programmed cell death. Cells that grow unchecked can lead to cancer.

Lignans, folate, quercetin, and other cancer fighters

Clean, whole foods contain many substances that help fight cancer by keeping your cells healthy, helping damaged cells heal, and protecting your body against damage from free radicals and carcinogens. Many of these compounds kill cancer cells by inducing apoptosis, which is the natural death cells should experience after a certain amount of time.

Eating lots of unprocessed fruits and vegetables is a good starting point for getting the substances your body needs to fight cancerous cells. These foods are rich in phytochemicals, such as quercetin, curcumin, and carotenoids, along with vitamin C and folate, which protect your cells against carcinogens and cancer development.

Here are just some of the phytochemicals (and the foods that contain them) that you need to include in your diet to help decrease your cancer risk:

>> **Lignans:** These phytoestrogens mimic the hormone estrogen in the body. They may prevent certain cancers, especially breast, skin, and colon cancer, from forming. Lignans can block estrogen from binding cells, thus limiting the formation of cancers that use estrogen to start growing. Those who eat foods containing lignans have a lower incidence of breast and colon cancer.

   You find lignans in flaxseed, sesame seeds, pumpkin seeds, whole grains, beans, berries, and green or black tea. But remember that too much flaxseed can actually increase the risk of prostate cancer in men, so men need to avoid more than small amounts of that particular food.

>> **Isoflavones:** There's a very strong correlation between isoflavone consumption and reduced risk of endometrial and breast cancer. Isoflavones are antioxidants, which means they stop free radicals from damaging your DNA; they work the same way the drug tamoxifen does to stop cancer recurrence. However, isoflavones, eaten regularly, can fuel the growth of pre-existing breast cancers. Some doctors warn against getting isoflavones in supplement form because supplemental isoflavones are much more concentrated and powerful than the phytochemicals you get in food.

   You find isoflavones in soy products, including soybeans, soy flour, soy milk, tofu, and tempeh, sesame seeds, and legumes. Navy, red, pinto, and garbanzo beans are also good sources of isoflavones.

>> **Curcumin:** Studies have shown that this substance can kill cancer cells by inducing apoptosis, or the self-destruction that cancer cells lack. In other words, it forces cancerous cells to commit suicide. It blocks estrogen-mimicking chemicals that promote cancer growth as well as enzymes that increase inflammation in the body. Curcumin is also a powerful antioxidant that protects DNA from carcinogens.

   You find curcumin in the spice turmeric, which is an ingredient in most curry powder blends. Enjoy lots of Indian food made with curry powder and add turmeric to relish and sauces to make sure you get plenty of it in your diet.

>> **Capsaicin:** This compound is the active ingredient that makes chile peppers spicy. Studies have shown that it can kill prostate cancer cells in vitro and human lung cancer cells. It can also slow the growth of leukemia. Capsaicin may help neutralize nitrosamines found in processed meats, too.

You find capsaicin in all chile peppers, especially in their seeds and inner membranes.

>> **Quercetin:** This flavonoid is a powerful tool in the cancer prevention battle because it promotes apoptosis in cancer cells. Population studies have found that people who consume lots of foods with this phytochemical have lower risks of breast, lung, and pancreatic cancer.

Find quercetin in broccoli, red onions, apples, red grapes, red wine, green vegetables, and citrus fruits.

Here are the main vitamins and minerals you need to include in your diet to decrease your cancer risk:

>> **Folate:** Folate and vitamin B12 work together to make DNA, which is the central control system of your cells. These nutrients can prevent changes to DNA that can lead to cancer. Focus on consuming folate-rich foods rather than supplements, because some studies have shown that getting too much folic acid (which isn't found in foods as folate is) can increase the risk of cancer. If you choose a supplement, look for folate rather than folic acid.

You find folate in black-eyed peas, spinach, asparagus, green peas, broccoli, wheat germ, and fortified breakfast cereals.

>> **Vitamin C:** Vitamin C helps fight cancer development by interfering with the cancer cell's ability to grow in low-oxygen conditions. Although vitamin C has a valuable antioxidant role as well, researchers at Johns Hopkins think that the interfering role may be more important in terms of cancer prevention.

You can get vitamin C from all citrus fruits, berries, broccoli, bell peppers, kale, papaya, cantaloupe, and cauliflower. Even so, doctors point out that getting enough vitamin C for optimal health from food sources alone is difficult, so some supplementation is necessary.

>> **Vitamin A:** This vitamin helps keep your immune system strong so that it can detect and kill precancerous cells. Vitamin A comes from animal sources like egg yolks, liver, and fish oils. Its precursor, beta carotene, comes from fruits and vegetables like carrots, broccoli, peaches, and spinach. Both types may help prevent cells from becoming cancerous. It's most valuable when you consume it in concert with other vitamins and phytochemicals in whole foods.

>> **Selenium:** This trace mineral may kill cancer cells before they can replicate. Studies have shown that people with low selenium levels in their blood are more likely to develop bladder cancer.

You find this powerful antioxidant in Brazil nuts, mushrooms, tomatoes, tuna, brown rice, eggs, and chicken. Pair selenium-rich foods with foods high in vitamin C, vitamin E, and beta carotene for even more antioxidant effects.

>> **Calcium:** This mineral helps your body repair damaged DNA, which, if left untreated, can cause mutations in cells that may lead to cancer. Get calcium from leafy green vegetables, dairy products, and fortified products. You may also want to take a calcium supplement; if you do, remember to include magnesium, too.

>> **Zinc:** Women who are deficient in zinc are at greater risk for breast cancer, because breast glands need a lot of this mineral for lactation. This mineral is also important in the prevention of prostate cancer and for wound healing.

Foods rich in zinc include oysters, beef, lamb, pork, clams, salmon, and egg yolks. Pumpkin seeds are the most concentrated vegetable source of zinc. Other nonmeat sources include dairy products, like milk, cheese, and yogurt, peanuts, beans, whole-grain cereals, brown rice, whole-wheat bread, potatoes, legumes, mushrooms, pecans, wheat germ, and brewer's yeast.

Stocking your cancer-fighting arsenal

You need to include many whole foods in your clean diet to reduce cancer risk. Brightly colored fruits and vegetables are the obvious first choice. Try to eat at least five servings of vegetables and at least three servings of fruit a day. It's not as hard as it sounds! A serving of vegetables or fruit is only ½ cup (which is about the size of a small apple or banana).

SUPPLEMENTS TO REDUCE CANCER RISK

Scientists are conducting thousands of studies to see whether taking supplements reduces the risk of developing cancer. Here's what they've found so far:

- Vitamin D reduces the risk of many cancers, most notably prostate, breast, and colon.

- Folate reduces the risk of cancers of the gastrointestinal tract.

- Omega-3 fatty acids can provide powerful protection against breast cancer.

- Di-indolylmenthane (DIM), a substance found in cabbage, broccoli, cauliflower, broccoli, Brussels sprouts, and other *Brassica* vegetables, reduces breast, cervical, and prostate cancer risk.

- Long-term use of certain supplements, especially beta carotene, can increase the risk of lung cancer in smokers.

Talk to a doctor skilled in nutrition about whether a supplement is right for you.

Eating a wide variety of whole foods is also very important, especially if you aren't focusing on organic foods. The FDA calculates the so-called safe dose of pesticides (which are carcinogens) in the foods you consume based on how much of that food you include in your diet. So if you eat dozens of nonorganic apples every day, you're undoubtedly consuming more of that pesticide than what's considered safe. Vary the fruits and veggies you eat to reduce pesticide intake. For a list of fifteen foods to always buy organic, see Chapter 10.

Eating many different kinds of foods that have cancer-prevention properties may increase their efficacy. Phytochemicals, vitamins, and minerals interact in ways that scientists don't yet understand, and scientists haven't even identified all the phytochemicals out there yet. Eating whole foods is the best way to stock your cancer-fighting arsenal.

REMEMBER

Include the following foods in your diet if you're concerned about cancer or have a family history of the disease:

>> **Ginger:** This root promotes apoptosis and has anti-inflammatory properties. In fact, doctors can extract and purify the substance that gives ginger its potent and spicy flavor, called 6-gingerol, and use it as an anticancer medicine. Add ginger to stir-fries and sauces, and use it as a flavoring in soups. It's also delicious in hot tea.

>> **Mushrooms:** These vegetables contain polysaccharides, such as beta-glucan, that build up your immune system as well as the protein lectin, which stops cancer cells from multiplying.

>> **Berries:** Strawberries, blueberries, and other berries contain lots of ellagic acid, which is an antioxidant that deactivates some carcinogens. Blueberries also contain anthocyanins, which are very potent antioxidants. Eat berries in combination in fruit salads and snack on them in between meals.

>> **Cruciferous vegetables:** These vegetables, which include broccoli, cabbage, Brussels sprouts, kale, cauliflower, and bok choy, contain glucosinolates that initiate apoptosis. They're also rich in indole-3-carbinol, which converts estrogens into protective types, and lutein, which can decrease the risk of prostate cancer.

>> **Tomatoes:** The lycopene in tomatoes can decrease prostate cancer risk. Cooked tomatoes have more absorbable lycopene, so concentrate on tomato paste, sauce, and juice. Be sure to consume some fat along with your tomatoes (butter or olive oil, for example) to help your body absorb the lycopene.

>> **Carrots:** These vegetables contain beta carotene, which helps protect your body against cancer when you consume it in food. Carrots also contain falcarinol, a substance that can reduce cancer risk. Don't cook the carrots to get the benefits of this substance, though, because it's water soluble.

- >> **Garlic:** The allyl sulfates in garlic slow down tumor growth and can prevent carcinogens from getting into your cells. This potent vegetable may help prevent stomach cancer because of its antibacterial properties against *H. pylori,* a common bacteria that can cause cancer.

- >> **Oregano:** This herb is a good source of quercetin. In fact, one tablespoon of fresh oregano has as much quercetin as a whole apple. It also contains a lot of beta carotene, vitamin K, iron, manganese, and calcium, along with potassium and magnesium.

- >> **Legumes:** Beans have the phytochemicals saponins, protease inhibitors, and phytic acid, which can stop or slow cancer cell reproduction and make cell division more difficult for cancer cells. Legumes are also high in fiber, which can decrease the risk of colon cancer.

- >> **Curry powder:** The turmeric in curry powder inhibits the enzyme COX-2, which is present in colon and bowel cancers. It also contains curcumin, which initiates apoptosis.

- >> **Tea:** Both green and black tea have polyphenols that keep cancer cells from dividing. Scientists think that green tea has a higher level of these substances.

REMEMBER

Keep in mind that eating a healthy diet is not a guarantee against illness. Exercising regularly, avoiding carcinogens like cigarette smoke and alcohol, and seeing your doctor for frequent checkups along with eating a good diet are the best ways to increase your chances of staying healthy.

Eating Clean to Prevent Diabetes

Type-1 diabetes is an autoimmune disorder with an inherited predisposition that appears mostly in children. Research observations of more than 10,000 children born in 1966 found that those whose mothers gave them vitamin D 2,000 IU every day for the first year of their lives had almost 80 percent less type-1 diabetes by 1997 than children whose mothers gave them no vitamin D during their first year.

Type-2 diabetes, which has a strong connection to diet in individuals with a genetic predisposition, appears mostly in adults who have become overweight and sedentary. Type-2 diabetes is one disease that you can help prevent with a clean and healthy diet.

In this section, we look at how eating a lot of sugar can disrupt your blood sugar and cause problems in your pancreas. We also give you tips for how you can break a sugar addiction and take a quick look at the glycemic index and the insulinemic index. The goal of diabetes prevention is to stabilize blood glucose, protect the pancreas against damage from free radicals and overuse, and improve your body's insulin sensitivity. Whole fruits and vegetables, whole grains, and healthy fats play an important role in achieving this goal.

Understanding your pancreas

Your pancreas is an organ located in your abdomen. It has two basic functions:

>> To regulate the level of sugar in your blood

>> To produce digestive enzymes that work in your intestines to help break down cellular debris, clean up cellular debris, and fight inflammation in your blood

Beta cells in the Islets of Langerhans (don't you just love that name?) in the pancreas produce insulin (which lowers the *blood glucose level*, or the level or sugar in your blood) and glucagon (which raises the blood glucose level).

REMEMBER

When your pancreas doesn't produce enough insulin (which leads to type-1 diabetes) or your cells don't respond to insulin (a state called *insulin resistance*, which leads to type-2 diabetes), the cells in your body don't get enough glucose for energy and can't work properly.

One of the big food culprits that can damage your pancreas is sugar. Sugar intake prompts the pancreas to release more and more insulin. Over time, your cells can become resistant to the insulin your pancreas puts out. When your body doesn't respond to insulin, type-2 diabetes develops.

SUGAR SUBSTITUTES: A BAD IDEA

If you're trying to kick a sugar addiction, don't turn to artificial sugar substitutes. In fact, stay away from sugar substitutes on the eating clean diet plan. These fake foods, which aren't found in nature, aren't good for you. Sugar substitutes taste sweet (obviously) and activate those same receptor sites in your brain that keep your sugar addiction alive. But scientists don't even know if sugar substitutes are really safe! Some studies show that artificial sweeteners can damage the thymus glands, liver, and kidneys in rats, but those studies haven't been conducted on humans. Scientists haven't done any large, long-term studies on the effects of products with artificial sweeteners.

Approximately one-third of all Americans (100 million) have a genetic predisposition to make a lot more insulin than the other two-thirds do in response to the same amount of sugar and carbohydrate intake. For this reason, this group is much more likely to develop insulin resistance and ultimately type-2 diabetes. If you have a family history of type-2 diabetes or low blood sugar, you're likely a part of this group and need to be a lot more careful about your sugar and carbohydrate intake.

TIP

Although both types of diabetes have a strong genetic link, lifestyle can play a part in developing either type of the disease. You can help prevent type-1 diabetes with vitamin D supplementation, especially if you start very early in life, and by avoiding gluten and dairy products, which have been found to be auto-immune "triggers" for type-1 diabetes in genetically susceptible individuals.

You may be able to prevent type-2 diabetes by avoiding refined foods, eating a clean diet, partaking in moderate exercise, and supplementing the diet according to your doctor.

An experiment conducted by Professor John Yudkin of the University of London demonstrated that individuals with a family history of type-2 diabetes gained three times as much weight on exactly the same high-sugar and high-carb diet as individuals with no family history of this disease. His experiment proved that the belief that "obesity causes type-2 diabetes" had to be modified to "the genetic tendency to type-2 diabetes causes obesity, which — if not reversed by diet and exercise — can proceed to type-2 diabetes."

Winning the fight against your lifelong love of sugar

Unfortunately, everyone is born with a sweet tooth. Sugar pleases the human palate. As many people grow, they lose their taste for sugar and learn to appreciate more complex flavors. But some people never outgrow the craving for sweetness. (See Chapter 13 for more information about your sweet tooth and tips for how to live with it.)

Eating foods high in sugar has a direct effect on your mood. When you consume simple sugars, your blood sugar skyrockets. Your pancreas pumps insulin into your body, dropping your blood sugar level and making you hungry and irritable. When you eat more sugar, your blood sugar levels increase — and the roller coaster keeps on moving.

REMEMBER

Keeping your blood sugar levels stable is the key to reducing cravings, and the eating clean diet is one of the best ways to accomplish this balance. Consuming six meals a day, each made up of satisfying whole foods, keeps your blood sugar levels, well, level. Level blood sugar levels greatly reduce your cravings and give you more energy throughout the day.

Making sure you eat when you get hungry is also important to breaking the sugar habit (see Chapter 5 for more information about the physical signs of true hunger). Hunger is a signal from your body that your blood glucose levels are dropping and that you need to replenish them. Train yourself to recognize true hunger signals. Eat when you get hungry, eat mindfully, and stop when you're full. Although doing so takes a lot of thought and planning, it's key to breaking a sugar addiction and reducing your chances of developing type-2 diabetes.

Eating a lot of sugar means taking in empty calories, which can lead to weight gain and excess belly fat. If your family has a history of type-2 diabetes, this weight gain can lead to metabolic syndrome, which is a direct forerunner of diabetes development. If you do choose to eat some refined carbohydrates, eat them with protein or fat to slow down the digestion of simple sugars.

ADDICTED TO SUGAR?

Can you be addicted to sugar? Some scientists think so. The type of sugar you're used to eating (refined sucrose) isn't found in nature. Table or granulated sugar is a very refined food, which you should avoid on the clean diet. Studies have shown that sugar can affect your brain chemistry and cause addiction symptoms. In fact, the taste of sugar activates the same receptor sites in the brain that are affected by heroin. Heroin! No wonder some people can't stop eating sugary foods.

One of the best ways to combat a sugar addiction is to deliberately add many more whole foods to your diet. If you fill up on carrots, celery, leafy green vegetables, and citrus fruits, you won't have a lot of room in your tummy for chocolate-covered caramels and malted milk balls!

Research demonstrates that chromium supplementation can significantly reduce sugar cravings. According to chromium expert Richard Anderson, MD, and the EPA, the toxic upper limit for nutritional chromium is 70,000 micrograms daily, so taking 3,000 micrograms (3 milligrams) daily until your sugar craving subsides is quite safe — and very frequently effective. Kicking your sugar habit can take weeks to a few months, so don't give up on this supplement too soon.

Consuming the right nutrients and food to prevent diabetes

Following the Paleo diet of nutrient-dense whole foods low on the glycemic and insulinemic indices may be one of the best weapons in your diabetes-prevention arsenal. And the best part is that those foods contain the phytochemicals, vitamins, minerals, and fiber you need for the best health.

If you're trying to prevent diabetes, try to get plenty of these phytochemicals:

>> **Lignans:** These phytochemicals are antioxidants that protect the pancreas against damage from free radicals. Lignans may also help prevent diabetes by improving glucose control in the blood. You find lignans in legumes, flaxseed, vegetables, and other seeds.

>> **Saponins:** Some saponins have insulin-like activity, which may help regulate blood glucose and stop cells from losing their insulin sensitivity, thus reducing the need for insulin and balancing blood sugar. Saponins are also powerful antioxidants, which help prevent damage from free radicals. Cells in your pancreas are as susceptible to free radical damage as any other. Find saponins in soybeans, peas, asparagus, spinach, and fresh herbs.

>> **Anthocyanins:** These compounds can help increase insulin production in your pancreas and are strong antioxidants. They can also help reduce the risks of metabolic syndrome. Find these compounds in sweet and sour cherries, red grapes, strawberries, and blueberries.

>> **Quercetin:** This antioxidant helps prevent damage to cells and can also help restore normal insulin function. Quercetin can interact with your DNA to reduce inflammation that can cause insulin resistance. Find it in apple skins, green tea and chamomile tea, red wine, citrus fruits, onions, grapes, and dark berries.

>> **Resveratrol:** This important antioxidant can improve insulin response in your cells and protect the pancreas from damage. It can also lower glucose levels in the blood and activate an enzyme in the body that increases insulin secretion and sensitivity. Find resveratrol in apple skins, red wine, cranberries, red and purple grapes, peanuts, and strawberries.

Vitamins and minerals are also important in the fight against diabetes development. Try to include these in your diet:

>> **Chromium:** This trace mineral helps insulin lower blood sugar levels. Many Americans are chromium deficient, probably because the foods they eat are grown in depleted soils. Good food sources of chromium include brewer's yeast, mushrooms, onions, romaine lettuce, eggs, and tomatoes.

» **Vitamin K:** People with insufficient levels of vitamin K have problems with insulin resistance and an abnormal response to glucose. Good sources of this vitamin include green vegetables such as broccoli and spinach.

» **Vitamin E:** This vitamin is another powerful antioxidant. Researchers have found that people with the highest vitamin E intake have a reduced risk of type-2 diabetes. You find vitamin E in eggs, meat, poultry, fish, spinach, nuts, seeds, tomatoes, and avocados.

» **Magnesium:** This mineral improves insulin sensitivity and is necessary for insulin production. People with diabetes have lower levels of magnesium in their blood. In fact, insulin resistance is directly associated with a magnesium deficiency. Good sources of magnesium include leafy greens like spinach and Swiss chard, soybeans, salmon, pumpkin and squash seeds, legumes, and nuts.

» **Biotin:** This vitamin, also known as vitamin B8 or vitamin H, helps the body efficiently metabolize glucose and reduce insulin resistance even in people who have diabetes. Biotin and chromium work synergistically to lower blood sugar levels. You find biotin in liver, yeast, egg yolks, brown rice, and peanut butter.

» **Niacin and niacinamide:** These forms of vitamin B3 help insulin lower blood glucose levels. However, very large doses of niacin can actually increase blood sugar levels in some people who have already developed diabetes. Niacinamide helps protect the Islets of Langerhans against damage from overuse, and also stimulates pancreatic islet stem cells, which can form new islet cells. Get niacin from red meats and lean meats, enriched cereals, whole grains, mushrooms, salmon and other fatty fish, peanuts, and seeds. Get niacinamide from fish, poultry, eggs, and meat.

THE IMPORTANCE OF EXERCISE

We can't write a chapter on preventing disease without mentioning exercise. Doctors and nutritionists all say that getting regular, moderate exercise is one of the best things you can do for your body and your mind. Thirty minutes of exercise five times a week is the goal. For diabetics, exercise can lower blood glucose levels and increase insulin sensitivity. Research shows that short bursts of intense exercise (interval training) are much more effective than aerobic exercise for reversing the tendency toward type-2 diabetes. Interval training three to five times a week for 12 to 15 minutes is sufficient. Plus, exercise is a great way to manage weight. No matter what disease you're trying to prevent, try to add exercise to your daily routine. Walking, swimming, yoga, or any sport can help make your life better, no matter what condition your body is in!

Incorporate the following foods into your diet to help prevent diabetes:

>> **Cinnamon:** Surprisingly, this common spice may help prevent diabetes. It contains a flavonoid called MHCP that mimics insulin activity, which helps regulate sugar metabolism. Sprinkle cinnamon on hot cereals, use it in recipes, and add it to your morning tea. Consuming just ¼ teaspoon a day can help.

>> **Cherries:** These delicious fruits — especially the tart Montmorency cherries — are a good source of anthocyanins, which can increase insulin production. (Note that maraschino cherries are not part of the clean eating diet plan!)

>> **Apples:** These fruits are high in quercetin, one of the phytochemicals that can help restore insulin function. People who eat lots of apples tend to have less diabetes.

>> **Tomatoes:** Tomatoes are a good source of lycopene and vitamin C. Some studies show that diabetics have low blood levels of vitamin C. The lycopene in tomatoes can stimulate the immune system.

>> **Fatty fish:** Omega-3 fatty acids are critical in the fight against diabetes. They reduce inflammation and protect cells in the pancreas. Studies show that people who eat large quantities of fatty fish like salmon have a lower risk of developing diabetes.

>> **Green tea:** The catechins and tannins in green tea can help lower blood sugar levels. One catechin in green tea called epigallocatechin gallate can mimic the effects of insulin, reducing insulin resistance in cells. Sip tea with your meals to reduce the amount of glucose your body absorbs.

>> **Vinegar:** This surprising addition to the list can help lower blood sugar levels. Research in Italy and Japan has found that taking a couple of spoonfuls of apple cider vinegar with meals reduces blood sugar levels and slowly reduces weight independent of diet changes.

>> **Nuts and seeds:** People who eat five or more servings of nuts weekly have a reduced chance of developing type-2 diabetes. Enjoy 1.5 ounces of almonds, pistachios, and walnuts every day.

>> **Lean meats:** These foods are good sources of protein, which helps keep you feeling satisfied longer and slows down the digestion of simple sugars. Eating more protein helps reduce blood sugar spikes, too.

>> **Leafy dark-green vegetables:** These foods are high in vitamin C and other antioxidants that protect your body against free radical damage. Dark greens are rich in B vitamins, which can help lower blood glucose levels.

TIP

Some studies indicate that the Paleo diet is the best one for people who may be prone to type-2 diabetes. This diet is relatively high in animal protein and fat and low in simple sugars and carbohydrates; it's the diet that your ancestors ate. Be sure to eat wild game, grass-fed beef, wild fish, and free-range chickens to get more omega-3 fatty acids. Eat lots of vegetables, lean meats, fish, seafood, nuts, and seeds, and reduce or eliminate sugary foods like fruit juices. Dr. William Douglass has found that eating a high-fat breakfast does not increase symptoms of metabolic syndrome, so try eating a higher-fat breakfast, including eggs and meat. See Chapter 6 for more on the Paleo diet.

Eating Clean to Help Prevent Autoimmune Diseases

Since no one really knows what causes autoimmune diseases, determining what diet you should follow or what specific nutrients you should eat to reduce your risk of these disease is a difficult task. But if you follow the eating clean diet plan and avoid processed foods, foods that have been highly refined, and foods heavily sprayed and treated with chemicals, you may be able to reduce your risk of developing an autoimmune disease. Development of these diseases does seem to have a strong genetic component, so if these diseases run in your family, you may be able to delay their onset with a clean diet.

In this section, we look at the foods that can help support your immune system and explain how to help keep it in control, such as through allergy testing. We discuss which phytochemicals, vitamins, and minerals you should add to your diet and why organic foods are so important for fighting autoimmune diseases.

Decoding the causes of autoimmune diseases

Autoimmune diseases are basically diseases of self-immunity. In other words, something triggers your immune system to attack normal body tissues.

Some researchers think that gluten and its companion protein gliadin are two of the triggers for autoimmune diseases, including type-1 diabetes. Researchers have also found that specific milk proteins can be autoimmune disease triggers if you have type-1 diabetes. Microorganisms can likely also trigger the body to attack itself. (Long ago, doctors found that strep bacteria can cause rheumatic fever and rheumatic heart disease, in which heart damage is caused by human antibodies against the streptococcal germ. Those antistrep antibodies also attack heart cell membranes.)

REMEMBER

Many people who suffer from autoimmune diseases also have food allergies. So if you have an autoimmune disease, get an allergy screening to make sure you're not eating foods that aggravate your condition. In general, you may want to avoid gluten, dairy products, yeast, and other possible allergens that can aggravate autoimmune conditions. See Chapter 14 for more information about controlling food allergies with the clean eating plan.

Since most physicians don't specialize in the diagnosis and treatment of food allergies, if you have an autoimmune disease or a food allergy, find a physician who does.

Getting the right nutrients

Which foods you should eat and which ones you should avoid depend on the autoimmune disease you're trying to prevent. Of course, you need to avoid processed foods and refined foods, as well as foods with empty calories that are high in sugar. After all, those foods are very low in the phytochemicals and other nutrients your body needs to stay healthy.

Concentrate on these foods and nutrients to help support your immune system:

>> **Lean meats:** Protein is important for your immune system because it helps your body make antibodies and other immune cells. Your body uses protein to repair cells and to keep tissues and organs in good shape.

- » **Choline:** This nutrient helps support a healthy intestinal lining and mucosa, which can help your body keep chemicals and additives from crossing the intestinal barrier into your bloodstream. Choline-rich foods include beef, seafood, eggs, soy, nuts, and flaxseed. However, do not take supplemental choline unless you're using olive oil regularly. Research has found that without a substance found in olive oil, choline can actually cause atherosclerotic problems.

- » **Fruits and vegetables:** Bioflavonoids, which you find in fruits and veggies, protect cell membranes and make the immune system more efficient. These colorful compounds have an antibacterial effect and are essential to cell health.

- » **Fiber:** Foods high in fiber help keep your intestinal immune system strong by removing chemicals and toxins that could damage your cells. When your colon ferments fiber, it also produces short-chain fatty acids, which your GI tract cells use to keep mucosa healthy.

- » **Essential fatty acids:** These fats, especially omega-3 fatty acids, are important for membrane health. Find them in cold-water fatty fish, olive oil, and nuts.

- » **Vitamin C:** This vitamin is essential to keeping your immune system functioning well. It acts as an antioxidant to help support the healing functions of your body and makes your immune system more efficient.

Understanding the importance of organic foods

Pesticides, food additives, and herbicides can aggravate the conditions that cause autoimmune diseases (namely, high levels of inflammation and the presence of triggers that lead the immune system to attack human tissue). In fact, the pesticides and herbicides in many nonorganic foods accumulate in the tissues in your body. These chemicals can reduce white blood cell counts and alter the effectiveness of many organs, including the thymus and spleen. So try to eat as many organic foods as possible.

Most fruits and vegetables grown in the conventional manner, with pesticides, fungicides, insecticides, and herbicides, grow in soils that are deficient in many nutrients. Organic farming replaces those nutrients, using several different methods, including crop rotation, supplementation with compost, and other natural fertilizers. As a result, organic foods can be a better source of the phytochemicals, vitamins, and minerals that are necessary to prevent and fight autoimmune diseases. Check out Chapter 10 for more information about organic foods.

In a 2009 study of 75,000 postmenopausal women, researchers found that those who used consumer insecticide sprays at least six times a year had a much greater risk of developing rheumatoid arthritis and lupus. The longer the exposure to these chemicals, the greater the risk. This research bolsters the theory that factors in the environment can trigger autoimmune diseases in many people. (*Note:* The study focused on women because 75 percent of all patients with autoimmune diseases are women.)

Pesticides and other chemicals like bisphenol A can act like hormones in the body, disrupting the endocrine system and changing the way your body reacts to inflammation and infections. These changes can trigger the over-response of the immune system that heralds an autoimmune disease.

So what does all this mean to you? Think about all the pesticides you consume when you eat fruits and vegetables that have been routinely sprayed with these chemicals. Add to that all the meat that has been fed grain sprayed with pesticides and the milk produced by cows grazing on treated fields; the list goes on and on. If there is autoimmune disease in your family, the best way to reduce your risk of developing it may be to eat a clean diet of whole organic foods.

SUPPLEMENTS TO STRENGTHEN THE IMMUNE SYSTEM

The supplements you may want to add to your diet to strengthen your immune system include

- **Vitamin C:** Vitamin C helps your body produce white blood cells and protects your cells against viruses.

- **Vitamin E:** Vitamin E also improves your body's ability to make white blood cells and is crucial in the production of *B-cells,* the cells that seek out and destroy bacteria.

- **Zinc:** Zinc is critical in the production of white blood cells and helps make them stronger. Without enough zinc, the thymus gland (the "master regulator" of the immune system) can deteriorate much more rapidly.

- **Selenium:** Selenium reduces the risk of immune system disorders.

- **Fish oil:** Fish oil is rich in the omega-3 fatty acids that help make phagocytes, which destroy bacteria. Those fatty acids also help calm your immune system so that it doesn't overreact to infection and inflammation.

Chapter 8

Eating Clean to Manage Diseases

I f you already have a chronic or acute disease, changing your eating habits (to, say, the eating clean plan) can help you feel better and may even help reduce your risk of complications and the overall effects of the disease. After all, what you put into your body directly affects how efficiently your body heals itself and how it fights infection and invaders like bacteria and viruses.

Becoming aware of what you eat and how it's prepared is the first step toward a healthier you. Then you can fine-tune your diet to help manage your particular condition and improve your life. The one big difference between eating clean to reduce your risk of disease and eating clean after a disease has developed is that you have to be a lot more diligent about following a healthy diet when you have a diagnosed disease. You don't have any margin for error anymore. But you can still eat delicious and satisfying food!

In this chapter, we take a look at some powerful nutrients that you can get from clean food and that can act to promote health in the body. We also discuss ways to fight heart disease, manage diabetes, fight cancer, and battle autoimmune diseases, like arthritis and multiple sclerosis.

Eating Powerful Nutrients to Improve Health

Nutraceuticals are food concentrates, isolates, or supplements that may provide health benefits in different ways than pharmaceutical medicines. In other words, nutraceuticals are the phytochemicals found in whole foods — the focus of the eating clean diet plan.

Proponents of nutraceuticals view dietary supplements as being capable of promoting health by using "Nature's tools." When taken in supplement form, these bioactive chemicals are in much higher concentrations than you could get from food. But the eating clean plan focuses on the food sources of these chemicals.

In this section, we look at the relationship between food and disease management and examine some proven helpful nutrients. We consider whether they really work and whether the eating clean diet has a place for these supplemental nutrients.

Clean food's healing properties

Food is essential to life; that's a fact. If you don't get enough of the basic nutrients and micronutrients, you'll develop deficiency diseases like scurvy or beriberi. But can food actually help you recover from disease or trauma? Thousands of years of traditional Chinese, ayurvedic, and folk healing say yes, and modern research is starting to agree.

REMEMBER

Because the foods you eat on the clean diet plan are, for the most part, whole, unprocessed (and possibly organic) foods that are cooked in healthy ways, you're already consuming many of the vitamins, minerals, and nutrients that help prevent and fight disease. You can add nutraceuticals in the form of supplements to your diet to strengthen your immune system or fight specific disease symptoms. Just be sure to talk to a doctor skilled in nutritional medicine before adding any nutraceutical supplement to your diet.

You can also eat more *functional foods,* which are foods that have been enhanced with vitamins and minerals. (For instance, manufacturers often add vitamin D to milk and calcium to orange juice without changing the looks and tastes of either drink.) The purpose of these enhancements is to provide increased nutrition. Although functional foods are processed, they're perfectly acceptable on the eating clean plan because the processing is minimal and adds healthy ingredients rather than artificial chemicals.

Proven nutrient solutions

Illness and disease weaken your immune system. Fortunately, though, some nutrients help strengthen your immune system and help your body fight off damage from illness and disease. To reduce contagious diseases, which could aggravate your underlying disease, and to help boost your immune system, focus on eating plenty of these foods and nutrients (which just so happen to be major players in the eating clean plan):

» **Foods rich in vitamin C:** This vitamin, which is also known as *ascorbic acid,* helps strengthen your immune system by increasing the production and activity of white blood cells. Foods rich in vitamin C include kiwi fruit, berries, and all citrus fruits.

» **Foods rich in vitamin E:** Because this vitamin is so efficient at neutralizing free radicals, it takes over some of your immune system's job and lets it concentrate on healing. Find this vitamin in nuts, tomato products, spinach, and fortified cereals.

» **Foods rich in allicin:** This pungent compound is a natural antibiotic. It can kill bacteria and fight infection. The best source of allicin is freshly chopped or crushed garlic.

» **Foods rich in beta carotene and other carotenoids:** These powerful antioxidants mop up free radicals that can damage cells and lead to a number of diseases. Find them in apricots, carrots, mangoes, nectarines, pumpkin, sweet potatoes, tomatoes, and watermelon.

» **Foods rich in zinc:** This important mineral plays a starring role in wound healing and immune function. It aids enzymes that help tissue grow and heal. Find zinc in wheat germ, liver, sesame and pumpkin seeds, chocolate, and peanuts.

These nutraceuticals are widely accepted as being effective in battling disease:

» **Oats:** The soluble fiber in oats reduces cholesterol counts in your blood. Beta-glucan, a unique fiber, forms a solution in the intestines that absorbs cholesterol and removes it from the body.

» **Lycopene:** This phytochemical, which you find in tomatoes and orange vegetables, reduces the incidence of prostate cancer. It's more bioavailable in cooked tomatoes.

» **Omega-3 fatty acids:** These essential fatty acids lower triglyceride levels in the blood. They are very important for brain formation and maintenance. You find them in fatty fish and in a prescription form called omega-3-acid ethyl esters (Lovaza). Fish oil supplements and flaxseed are good nonpharmaceutical sources of this nutrient. Look for high amounts of EPA and DHA in any supplement.

>> **Berberine:** Controlled trials have shown that this component of the herbs goldenseal, Oregon grape, and Coptis chinesis helps regulate blood sugar as well as the number-one prescription drug for type-2 diabetes, metformin. Researchers also reported that berberine controlled lipids (cholesterol and triglycerides) in people with type-2 diabetes better than metformin. If you have type-2 diabetes or are prediabetic, check with a physician knowledgeable in nutritional and natural medicine about how to use this nutraceutical in your circumstances.

>> **Cinnamon:** Polyphenols and compounds called cinnamaldehydes are the active ingredients in this delicious spice; they help remove glucose from the blood. In fact, doctors often advise people with type-2 diabetes to consume some cinnamon every day because it helps improve glucose and lipid levels.

>> **Probiotics:** Your intestines need good bacteria to help keep you healthy and to guard against the bad bacteria that you encounter every day. Probiotics provide good bacteria, may help your body use calcium, and may be heart healthy. You find probiotics in yogurt, miso, sauerkraut, tamari, and aged cheese. Just be sure to look for the key phrase *active cultures* on the food labels.

>> **Vitamin D:** The sunshine vitamin is critical to bone health; people who take vitamin D supplements have a reduced bone fracture risk. Many research studies have also found that adequate vitamin D reduces risk of breast, prostate, and colon cancers, as well as cardiovascular, autoimmune, and many other diseases. You find vitamin D in cod liver oil, salmon, and mackerel. (For more details, check out www.vitamindcouncil.org.)

Sunshine is the best source of vitamin D. People living away from the equator have a hard time getting enough vitamin D, so they usually need to take a supplement. You can take too much vitamin D, though, so check with a physician to find out the amount that's right for you and your family.

>> **Vitamin C:** This vitamin may help prevent stomach cancer and reduce the risk of other cancers. It also lowers the risk of stroke, diabetes, and heart disease and reduces the risk of gallstones. You find vitamin C in citrus fruits, broccoli, bell peppers, strawberries, kale, and watermelon.

>> **Beta carotene:** This phytochemical may help prevent stomach cancer and reduce the risk of other cancers, as well as heart disease, high blood pressure, arthritis, and Alzheimer's. Your body turns it into vitamin A. If you take a beta carotene supplement, make sure it's a component of mixed carotenoids (the way it occurs in nature and in whole foods). Taken alone, it can occasionally cause problems. Foods rich in beta carotene include sweet potatoes, carrots, spinach, squash, and broccoli.

Older people and people with weak thyroid function often have difficulty converting beta carotene into vitamin A, so check with a physician skilled and knowledgeable in natural medicine for a personal recommendation about vitamin A.

>> **Glucosamine:** Your body turns this amino sugar into collagen, which strengthens cartilage (the shock absorber in your joints). Most patients who take glucosamine sulfate supplements have a significant decrease in arthritis pain.

>> **Plant sterols:** These compounds are similar to cholesterol but are found in plants. Sterols include beta-sitosterol, stigmasterol, and campesterol. They can help lower cholesterol in the blood by competing with cholesterol for space in the fat clusters produced by bile. The plant sterol amounts in food are usually too low to be of physiological benefit, so manufacturers often add them to margarines and spreads. They're also available as dietary supplements.

>> **Curcumin:** This compound, which you find in the spice turmeric, is a powerful anti-inflammatory agent. It has powerful antitumor properties and may help reduce plaque buildup on artery walls. In fact, curcumin has actually slowed the growth of cancer cells in the lab and has been shown to reduce the risk of Alzheimer's disease.

Remember to rely as much as you can on whole foods rather than the refined single supplements of these nutraceuticals. In many double-blind, placebo-controlled medical studies, these substances have produced mixed results, although a lot of anecdotal evidence supports their effectiveness. However, what actually provides the health benefits seen in these studies may be the combination of these compounds with other substances in whole foods and not any one compound alone. Because human bodies and the interactions between nutrients are so complex, nutrients very likely work together to produce the good health you see when you eat a whole and healthy diet.

Also keep in mind that many nutrients and phytochemicals that scientists don't even know about yet exist in whole foods. Following the eating clean diet plan of consuming whole, unprocessed foods in a good variety is the safest way to take advantage of healing nutrients (both the known and unknown).

Eating Clean to Help Fight Heart Disease

Did you know that you can help fight heart disease just by what you eat? In this section, we look at the foods and nutrients that you can eat to help reduce inflammation and blood pressure, control cholesterol, and manage heart disease.

If you have heart disease, whether you have atherosclerosis or have had a heart attack, the first thing to remember is that you must follow your doctor's advice. Never stop taking any medication without talking to your doctor first.

Getting your antioxidants

Antioxidants found in whole foods are important to your body's fight against heart disease. For one, the phytochemicals and vitamins with antioxidant properties help fight inflammation, which many doctors think is a good way to treat those with congestive heart failure. In addition, those same nutrients can help reduce cholesterol levels. In fact, eating a combination of foods high in antioxidant phytochemicals, plant sterols, and fiber (especially soluble fiber) can lower cholesterol levels as effectively as statin medications — without the harmful side effects!

To manage heart disease on the eating clean diet, focus on eating the following vitamins, nutrients, and foods:

>> **Vitamin D:** Researchers have discovered a strong correlation between vitamin D deficiency and chronic heart failure. Doctors don't really understand this vitamin's protective role, but they do know that it helps counteract congestive heart failure and may slow the progression of arterial plaques.

>> **Pomegranates:** These ancient fruits stop the oxidation of LDL cholesterol, which can lead to plaque formation, and reduce oxidative stress on cells. The antioxidants in these fruits also stop the overgrowth of too many muscle cells in the blood vessels, which contributes to high blood pressure. Eating pomegranates may actually reduce atherosclerosis.

>> **Green tea:** This beverage can help dilate arteries, allowing blood to flow more freely within them. Just don't add milk to your tea because doing so negates the benefits.

>> **Blueberries:** These little berries help fight hardening of the arteries. Eating ½ cup of fresh blueberries every day may help reduce the size of lesions in the arteries.

>> **Broccoli:** A recent study at the University of Connecticut found that broccoli has phytochemicals that increase levels of a heart-protective protein in the blood.

>> **Resveratrol:** This phytochemical can increase blood flow through the arteries, stop the oxidation of LDL cholesterol, reduce platelet clumping, and improve blood vessel dilation.

>> **Nuts:** Eating a handful of nuts a day can lower LDL cholesterol levels, help keep the lining of arteries supple, and reduce blood clot risk. The best nuts to eat are walnuts, almonds, pecans, macadamia nuts, hazelnuts, and Brazil nuts.

>> **Whole grains:** Whole grains, as opposed to refined grains, are good sources of the B vitamin complex, folate, iron, magnesium, and selenium, all important nutrients for heart health. Insoluble fiber in whole grains can also slow the progression of cardiovascular disease.

>> **Cooked tomatoes:** The lycopene in tomatoes, made more available by the cooking process, eliminates free radicals that oxidize LDL cholesterol (the type that causes the most damage to arteries).

>> **Omega-3 fatty acids:** These compounds decrease the risk of abnormal heartbeat and slow the growth of plaque in the arteries. Even in people who have heart failure, eating two servings of fatty fish a week can help preserve heart function.

TIP

Refer to Chapter 4 for more information about antioxidants and phytochemicals. If you have heart disease, be sure to follow your doctor's recommendations. Talk to him or her about your diet and ask for suggestions about the best foods to eat and supplements to add to your routine.

Chewing the good fat

Nutrition and dietary science have been moving away from pointing out a single culprit in the development of heart disease and putting more focus on diet patterns. In other words, blaming saturated fat intake alone for heart disease may be incorrect. Instead, the typical Western diet of processed foods high in refined sugars, white flour, trans fats, processed meats, in addition to saturated fats may be to blame for the high incidence of heart disease in America. You need to look at the whole picture when deciding what to eat to manage heart disease.

REMEMBER

Focusing on eating whole foods, avoiding processed foods and trans fats, reducing or eliminating sugar and refined grains, and consuming lots of fruits and vegetables (that is, following the eating clean plan!) may be the key to better heart health, no matter what your fat intake is. In fact, a 2010 study in the *American Journal of Clinical Nutrition* found no evidence that saturated fat intake led to higher risk of heart disease.

Scientists do know that eating some types of fats can help reduce cholesterol levels, blood pressure, triglyceride levels, and inflammation. Specifically, studies have proven that the monounsaturated fats found in olive oil, nuts, and avocados, and the essential fatty acids found in fatty fish, flaxseed, and walnuts help protect your heart.

So you don't have to fear fat if you have heart disease; just choose the healthy types. Eat foods that fill you up, always combine proteins with carbohydrates, eat whole foods, avoid junk food, and enjoy foods that are good sources of healthy fats.

In fact, for some people — especially those at risk for type-2 diabetes (which increases the risk of heart disease) and those with metabolic syndrome (which involves excess belly fat, high blood pressure, insulin resistance, and high triglyceride numbers) — a high-protein, low-carbohydrate, and relatively high-fat diet may be best. But no one diet is best for everyone, so talk to your doctor about what eating plan best meets your needs.

Adding a few essential supplements: CoQ10 and L-carnitine

Many people take supplements of coenzyme Q10 (CoQ10) and L-carnitine to help reduce the effects of heart disease. Do these supplements work? What do studies say about their effects? Should you take them? Read on to find out.

CoQ10

CoQ10 produces the energy that makes your heart muscle (and other muscles) contract. It also decreases arterial plaque buildup, slows abnormal blood clot formation, and prevents the oxidation of LDL cholesterol. CoQ10 is a critical element in the production of adenosine triphosphate (ATP), an energy source for the mitochondria in your heart cells, and is a potent antioxidant.

A LITTLE BACKGROUND ON CoQ10 AND STATINS

In 1990, two patents were issued covering the use of CoQ10 in combination with statin drugs to prevent, treat, or ameliorate the complications brought on by the drugs. The first patent, issued to Jonathan A. Tobert and assigned to Merck & Company, Inc., clearly states that by lowering CoQ10, the statin drugs can cause predictable elevations of liver enzymes with liver damage. It also states that giving CoQ10 along with the drugs can prevent this complication or treat it if it already exists.

A month later, a second patent was issued to Nobel laureate Michael S. Brown, MD, well known in scientific circles for his work in fat and cholesterol metabolism. This patent, which was also assigned to Merck, states that statin drugs, by causing a reduction in CoQ10, can produce complications of muscle pain, weakness, and myopathy. The patent covers a combination product of CoQ10 added to a statin to prevent these complications, plus the use of CoQ10 for the treatment of these complications.

Your body naturally makes CoQ10, but the amount you make decreases drastically with age. People with heart disease and heart failure also have lower levels of CoQ10 in their heart muscle cells. For this reason, many people at risk for heart disease take CoQ10 supplements. In fact, one study found that people who take CoQ10 supplements after a heart attack have fewer repeat heart attacks and less chest pain. According to other studies, CoQ10 may also help reduce edema (swelling) in the legs and reduce fluid buildup in the lungs. Still other studies have shown no benefit. So be sure to talk to your doctor for advice.

Because study results have been inconclusive or contradictory, we can't provide a firm conclusion or recommendation about this supplement. But an increasing number of physicians make a special study of nutritional medicine and the use of nutraceuticals, so you may want to check with such a specialist before taking a CoQ10 supplement.

WARNING

If you're taking statins to lower cholesterol, talk to your doctor about supplementing your diet with CoQ10 pills to make sure they're right for you. Diabetics should use CoQ10 only under a doctor's supervision because it can lower blood sugar levels.

L-carnitine

Doctors prescribe L-carnitine to help reduce the symptoms of *angina,* or heart pain. This amino acid can help improve a heart patient's ability to exercise, which angina may limit. Some studies have shown that patients who receive L-carnitine after a heart attack suffer fewer repeat heart attacks, but other studies have not shown this effect.

Like CoQ10, L-carnitine works to provide energy to the mitochondria, which are the engines of your cells. Because heart cells use so much energy, any depletion in the mitochondria in your heart cells has a significant adverse impact on heart function.

For more information about vitamins and minerals for preventing and treating heart disease, check out *The Sinatra Solution: New Hope for Preventing and Treating Heart Disease,* by Stephen T. Sinatra, MD.

REMEMBER

Talk to your doctor about supplementing your diet with L-carnitine if you're fighting heart disease. Pairing this amino acid with CoQ10 has been of great benefit to some patients, demonstrating the synergy between nutrients. But not every person responds favorably to adding this supplement, which is why you need to work closely with your doctor and/or a physician who specializes in nutritional medicine and the use of nutraceuticals before you change your diet or start supplementation.

Eating Clean to Manage Diabetes

When you're diagnosed with diabetes, one of the first things your doctor tells you is that you must change your diet. After all, keeping your blood sugar as stable as possible is the key to diabetes management. With diabetes, either your body doesn't make enough insulin (type-1) or the cells in your body have become resistant to insulin (type-2).

If you have type-2 diabetes, you have an unusually vigorous insulin response to sugar and carbohydrate consumption. In other words, your body is more sensitive than usual to sugar and refined carbohydrates. Over time, because of this vigorous insulin response, your cells develop insulin resistance to a point where the insulin your pancreas secretes can't control blood sugar levels. When your insulin resistance reaches that point, you have a diagnosis of type-2 diabetes.

In contrast, if you have type-1 diabetes, the pancreatic cells that make insulin die, and insulin production fails and finally ceases. Without insulin to regulate your blood sugar, your blood sugar levels go too high.

In this section, we look at how a diet of clean foods can help you manage diabetes and reduce your dependence on insulin. As with heart disease, never stop taking any medication without first checking with your doctor.

Note: Eating clean can certainly help you feel better, but keep in mind that while you can sometimes reverse type-2 diabetes through diet and weight loss, especially in the early stages, type-1 diabetes has no cure.

REDUCING TYPE-1 DIABETES IN BABIES WITH VITAMIN D SUPPLEMENTS

A 31-year study of type-1 diabetes tracked more than 10,000 infants born in 1966. Researchers completed the study in 1997 and published the results in *The Lancet* in 2001. They found that vitamin D supplementation given in the first year of life reduced the incidence of type-1 diabetes by 80 percent.

If type-1 diabetes runs in your family, check with a physician knowledgeable in nutritional and natural medicine about giving a vitamin D supplement to your baby.

Eating enough fiber and whole foods

Fiber and clean, whole foods are the keys to managing diabetes. As you increase your intake of healthy foods, eliminate junk foods, processed foods, and refined flour and sugar from your diet.

As soon as you know you have diabetes, talk to your doctor about which foods you can eat and how you can manage your blood sugar.

Fiber

Fiber-rich foods not only fill you up but also can help lower blood sugar levels. Fiber is considered a "free food" for people with diabetes. Because your body doesn't digest much of it, even though it's a carbohydrate, it doesn't affect your blood sugar.

Most Americans don't get enough fiber. A new study published in the *New England Journal of Medicine* found that people with type-2 diabetes can lower blood sugar levels by eating more fiber — up to 50 grams a day. The trick is to increase fiber intake gradually so that you can avoid digestive problems.

When adding fiber to your diet, focus on eating soluble fiber to manage diabetes. Soluble fiber forms gels in the stomach and intestines, and these gels help feed friendly bacteria and delay the emptying of your stomach so that you feel full longer. Soluble fiber also slows down the digestion of carbohydrates and sugars by trapping them in the gels so that your blood sugar levels don't spike after a meal or snack. It can also increase your cell's insulin sensitivity, which may reduce the need for added insulin. In addition, soluble fiber can remove cholesterol from the foods you eat, which may help prevent heart disease, a major risk for those with diabetes.

Try to get soluble fiber from as many different whole foods as possible:

>> **Whole grains:** People who get lots of fiber from whole-grain sources have lower blood pressure and a lower body mass index (BMI). Oats are a very good source of soluble fiber. However, many doctors specializing in nutritional medicine recommend that people with type-2 diabetes follow the Paleo (caveman) diet, which excludes grains and dairy products (see Chapter 6 for details). Fortunately, you can find many excellent nongrain sources of fiber, too (just read the rest of this list for details!).

>> **Whole vegetables:** Try to eat vegetables unpeeled for more fiber content. The vegetables with the highest soluble fiber content include artichokes, broccoli, tomatoes, carrots, cucumbers, and celery.

>> **Fresh fruit:** Eat the skin of apples and pears for the most soluble fiber content. Other fruits high in soluble fiber include oranges, strawberries, blueberries, and other berries. But remember that many people with diabetes have to cut down on fruit because this food category is high in sugars.

>> **Dried fruit:** Like fresh fruit, dried fruit is high in fiber, vitamins, and minerals, but it's also high in sugar. Talk to your doctor about adding dried fruit to your diet.

>> **Nuts and seeds:** These foods have lots of good fats that can help you feel satisfied longer, along with a good dose of soluble fiber. Include walnuts, Brazil nuts, pistachios, and almonds in your diet, along with sunflower seeds and sesame seeds.

>> **Legumes and beans:** Kidney beans, soybeans, and lima beans all have three grams of soluble fiber per ½-cup serving. Other types of beans have about two grams of fiber per serving.

TIP

As you increase your fiber intake, remember to drink more water to prevent constipation and to help the digestive process.

Whole foods

Eating plenty of whole foods that are rich in vitamins, minerals, and phytochemicals is crucial when you're managing diabetes. After all, the nutrients in whole foods can help regulate blood sugar to avoid spikes and dips, help you lose weight, and help fight oxidation and free radical damage that can harm your pancreas, heart, kidneys, and other organs. Because your wound healing is slower and you're more prone to infections when you have diabetes, keeping your immune system as healthy as possible is important.

Many people with diabetes also want to lose weight. The best approach is to get as many nutrients as possible from the calories you consume. Focus on nutrient-dense foods — which just happen to be the whole foods on the eating clean diet plan — rather than empty-calorie foods.

WARNING

AVOIDING JUICES

Diabetics and people who are at risk for developing diabetes should avoid juices, especially fruit juices. These products, while natural, are very high in simple sugars and don't have the fiber of whole foods to stop the sugar from entering your bloodstream very rapidly. In fact, when coauthor Linda's husband was diagnosed with heart disease, he turned to drinking fruit juices instead of soda pop. Within a few months, his blood sugar was in the diabetic range. Eliminating most juices and eating whole foods instead brought it down to a normal level — to Linda's great relief!

Don't be afraid of good fats. In people with diabetes, excess insulin makes the liver manufacture more cholesterol (especially LDL cholesterol) and triglycerides, and carbohydrates (particularly simple carbs) — not fats — overstimulate insulin production. Good fats, found in lean meats, nuts, and seeds, are satisfying, help slow the release of sugars into your system, and make you feel full longer. Plus, the lower-carb diet is naturally higher in fats (because you have to eat something and the triad of carb-fat-protein will change), so enjoy eating the healthy fats. They're good for you!

REMEMBER

Diabetes weakens your body and its immune system, so try to avoid any foods (or food products) that could increase the risk of developing other diseases. Make sure to read about organic foods and the so-called filthy fifteen nonorganic foods you should avoid in Chapter 10. Most people can't afford to eat an entirely organic diet, but try to avoid the foods that are most highly contaminated with pesticides and herbicides to help you keep your exposure to a minimum.

Making the best clean food choices

This section is all about the foods you should and shouldn't eat when you have diabetes. But keep in mind that every person with diabetes is different. Focus on the goals you want to reach. If you want to lose weight, read about using the eating clean diet to trim pounds in Chapter 6. If you want to eat to strengthen your heart, read about the phytochemicals and nutrients you need to concentrate on in Chapter 7. And remember to choose healing foods that promote health and help your body heal from the damage this disease causes (see Chapters 3, 4, and 6 for details).

REMEMBER

Before changing your diet to meet any of your goals, talk to your doctor, nutritionist, and perhaps a doctor specializing in natural and nutritional medicine about the foods you want to add to your daily menu and your overall diet plan. And don't forget to get some exercise! For people with diabetes, even mild to moderate exercise can make a big difference in overall quality of life. Plus, exercise is an important part of the eating clean plan.

Knowing what foods to eat the most of

If you have diabetes, follow these tips to get the most benefit from the foods you eat:

>> **Eat plenty of high-fiber foods.** Whole grains, legumes, vegetables, nuts, seeds, and a judicious amount of whole fruits pack fiber into your diet. Try not to peel vegetables and fruits to get the highest fiber content.

>> **Combine carbs with fiber, protein, and fat.** If you eat carbs, make them whole grain, and eat them with foods high in fiber and good fats. This combination of foods helps slow down the absorption of sugars into your blood stream and prevents those dreaded glucose spikes.

>> **Add cinnamon to your diet.** This fragrant spice helps control blood sugar levels. Use whole cinnamon when possible; boil about ½ teaspoon of whole cinnamon in water and then use the water in recipes and hot drinks. Discard the solid remainder.

>> **Consider following the Paleo diet.** Eat more protein, especially organic meat from grass-fed beef. Search out the least processed foods and focus on eating a diet relatively high in protein and good fats. (See Chapter 6 for details on what to eat as part of this diet, and about the Kraft pre-diabetes test, which will tell you if the Paleo diet is best for you.)

>> **Think of your daily diet like an inverted pyramid.** Eat your largest meal in the morning, eat a moderately sized lunch, and eat a small dinner, with some healthy snacks in between. Studies on mice have found that eating on this type of schedule can improve control of high cholesterol, high triglycerides, and high blood pressure, which are all concerns for people with diabetes.

>> **Use sweeteners like stevia or lo han for a sweet taste.** These sweeteners have little to no impact on blood glucose levels.

Remember that you can still enjoy your food! Being afraid of food is only natural after a serious diagnosis. But clean, whole foods can be your partner as you manage diabetes. Include foods you really love in your diet as long as they're clean and unprocessed, and make mealtime an enjoyable experience by adding flavor to your food with natural herbs and spices.

Knowing what to do if you do eat processed foods

When you have diabetes, reading food labels is more important than ever. The best way to get the right balance in your diet is to avoid processed foods and use whole foods instead. But if you do consume some processed foods, keep the following guidelines in mind:

>> Count your carbs and/or focus on avoiding simple sugars and refined carbs if your doctor tells you to do so.

>> Avoid trans fats or anything with the word *hydrogenated* attached to it. Trans fats are bad for everyone, but people who eat more trans fats have a higher risk of developing diabetes. These fake fats also have strong ties to the development of heart disease.

>> Do your best to completely eliminate refined sugar. This product (we can't call it food) removes nutrients, such as magnesium, the B-complex vitamins, and

chromium, from your body. For information about breaking a sugar addiction (and it is an addiction), see Chapter 6.

>> Watch out for sugars that can hide in foods. Food labels use quite a few words for *sugar*. Look at the carbohydrate amount on the label and choose foods with the lowest number.

>> Be careful about salt intake. Because diabetes can weaken your kidneys, reducing your sodium intake is critical. Sodium hides in many processed foods, so read labels carefully.

Eating Clean to Fight Cancer

Cancer is one of the scariest diseases out there. Just hearing a doctor mention the word can be terrifying. But more and more people are surviving cancer and even living with it for years. Your diet is an important tool in the fight against cancer. It needs to support your treatment, helping you maintain your weight, control infection, and improve your quality of life.

In this section, we look at which foods (and food products) to avoid when you're fighting cancer and which ones to eat more of to make your body and immune system as strong as possible. We look at the foods that may cause cancer and the foods that help reduce your risk for it. (If the foods can reduce your risk for cancer, they may help your body fight it, too.) These foods may also help reduce the side effects of traditional cancer treatments.

REMEMBER

The exact nutrients you need to focus on depend on the type of cancer you have. So be sure to contact a physician skilled in nutritional medicine for more specific details before you change your diet or add supplements.

Avoiding sugar and artificial ingredients

One of the main precepts of the eating clean diet plan is avoiding processed and refined foods, and it should be your first step in designing a diet to help you fight cancer. After all, if switching to a clean diet could prevent more than half of all cancers, eating a clean diet could very well help you fight the disease, too.

Consider this: The average American consumes 14 pounds of additives, preservatives, artificial flavorings and colorings, and emulsifiers every single year. Although these materials aren't considered carcinogenic in and of themselves, no one really knows the long-term effects of ingesting all these chemicals, especially in combination. Just as phytochemicals, vitamins, and minerals work together to help make you healthy, many people who eat clean believe that artificial chemicals may work together to make you sick. So try to avoid processed foods, synthetic ingredients, nonorganic foods, and genetically modified foods. In particular, if you've been diagnosed with cancer, do your best to avoid these foods:

>> **Saturated fats:** Avoid these fats as much as possible, especially in meat products from grain-fed beef, caged chicken, and factory-farmed pork.

>> **Sugar:** This product promotes the growth of existing cancer cells. In fact, researchers have found that consuming just one teaspoon of sugar can impair your immune system by 50 percent for several hours. Simple sugars can reduce your white blood cells' ability to destroy bacteria and viruses by 50 percent.

>> **Milk from cows given BGH:** Bovine growth hormone (BGH) has been found to increase all kinds of cancer risk. In fact, some researchers recommend that you don't drink milk at all because they've found a link between cow's milk consumption and prostate cancer development. The studies done so far don't offer direct proof, but choosing almond or soy milk rather than dairy milk may be better for your health.

>> **Trans fats:** Some studies have shown that trans fats may increase the risk of some kinds of cancers, especially breast cancer and colon cancer. Everyone, especially cancer patients, should avoid this fake food. It becomes part of your cells, making the cell walls flabby and less responsive to nutrients, which is the last thing your body needs when you have cancer.

>> **Processed meats:** Manufacturers add sodium nitrite and nitrates to foods as preservatives. These preservatives also make processed meats pink and provide a lot of the flavor you're used to. But your body transforms these compounds into nitrosamine, which is a carcinogen.

>> **Soy:** Although soy can be good for you, the isoflavones in this product can act like estrogen in the body. Getting too much soy can increase the risk of breast cancer recurrence. Anyone who has had estrogen-sensitive breast cancer should avoid soy products.

>> **Omega-6 fatty acids:** These compounds can speed up the growth of cancer cells. In lab tests, these fatty acids promoted the growth of prostate cancer cells. In most Americans, the omega-3:omega-6 fatty acid ratio is too slanted toward omega-6, so avoid foods that contain this fat, such as polyunsaturated vegetable oils.

In addition to avoiding these particular ingredients, take a close look at how you prepare your foods. Read through Chapter 11 to understand the cleanest types of food preparation. Avoid fried foods, grilled foods, and any foods cooked at high heat. These techniques increase the amount of acrylamides and aromatic polycyclic hydrocarbons, both of which are carcinogenic.

SUPPLEMENTS TO FIGHT CANCER

Some supplements you may want to include in your fight against cancer are fractionated citrus pectin, which supports the immune system and may help reduce metastasis, and melatonin, which helps your body produce red blood cells, maintain body weight, and slow the growth of some cancer cells. A vitamin D supplement may be a good idea, too, since even with good sun exposure, your body's ability to synthesize vitamin D precursors declines with age. Also consider supplementing with folate, vitamin B12, vitamin A, zinc, and vitamin C.

Before you add any supplements to your diet, check with your oncologist. Make sure that he or she knows and approves exactly what you plan to take. Some physicians, particularly naturopathic physicians (NDs), specialize in providing nutritional support for individuals undergoing conventional cancer treatment.

Knowing which foods can help fight cancer

Cancer is the abnormal, out-of-control growth of cells that takes nutrients and energy away from normal cells. So the goal of cancer prevention and/or management is to prevent abnormal cell growth and transformation. The nutrients that accomplish this task are phytochemicals, vitamins, and minerals. The eating clean diet is a wonderful plan for everyone, but it's especially important for those who are fighting cancer.

Choose these foods to help you in your fight against cancer:

>> **Fatty fish:** Fatty fish is the number-one source of omega-3 fatty acids, which are some of the best nutrients to fight breast cancer and slow the growth of most cancer cells. Just be sure to choose smaller fish that have lower mercury contents, and avoid tuna, swordfish, shark, king mackerel, red snapper, and orange roughy.

>> **Organic, grass-fed meats:** Organic and free-range meats have fewer omega-6 fatty acids and more omega-3 fatty acids. The pesticides and herbicides present in the fat of traditionally raised meats have been linked to cancer development.

>> *Brassica* **vegetables:** These veggies, which include broccoli, cauliflower, kohlrabi, Brussels sprouts, and cabbage, contain indole-3-carbinol (I3C), which is a tumor risk–reducing compound. They also have isothiocyanates, which have shown anticarcinogenic properties in cell cultures and animal studies. As a bonus, they contain lutein and xeaxanthin, two powerful antioxidants.

- >> **Organic fruits and vegetables:** Avoid pesticides, herbicides, and other toxins by choosing organic fruits and vegetables whenever possible. If you can't afford to purchase all organic produce (which is the case for many people), take a look at Chapter 10 for a list of the fifteen foods you should never buy nonorganic and a list of the foods that are okay to buy nonorganic.

- >> **Citrus fruits:** Citrus fruits contain a compound called limonene, which is being tested as a cancer treatment. They're also a rich source of monoterpenes, which can help remove carcinogens from the body.

- >> **Green tea:** This classic beverage contains epigallocatechin, a phytochemical from the catechin family that has proven antitumor activity.

- >> **Garlic:** The allium compounds in garlic can help destroy cancer-causing substances in the body. Diallyl sulfide can destroy carcinogens that reach your liver.

- >> **Turmeric:** The curcumin in turmeric has been found to inhibit breast cancer in mice. It also halts production of an enzyme found in people who have bowel and colon cancer. In fact, this nutrient may someday be a cancer treatment.

- >> **Flaxseed oil:** The lignans in flaxseed act as antioxidants and may block cancerous changes in your cells. This oil also has a lot of omega-3 fatty acids. However, more than a little flaxseed oil has been found to increase prostate cancer risk.

- >> **Water:** Remember to drink plenty of water, especially when you're undergoing chemotherapy treatment. Drinking enough water every day is crucial to reducing constipation, which is found to increase cancer risk.

Eating Clean to Battle Autoimmune Diseases

When you've been diagnosed with an autoimmune disease, the foods you eat become especially important. After all, you can ease the symptoms of lupus, ulcerative colitis, rheumatoid arthritis, multiple sclerosis, and other autoimmune diseases by eating a clean diet of whole, unprocessed foods and paying attention to food allergies.

In this section, we look at how the foods you eat and the nutrients you focus on can improve the symptoms of these devastating diseases. Diet isn't a substitute for healthcare and medication, but you can become a partner in your own care by carefully choosing the foods you eat and the foods you avoid.

Lupus

Lupus tends to affect women in their childbearing years, since estrogen levels are highest at that time. However, research has shown that not all estrogens aggravate lupus; in fact, estriol can help women achieve major relief from lupus symptoms. Women with this disease tend to have higher levels of an estrogen called 16-hydroxyestrogen and lower levels of 2-hydroxyestrogen. Adding *Brassica* vegetables to the diet can help improve this ratio.

To help manage the symptoms of lupus, focus on getting plenty of these nutrients:

>> **Fish and fish oil:** The fatty acids DHA and EPA in fish and fish oil have anti-inflammatory properties, which can help improve symptoms of lupus.

>> **Di-indolyl Methane (DIM):** This compound, which you find in *Brassica* vegetables, such as Brussels sprouts, bok choy, broccoli, and cabbage, can help improve your 2- to 16-hydroxyestrogen ratio by increasing the production of 2-hydroxyestrogen.

>> **Vitamin D:** The sunshine vitamin is critical to lupus prevention and management. Many people who suffer from this disease are deficient in vitamin D. The best way to get this vitamin is to get some direct sun exposure on unprotected skin as often as possible. But because many people with lupus develop rashes when exposed to the sun, supplements are sometimes necessary. Talk to a doctor proficient in nutritional medicine about vitamin D supplements.

>> **Flavonoids:** These powerful antioxidants help reduce inflammation in people with lupus. They can also mitigate the effects of an overactive immune system. Find flavonoids, especially apigenin, in apples, cherries, grapes, parsley, artichokes, nuts, tea, and wine.

>> **Ellagic acid:** Found in raspberries, strawberries, pomegranates, and walnuts, this phytochemical acts as an antioxidant in the intestinal tract — just where you need it! It also blocks enzymes that are necessary for cancer cell growth.

>> **Vitamin B6:** The pyridoxal phosphate form (P5P) of this vitamin is most effective. Many drugs and chemicals known to dramatically increase the risk of lupus inhibit vitamin B6-dependent enzyme systems. Although no controlled studies have been done yet, over the past 40 years, many people with lupus have told coauthor Dr. Wright that they definitely feel better with extra vitamin B6. Good food sources of vitamin B6 include bananas, celery, cabbage, asparagus, tuna, garlic, cauliflower, Brussels sprouts, kale, and collard greens.

>> **Lycopene:** You find this phytochemical, along with other antioxidants that fight inflammation by neutralizing free radicals, in red-colored fruits and vegetables, specifically in tomatoes.

In addition to consuming the nutrients we list here, try to minimize or eliminate all sources of gluten from your diet. Gluten sensitivity and lupus (as well as many other autoimmune diseases) are very closely related. In fact, they're so closely tied that if you have autoimmune diseases in your family, you should eliminate gluten as a precautionary measure. Gluten isn't an essential nutrient in the human diet, so don't worry about eliminating it.

Also consider eliminating milk and dairy products; components of milk and dairy have been proven to trigger type-1 diabetes, which is actually an auto-immune disease. Antibodies to gluten and dairy proteins are often found in tests of individuals with auto-immune disease of all types.

Ulcerative colitis

People with ulcerative colitis need more good gut bacteria to help their bodies prevent an immune system attack. Reducing processed foods is an essential first step in managing this disease, but eliminating foods that contain gluten, dairy products, and yeast is also important.

Eating lots of raw, clean, whole fruits and vegetables is one of the best ways to help balance the bacteria in your intestines. But you need to avoid cruciferous vegetables, along with garlic, onions, and dried fruit, because these foods contain sulfur, which may increase the bad bacteria in your gut. Also try to reduce your intake of fat and protein if you have ulcerative colitis.

Dr. James Breneman, former Chair of the Food Allergy Committee of the American College of Allergists (now the American College of Allergy, Asthma, and Immunology) reported in his book *Basics of Food Allergy* (Breneman) that ulcerative colitis sufferers had noticeable improvement when they eliminated all milk and dairy products from their diets. Dr. Wright's observations have revealed the same results and have actually found that elimination of all gluten helps even more.

REMEMBER

The eating clean diet plan is ideal for people with ulcerative colitis because eating several small meals throughout the day makes for much easier digestion than eating two or three larger meals. Plus, nutrient-dense foods are very important for dealing with ulcerative colitis, since irritation in the intestines or colon can reduce nutrient absorption. Eating mostly bland and smooth foods may also help reduce symptoms; however, you may need to follow an elimination diet to determine which foods trigger your condition.

To help prevent and treat ulcerative colitis, focus on getting lots of these nutrients:

>> **Vitamin D:** This nutrient is relevant to both prevention and treatment of most autoimmune conditions, including ulcerative colitis. Consult a physician proficient in nutritional medicine to find out how much supplemental vitamin D is right for you.

>> **Fish and fish oil:** These foods can improve symptoms of ulcerative colitis because the fatty acids DHA and EPA in fish and fish oil have anti-inflammatory properties.

>> **Flavonoids:** By helping to reduce oxidation of fats and neutralizing free radicals, all the flavonoids can help soothe an irritated digestive system. Specifically, the flavonoids in olive oil and fish oil can help reduce colon inflammation. Get flavonoids from fruits, vegetables, herbs, such as basil and thyme, and spices, such as turmeric and cumin.

>> **Pectin:** This complex carbohydrate can help regulate digestion and enhance the good bacteria in your intestines. Find it in apples, carrots, peas, beans, and potatoes.

>> **Quercetin:** As an antioxidant, this phytochemical helps battle free radicals that can lead to inflammation. It's also a natural anti-inflammatory agent that can help improve the efficacy of any drugs you may be taking to combat the symptoms of ulcerative colitis.

>> **Beta-glucan:** This nutrient helps regulate the immune system and can reduce the risk of colon cancer. (The risk of developing colon cancer increases in people with irritable bowel syndrome, or IBS, and Crohn's disease.) Find beta-glucan in mushrooms and tea.

>> **Calcium:** Calcium-rich foods can help regulate your colon and prevent diarrhea. Because dairy products are one of the primary dietary sources of calcium and because you may need to avoid them as part of your disease management, a supplement may be your best bet for getting enough calcium. Also consume spinach, legumes, and nuts to get more calcium. Remember to always take magnesium with calcium, but work closely with your doctor to find the right combination for you as excess magnesium can cause loose bowels and diarrhea.

Rheumatoid arthritis

The cause of rheumatoid arthritis (RA) is officially unknown, although many experts believe that it's an autoimmune disease. It results in considerable body-wide inflammation. Although RA has no widely known cure, eating the right kinds of foods — especially foods with antioxidants and other phytochemicals that help reduce inflammation — can provide some relief from its devastating symptoms.

Eating a diet of nutrient-dense foods, especially fruits and vegetables, can help make your joints and muscles healthier. An elimination diet that focuses on allergenic foods is a good starting point for treating RA because food elimination often reduces symptoms. The foods that cause allergies may include dairy products, chiles, among others. In addition, omega-6 fatty acids in grain-fed red meats and nearly all vegetable oils are pro-inflammatory, so people with RA may need to reduce their intake of those foods as well. Reducing or eliminating the amount of refined sugar you eat is also a good idea, since sugar can be inflammatory.

REMEMBER

The important thing to remember about RA is that different people react differently to different foods. Some people benefit from eliminating dairy products, while others aren't bothered by that group of foods in the first place. Likewise, eating grain-fed red meat may increase inflammation in one group of patients but not in others. Fish oil supplements can help relieve symptoms in most people but not all. So work with your doctor to fine-tune your clean eating diet to include the foods best for you.

To help reduce the effects of RA, focus on eating these nutrients and foods:

>> **Omega-3 fatty acids:** These polyunsaturated fats are anti-inflammatory. Studies show that consumption of these fats can help relieve some of the symptoms of RA. Get them from wild salmon, sardines, and trout, as well as walnuts. Also consider taking a fish oil supplement.

>> **Gamma-linolenic acid (GLA) and alpha-linolenic acid (ALA):** These natural oils can help reduce inflammation and swelling in affected joints. You find GLA in seeds and seed oils, particularly borage, black currant, and evening primrose. You find ALA in wheat germ oil, fatty fish, and leafy green vegetables.

>> **Zinc:** Most, though not all, research with zinc has found it helpful for reducing the effects of RA. The best food sources of zinc include pumpkin seeds, beef, pork, beans, brown rice, yogurt, and whole grains.

>> **Copper:** This mineral is a known anti-inflammatory agent. Research has found that wearing copper bracelets can reduce pain in RA patients. The best food sources of copper include legumes, oysters, cherries, mushrooms, dark leafy greens, and tofu.

>> **Ginger:** This root vegetable is anti-inflammatory and can help reduce the pain of osteoarthritis. Stir it into stir-fries and sauces, and add it to tea.

>> **Beta carotene:** This vitamin A precursor acts as an antioxidant, which reduces inflammation and therefore helps improve joint health. It can also help reduce swelling. Eat more carrots, cantaloupe, pumpkin, spinach, kale,

parsley, and sweet potatoes to get more beta carotene in your diet. Be sure to get beta carotene as part of your mixed carotenoids.

» **Vitamin C:** This vitamin is a powerful antioxidant that helps fight infection. It may also protect against inflammatory polyarthritis, which is RA in two or more joints at the same time. Since arthritis patients should avoid tomatoes, peppers, and potatoes, which are good sources of this vitamin, find it in broccoli, cabbage, asparagus, raspberries, bananas, and strawberries.

» **Di-indolymenthan:** Also known as DIM, this nutrient, which is found in *Brassica* vegetables like Brussels sprouts, bok choy, broccoli, and cabbage, can help improve the symptoms of RA.

» **Vitamin E:** Another antioxidant, this vitamin helps stabilize cartilage that serves as the connection between muscles and bone. Good sources for this vitamin include peanut butter, nuts, seeds, whole grains, and avocados. If you use a supplement, look for mixed tocopherols.

» **Calcium and vitamin D:** These nutrients are important for bone and joint health. Supplements of these vitamins may be necessary, since dairy products, which are a good source of calcium, may be eliminated from the RA diet. Nondairy sources of calcium include leafy greens, almond milk, soy milk, fortified cereals, and soybeans. Nondairy sources of vitamin D include cod liver oil, mackerel, and egg yolks. If you use a calcium supplement, make sure to get magnesium also.

Keeping your weight at a normal level is also very important for arthritis sufferers. Extra weight puts stress on your already damaged joints. Many prescription medications can cause weight gain, so try to stay active, eat a good diet, and follow the eating clean plan.

WARNING

Get your 2-hydroxyestrogen:16-hydroxyestrogen ratio checked if you have RA. Urinary loss of 2-hydroxyestrogen is ten times higher in individuals with RA than in healthy individuals; urinary loss of 16-hydroxyestrogen remains the same. While still in the body, 2-hydroxyestrogen can slow overly aggressive tissue growth and inflammation that occurs in people with RA, so using foods and supplements to slow the abnormally high loss of 2-hydroxyestrogen can be helpful.

Irritable bowel syndrome

Doctors don't know exactly what causes irritable bowel syndrome (IBS), but it may be an immune system illness. Symptoms of IBS include abdominal pain and cramps that are relieved after a visit to the bathroom, and are associated with a change in stool frequency and appearance. Sufferers of this syndrome may have restricted lives because they can never be too far away from a restroom.

Medications can help control this disorder, but you can also help relieve symptoms with your diet. The elimination diet is a good place to start. You eliminate all gluten, cereal grains, soy, dairy, and fast food for at least three weeks. Keep a food journal. Then gradually reintroduce one food group at a time into your diet. If you experience symptoms, that food is a trigger for you and should be eliminated from your diet permanently.

Stress management may help control IBS symptoms. Many people with IBS are diagnosed with general anxiety disorder. Relaxation techniques, journaling, meditation, and gentle exercise such as yoga can help.

The foods you should avoid if you are diagnosed with IBS may include the following:

>> **Greasy foods:** French fries, fried chicken, sausages, and pizza can trigger IBS symptoms. But healthy fats, found in nuts and fatty fish, are good for you.

>> **High-FODMAP foods:** This acronym stands for "fermentable oligo-, di-, monosaccharides, and polyols" (hence, the need for an acronym). These are carbohydrates that are poorly absorbed in the intestine. Some of the high-FODMAP foods include apples, grapefruit, pears, nectarines, watermelon, artichokes, asparagus, Brussels sprouts, cauliflower, celery, onions, peas, and shallots.

>> **Beans and legumes:** The carbohydrates in these foods are difficult to digest. Your gut bacteria ferment them, which produces lots of intestinal gas.

>> **Spicy foods:** These foods, which include spicy peppers such as jalapeños, can cause pain in your abdomen. Studies show that some IBS patients have more nerve fibers in their guts that react to capsaicin, the substance in peppers that causes the pain sensation in your mouth.

>> **Wheat:** This grain contains gluten, which causes distress in those with celiac disease and may cause symptoms in people with IBS. Gluten-free foods are readily available on the market now.

Multiple sclerosis

Many people with multiple sclerosis (MS) have food allergies, so be sure to have a food allergy test with a doctor skilled in nutrition as the first step in your plan to battle this disease. If you're allergic to some foods, avoid them scrupulously. (For more information about dealing with food allergies, see Chapter 14.)

Another important step in battling MS is following a healthy diet. One diet in particular — the Swank diet, which was first developed by Professor of Neurology Roy Swank at the Oregon Health and Sciences University — can make a difference in long-term survival for people with MS. The Swank diet is a low-fat diet that focuses on organic vegetables, fruits, whole grains, nuts and seeds, fatty fish, and no processed foods. Sound familiar? It's actually very similar to the eating clean diet plan.

Although focusing on whole foods on the clean eating diet plan can help support the health of people with MS, the Swank diet goes a bit further by advising you to completely avoid these products:

>> Saturated fat

>> Trans fats

>> Food additives

>> Preservatives

>> Colorings

>> Artificial flavorings

>> Refined flour

>> Refined sugar

The Swank diet is high in unsaturated fatty acids, specifically oleic, linoleic, linolenic, and arachidonic acids. The oils that are high in these fats include olive oil, sesame seed oil, and flaxseed oil. Avoiding hydrogenated oils, fake fats, margarine, and shortening is very important on this diet.

Improving your omega-3:omega-6 ratio is also critical when dealing with MS. Omega-3 fatty acids help suppress an overactive immune system and reduce inflammation in the body. For more on this crucial ratio and tips for how to move it toward optimal levels, see Chapter 3.

Research reported in 2002 by UCLA scientists found that estriol (one of three "major" estrogens) very significantly reduced symptoms of multiple sclerosis. To investigate this further, check with a physician skilled and knowledgeable in natural medicine.

SUPPLEMENTS TO HELP FIGHT AUTOIMMUNE DISEASES

Anyone who's at risk for autoimmune diseases should add a good multivitamin to their diet. Reduced nutrient absorption is a risk factor for those with lupus, so increasing available nutrients may help prevent malnutrition. You may want to consider taking extra vitamins, especially vitamin D, which is important in the prevention and treatment of autoimmune diseases. Consider taking supplements of vitamins C and E, as well as calcium and magnesium, since getting enough of those nutrients can be difficult on an RA diet.

Because inflammation is a major feature of any autoimmune disease, natural anti-inflammatories can be very helpful. The omega-3 fatty acids in fish, especially fish oils, are essential nutrients with important anti-inflammatory properties. Consider adding fish oil to your supplement program if you have an autoimmune disease.

Researchers have found that the B vitamin PABA (para-aminobenzoic acid) can be a significant help for several autoimmune diseases. However, quantities required are relatively large, so be sure to consult with a doctor skilled and knowledgeable in nutritional medicine about use of this supplement.

3

Planning and Preparing Your Eating Clean Adventure

Chapter 9

Planning and Stocking the Eating Clean Kitchen

How often do you clean your kitchen? If you're like most people, you go through your fridge about once a week, your pantry about once every few months, and your freezer once every few years. Even if you clean more often, cleaning your kitchen to start your eating clean lifestyle is a whole new concept.

When you make the decision to switch to a clean eating lifestyle, one of the first things you need to do is clear your kitchen of certain foods. Even if you've been eating healthy food lately, you'll be surprised by the number of processed foods hiding in your fridge, pantry, and freezer. Now's the time to read labels and closely examine the food you've been putting on your table — and get rid of the bad stuff.

The two places that have the biggest effect on your diet are your kitchen and the grocery store. When you're hungry, you eat what you can find in the kitchen, and what's in your kitchen comes straight from the grocery store. Thus, you can immediately improve your diet just by making a few changes in your shopping habits.

In this chapter, we look at what foods you should keep and what foods you should throw out or donate. We look at how to stock your kitchen with clean foods and how to store those foods for maximum freshness. We explain how to navigate the grocery store and help you stick to your eating clean plan (despite the many processed foods you encounter there). Finally, we look at farmers' markets, food cooperatives, and Community Supported Agriculture (CSA) as alternatives to the big chain supermarkets.

Organizing Your Kitchen

As all Type A people know, organization is next to godliness. Well, not really. But embarking on the eating clean lifestyle does mean you have to get organized in your kitchen. In other words, you have to know what's in your kitchen and get rid of foods that are no longer part of your diet.

The first step to creating a clean kitchen is unearthing foods that need to go. Yes, we mean going through each and every food (or food-like) item in your house, deciding whether you should keep it, throw it out, or donate it, and then taking action.

Cleaning out your cupboards is a great place to start. Many people have products well past their expiration dates still on their shelves, as well as products they just don't use anymore. In this section, we tell you which products to keep and which ones to discard and what to do with the foods you get rid of.

Sorting through your food

As with all lifestyle changes, the first real step in switching to the eating clean plan is creating an environment that supports your goal. If the house is full of junk food and you're a junk food junkie, those cheese curls and sour cream potato chips won't just sit there until they're soggy and past their expiration date. So you need to get rid of all that junk food and replace it with clean, healthy, and delicious foods and snacks.

Start by removing all the food items from your pantry or kitchen shelves. Place everything on the kitchen counter and gather a few sturdy boxes for sorting. While the shelves are empty, wipe down the pantry with a clean cloth dipped in a non-toxic cleaner. (You can find green cleaners at the grocery or hardware store or make your own by mixing water with a little lemon juice or vinegar.) As a matter of fact, clean off any cans or unopened packages, too. Everything you put back into your pantry should be as clean as possible in every way!

After you have all the food out of the pantry, you need to sort it into three different boxes: keep, donate, and throw out. Mark the boxes with a marker or pen so you don't get mixed up as you're sorting.

Foods to keep

The first box or category consists of the foods you've decided to keep eating. Which foods you include in this first category is totally up to you. When you're first getting started, think about which clean eating properties and qualities are most important to you. If you're not going all-out into this new lifestyle but are trying to ease into it, don't get rid of everything all at once. For example, you may want to keep pastas that aren't whole grain, some condiments, favorite breakfast cereals, or certain canned fruits and vegetables that you really like. From there, just keep the cleanest foods; you can supplement them with new purchases as you go.

In general, you can keep foods that are

>> **Minimally processed:** Like maple syrup, soy milk, whole-wheat flour, and canned beans

>> **Organically grown, according to the label:** Like foods with labels that say *100% organic, organic* (meaning that the food contains at least 95 percent organically grown and produced ingredients), or *made with organic ingredients* (meaning that the food contains at least 70 percent organically grown and produced ingredients)

>> **Made from whole grains:** Like whole-wheat breads and whole-grain pastas

>> **Raw or unprocessed:** Like brown rice, whole nuts, quinoa, lentils, dried legumes, and honey

>> **Low in sugar and salt:** Like dried fruits and mushrooms and certain clean canned foods

>> **Free of preservatives or additives:** Like plain oils, vinegar, and tea

Foods to donate

You can donate any food that's not in your "keep" box but is still wholesome to a charity or food pantry. Food banks and many charities accept unopened and undamaged packages of food, and many grocery stores have drop boxes or areas where you can leave food. You can also check in your phone book for donation locations. You may want to call ahead to ask whether the foods you intend to donate are things they can use.

You can donate foods that are

>> **Not past their expiration date:** If an item doesn't have an expiration date, play it safe and just discard it unless you're sure you bought it within the past week or two.

>> **In undamaged packaging with no broken seals or caps:** Most food pantries don't accept products that have been opened, but you can double-check before you throw those products away.

>> **No longer a part of your diet but are still edible:** You may not want to eat that box of macaroni and cheese mix, but it may keep someone else from going to bed hungry.

Remember to ask for a receipt when you make your food donations because most donations to food pantries or other charities are tax-deductible. Plus you can feel good about helping less fortunate members of your community.

Foods to throw away

Be fairly ruthless about the foods you throw away. Most people have a few mystery packages in their freezer or fridge, usually pushed to the back or the bottom, that have gone long past the point of being wholesome, let alone appetizing. Remember the basic rule of food safety: When in doubt, throw it out.

Throw away any food that

>> Is past its expiration date

>> Has freezer burn

>> Is moldy, has strange smells, or is discolored

>> Doesn't have a strong aroma when it should, like dried herbs and spices

>> Has a damaged package or a broken seal

Repeat this sorting process with all the foods in your fridge and freezer. If you have perishable items from the fridge and freezer that you want to donate, be sure to get them to the food bank quickly. Don't leave any perishable foods out of refrigeration for two hours or they can become unsafe. Be sure to tell the staff at the food bank when you took the items out of the fridge or freezer.

Dumping the junk: Can't pronounce it? Get rid of it!

After you collect all the food that's still good in your kitchen, you need to decide which of those items fit into your new eating clean lifestyle. To get an idea of which foods are good for you and which ones aren't, you have to start reading labels. Every food that has been manipulated in some way has an ingredient list on the label. That list can be as short as one ingredient (such as the list you see on a package of frozen organic raspberries) or as long as your arm (such as the list you see on a pack of low-fat artificially flavored snack cookies).

TIP

If you can't pronounce an ingredient on a food label, don't eat that food. The American food supply contains more than 14,000 artificial chemicals. You may not be able to avoid all of them, but you can certainly cut down on their presence in your kitchen — and your stomach.

Junk food really has no place in any healthy diet. You know what junk food is: flavored potato and tortilla chips, candy bars, artificial dips and spreads, packaged cookies, soft drinks . . . the list goes on and on. These foods provide little to no nutrients for every calorie, and they contain tons of artificial everything.

WHAT DO EXPIRATION DATES REALLY MEAN?

Several different types of expiration dates appear on products you see in the grocery store; they all mean something slightly different.

- *Sell-by dates* mean the last day the store should offer the item for sale. If you see a product on the store shelf beyond this date, tell the manager about it.

- *Best-if-used-by dates* refer to quality, not the wholesomeness of the product. The product is still safe to eat after that date, but the flavor or texture may have deteriorated.

- *Use-by dates* represent the last day that a product is at its best quality.

The only products that the law requires to have actual expiration dates are baby foods and infant formula. The dates on all other products are voluntary and not covered by federal regulations. These dates are more about food quality than food safety. However, food quality also depends on storage conditions. If you store a product in very high heat or humidity, for example, its quality may deteriorate before the date on the package.

Junk foods are generally high in sodium, high in simple carbohydrates (which raise blood sugar levels and then cause them to plummet), high in sugars, high in artificial substances, and low in nutrients. Really, follow the phrase made popular in the war against drugs and "just say no."

To eat clean, discard any foods that contain

>> **Bisphenol A (BPA):** This compound can induce early puberty and may cause obesity and attention deficit disorder. Manufacturers often use it in food packages. In fact, unless a label specifically states that the packaging was made without BPA, it most likely contains the substance. Any plastic bottle marked with a 7 on the bottom also contains BPA.

>> **Phthalates:** Some manufacturers use this form of plastic in buckets, conveyor belts, and plastic containers. Unfortunately, phthalates can migrate into food when the two substances come into contact. Foods can come into contact with these phthalate-containing products anywhere between the farm and the supermarket. Recent studies have shown that phthalates may cause reproductive damage and damage to the liver and kidneys and may be carcinogenic. To avoid products that contain phthalates, avoid foods with these terms on their labels: *DBP, DEP, DEHP, BzBP,* and *DMP.* Also beware of the term *fragrance,* since that ingredient can contain phthalates.

>> **A long list of ingredients:** As a general rule, the longer the ingredient list, the more processed the food. If the ingredient list is printed in type so small you need a magnifying glass to see it clearly, that item probably doesn't belong in your newly clean kitchen.

>> **Artificial flavors and colors:** If you see these exact phrases on the ingredient list, don't eat the food. Food manufacturers can use the umbrella terms *artificial flavors* and *artificial colors* as long as the chemicals used in the product are on the Generally Recognized As Safe (GRAS) list developed by the U.S. Food and Drug Administration (FDA). Some names for these chemicals include *Yellow No. 5, Red No. 5, ethyl propionate, diacetyl, ethylvanillin,* and *guanylic acid salts.*

>> **Preservatives and additives:** These ingredients are usually unpronounce-able and include butylated hydroxytoluene (BHT), butylated hydroxyanisole (BHA), polyethylene glycol, polysorbate 20, potassium bromate, inosinic acid — well, you get the idea.

>> **Thickeners and emulsifiers:** These chemicals help keep salad dressings in suspension and thicken soups and purees. They include xanthan gum, alginic acid, potassium alginate, polyglycerol ester, and lactylated monoglycerides.

>> **Added salt:** Manufacturers use many different terms for salt, including *sodium, MSG, soy sauce, broth, brine, disodium phosphate, sodium bisulfate, sodium alginate, sodium propionate,* and *sodium benzoate.* The terms *smoked, corned,* or *cured* also mean the food contains added salt.

» **Added sugar:** Words that manufacturers use on ingredient lists to mean sugar include *high fructose corn syrup, sucrose, saccharose, xylose, glucose, dextrose, fructose, maltodextrin, molasses, cane juice, sorbitol, maltitol, isomalt,* and *concentrated fruit juice.* Avoid products that contain these terms in the top places on their ingredient list.

» **Artificial sugars:** Artificial sugars include Splenda (also called sucralose), saccharin, Equal (also called aspartame), and acesulfame K (known under the brand names Sunett and Sweet One).

» **Artificial fats:** Any mention of the word *hydrogenated* in an ingredient list means the food contains trans fats — even if the label clearly says "0 trans fats." (That particular claim really means the food contains less than 0.5 grams of trans fats per serving, which can quickly add up when you eat more than one serving).

Your body incorporates this fat into its cell structure, resulting in a weakened immune system that leads to all sorts of diseases. So avoid it at all costs! Other artificial fats you need to avoid include Olestra, Simplesse, and Stellar.

» **Monosodium glutamate (MSG):** This flavor additive hides behind a plethora of words and phrases, including *hydrolyzed vegetable protein, natural flavors, glutamic acid, calcium caseinate, gelatin, monopotassium glutamate, yeast food, natrium glutamate, textured protein, soy sauce, malt extract, whey protein concentrate, stock, soy protein, barley malt, vetsin,* and any phrase containing the term *disodium.*

Whew. Looking at this list, which is by no means complete (because this book isn't big enough to contain all of them), you can see why disease and obesity rates are skyrocketing in America today. Even if you don't completely adhere to the eating clean lifestyle, think about avoiding products made with these chemicals.

A FEW JUNK FOOD TIDBITS

If you're still not convinced about the dangers of junk food, here are three key points to keep in mind:

- Pregnant women who eat junk food tend to have children who are born craving it.

- An unwrapped Twinkie placed outside on a window ledge for four days didn't change in color, texture, appearance, or flavor. Birds wouldn't eat it, although the product did attract flies.

- Rats fed a steady diet of junk food chose to starve for weeks when they were finally put on a healthy diet because they were addicted to the junk food.

TIP

Take some time to go over this list. You don't need to memorize all the words and variations, but you do need to be familiar with the basic terms. When you realize that *natural flavor* means that MSG is probably lurking in the food, that term will start to catch your eye. Read every single label on every single food that carries one, even if you purchase it frequently. Manufacturers can change product ingredients with no notice. Focus on buying and eating foods with short labels that contain easily understood words, and your eating habits will improve dramatically.

Classifying processed foods: Deciding which ones are okay to keep

Processed foods aren't unhealthy in and of themselves. To feed millions of people, farmers and manufacturers have to ship food around the world and across the country. To prevent bacterial growth, mold growth, and spoilage during the shipping time, manufacturers add some preservatives and additives to food, and that's okay — to an extent.

Using an absolutely pure definition, *processed foods* are any foods that have been

>> Canned

>> Bottled

>> Aseptically packaged

>> Freeze-dried

>> Frozen

>> Dehydrated

>> Refrigerated

So not all processed foods are unhealthy or banned from the clean diet. For instance, frozen vegetables that are processed without added chemicals are still processed, but they're perfectly fine for most clean diet plans. Canned beans, if you can find them made without added salt and packed in BPA-free cans, are certainly clean foods. Look for minimally processed foods with few ingredients, and make sure you can pronounce the ingredients on the label. Although trying to stick to unprocessed foods is best, eating a few processed foods over the course of a week isn't going to hurt.

Any food that manufacturers have added nutrients to is also processed, but that doesn't make it bad for you. For example, some orange juice brands now have added calcium, milk is often fortified with vitamin D, and cereals have added fiber and psyllium to help lower cholesterol. These foods are called *enhanced foods* because they have more nutrients than what naturally occur in that product or than what are removed during processing.

Enhanced foods aren't necessarily bad for you, but consider this: If you're eating a clean diet full of natural foods, with plenty of fruits and vegetables, whole grains, legumes, nuts, seeds, and lean meats, you really don't need these added nutrients. And you do pay more for them!

REMEMBER

Getting nutrition from whole foods is better than relying on processed foods because scientists haven't identified absolutely all the nutrients, particularly micronutrients, people need to stay healthy. Some compounds that are necessary to good health are found only in whole foods, so if you eat only processed and fortified foods, you're likely missing out on a currently unknown but still essential nutrient. (For more about micronutrients, see Chapter 3.)

Stocking Your Clean Kitchen

After you finish purging your kitchen of the foods you no longer want to include in your diet, you're ready to put food back into your pantry, fridge, and freezer. You have plenty of room now, so you need to fill it up with delicious, wholesome, whole foods.

Before you head to the store, though, you need to take inventory so you know which types of foods and other household items you need to replace and which ones you already have on hand. Taking inventory is especially important for the freezer, which most people clean out less frequently than the fridge or pantry.

In this section, we go over which clean staples are the best to keep on hand for your pantry, fridge, and freezer, and we explain how to store them so they stay fresh and wholesome as well as how to extend their shelf life.

TIP

Make sure you label all your foods and mark them with the date you purchase them. And enjoy the feeling of satisfaction you get from having a kitchen that's clean, organized, and full of yummy things to eat.

Clean staples for your pantry

Your pantry is a great place to keep clean staples that you can use for snack foods and meal ingredients. Some of these products do come in cans and jars. If you can afford to do so, look for organic varieties of these products. Also try to find environment-friendly packaging, like plain cardboard rather than plastic and bottles rather than cans.

TIP

You can stock some processed items, as long as they have no or very few artificial ingredients and include whole foods. For instance, some crackers and chips are made with whole grains and contain no hydrogenated fats. These foods make good quick snacks or supplements to homemade snacks when you're getting into the swing of the clean eating plan.

Your clean pantry may include the following foods:

- Apple cider vinegar, balsamic vinegar, and plain vinegar
- Baking soda and baking powder (made without aluminum)
- Brown rice and wild rice
- Canned tomatoes processed without salt or chemicals
- Canned water-packed fruits
- Canned wild salmon
- Dried herbs and spices
- Dried legumes like kidney beans, black beans, garbanzo beans, great northern beans, and lentils
- Garlic and onions
- Honey, agave nectar, brown rice syrup, and maple syrup
- Low-sodium broths and stocks
- Mustard and other clean condiments like chutney
- Olive oil and sesame oil
- Organic bottled salad dressings
- Organic dried fruits
- Organic peanut butter and other nut butters
- Pasta and marinara sauces made with only a few natural ingredients
- Potatoes and sweet potatoes
- Sea salt and peppercorns
- Seeds like pumpkin seeds, sunflower seeds, sesame seeds, and flaxseed
- Unsweetened, organic applesauce
- Variety of tea
- Whole, unsalted, unflavored nuts

» Whole grains like barley, oats, quinoa, wheat berries, oat bran, and millet

» Whole-grain cereals

» Whole-grain or multigrain pasta

» Whole-wheat flours and other specialty flours

REMEMBER

Your pantry list may be very similar to the one we include here, or it may be quite different, depending on the plan you've chosen and where you are in the eating clean transition. If your family is very resistant to change, for instance, look for foods that are similar to the foods they're familiar with but healthier. Buy organic pasta sauce instead of the type loaded with salt, sugar, and preservatives. Look for the pasta that's made with whole grains but still looks like regular white pasta. Buy some snacks that are made with natural ingredients but that offer similar tastes to the junk foods they love.

Most of these foods will keep for a year if unopened. Be sure to note expiration dates on these products. If a product's package doesn't include an expiration date, use a waterproof marker to write the date you purchased the product directly on the package. And don't forget to read the label instructions because you need to refrigerate some of these foods after opening them.

STORING TRICKY FOODS

Although food storage sounds simple (everything goes in the pantry, fridge, or freezer, right?), some foods, like potatoes, tomatoes, and nuts, require a little more thought before you store them.

- Store potatoes and onions well apart from each other. Each gives off gases that make the other ripen too quickly.

- Don't refrigerate potatoes, bananas, or tomatoes. If you refrigerate potatoes, they'll become sweet. If you refrigerate bananas, their skins will turn black, although the flesh is still fine. If you refrigerate tomatoes, they'll lose their flavor.

- Store potatoes away from light. Otherwise, they can develop green spots that contain solanine, a natural toxin.

- Store nuts in the freezer because they're high in oils that can go rancid over time. Just be sure to thaw them before chopping or they'll be mushy. You can store nut oils in the fridge for the same reason. You'll know when nuts have gone rancid when they taste very bitter; when they reach that point, discard them. *Note:* If you use the nuts frequently, you can store them at room temperature.

Perishable clean foods

Perishable clean foods belong in the refrigerator. You may already be buying many of the foods we describe in this section. You can keep purchasing the same items, or you can switch to organic or locally produced goods. Because some of these foods (like yogurt and cheese) are processed, look for varieties that have short ingredient lists and are made with as few artificial ingredients as possible.

Here are just some of the foods that belong in your fridge, along with their average lifespan:

>> **Butter:** Good for about a month

>> **Cottage cheese and sour cream:** Good until the expiration date

>> **Fresh fruits, such as oranges, grapes, berries, apples, strawberries, melons, lemons, limes, kiwi, peaches, pears, pineapple:** Usually good for 2 to 5 days

>> **Fresh herbs:** Good for 2 to 3 days

>> **Fresh vegetables, such as green beans, asparagus, broccoli, cabbage, carrots, cauliflower, cucumbers, greens, lettuce, mushrooms, peppers, and tomatoes:** Good for 2 to 6 days

>> **Milk, soy milk, rice milk, or almond milk:** Good until the expiration date

>> **Natural cheeses:** Good until the expiration date

>> **Opened condiments like mustard, clean ketchup, chutneys, and salsa:** Good until the expiration date

>> **Organic eggs, preferably free-range:** Good for a few weeks past the expiration date

>> **Organic meats, including beef, chicken, bison, wild salmon, pork, and ground meats:** Good for 2 to 3 days past the sell-by date

>> **Plain fruit juices:** Good until the expiration date

>> **Plain yogurt (especially Greek yogurt, which has a richer taste):** Good for about a week past the expiration date

When storing these foods, make sure you wrap them well. The refrigerator is a very dry place, and unwrapped delicate foods like berries, fresh herbs, and greens will wilt quickly. Another reason why you need to wrap your foods is to keep the flavors from transferring from one food to another. After all, you don't want your butter to taste like cabbage or your yogurt to smell like broccoli. Reusable containers (BPA and phthalate free, please) are a good choice for wrapping because they're clean and green.

As far as temperature goes, set the fridge to maintain a temperature between 32 degrees and 40 degrees. Keep a thermometer in the fridge to make sure it works properly.

TIP

Perishable foods keep well for only a few days, so be sure to plan your meals so that you use up all the food while it's still fresh. In other words, don't go overboard and buy more food than you can eat in a week. Follow expiration dates carefully, especially for fresh meats and dairy products.

Clean staples for the freezer

Even though most freezer foods have been processed, some of them, including frozen fruits and vegetables that are processed without sauces, cheeses, or artificial ingredients, still make good additions to your eating clean diet. Be sure to set your freezer at 0 degrees to keep your food safe and wholesome for as long as possible. If stored properly, your frozen foods should last for about a year. Choose frozen foods with few ingredients, no additives, and no added chemicals.

The foods you may want to add to your freezer include

>> Clean frozen fruits that are as unprocessed as possible, such as peaches, strawberries, mangoes, cranberries, and blueberries, among others

>> Clean frozen vegetables that are as unprocessed as possible, such as corn, green beans, snap peas, broccoli, peas, squash, edamame, Brussels sprouts, and spinach

>> Fish packaged for the freezer

>> Frozen fruit juice concentrates with no added sugar

>> Frozen homemade treats, like yogurt pops, fruit pops, and frozen fruit mixtures

>> Homemade meals packaged for the freezer and clearly marked

>> Meats packaged for the freezer

>> Minimally processed frozen vegetable blends

Just like the refrigerator, the freezer is a harsh environment. *Freezer burnt* food is actually frozen food that has dehydrated. Those rough patches of frost aren't unsafe to eat, but they are unpalatable. To prevent freezer burn, always use freezer wrap, bags, or packaging to protect the food before you place it in the freezer. Label everything, and be sure to rotate foods, using older products first, so that they don't get lost in the frozen depths.

Keep a small notebook near the freezer with a list of what's in it. That way, you can replenish items you're low on and remind yourself to use up that last pound of chicken before you buy some more.

Navigating the Grocery Store

Ah, the grocery store. Some people really like to shop, others view it as a necessary evil, and still others will do just about anything to get out of a trip to the store. But when you know how to shop with a purpose (thanks to a detailed list and a mind map of the store's layout), the grocery store can become less of an enemy and more of a friend.

In this section, we explain how to make out a grocery list before you leave your house and then how to stick to it when you get to the store. We also dissect the average grocery store layout and uncover some tricks grocers use to direct you to expensive, processed foods.

Sticking to your list

Your current grocery list may be a work of art, or it may be a few items scribbled on the back of your bank receipt. Either way, you likely have a few changes to make because the eating clean lifestyle demands a fairly rigorous devotion to an organized shopping list. Remember, you can't rely on fast food anymore, so you need to plan homemade meals, minimeals, and snacks for every day.

TIP

As you create your grocery list, consider keeping a magnet-backed notepad on your fridge or in another central location in your kitchen. Attach the list (and a pen or pencil) to something immovable so that nobody walks off with it. (Searching for a missing grocery list is not an efficient way to manage your clean eating lifestyle.) You can also make your grocery list on the computer, using a basic form that includes items you buy every week (such as milk, lettuce, or whole-wheat pasta). Then just print it out and fill in the other foods you need for any given week.

After you've established a good place for your grocery list, follow these steps to add items to it:

1. When you run out of a staple ingredient, whether it's milk, pecans, or olive oil, write it down on the list.

That way, you won't be in the middle of a recipe, reach for an ingredient, and discover you're all out.

2. **At the beginning of each week, plan the menus and recipes you want to eat that week.**

   Don't forget to pick out recipes for meals, snacks, minimeals, and treats.

3. **Write down the foods you need to make these recipes.**

4. **Compare these foods to the items you added in Step 1, and cross off any duplicates.**

5. **Write down all the foods (and quantities) you need to buy on a clean sheet of paper so that you have your whole list in one place.**

   Think about organizing your list according to the layout of the grocery store you frequent. For instance, you may choose to list fruits and vegetables first, then staples like rice and dried beans, meats, dairy items, and frozen foods. Then all you have to do is read down the list when you're at the store.

Until you get the hang of making good grocery lists, check out the many pre-printed grocery lists available online. Print out a few and try them out to see whether they match your eating clean lifestyle. Just type *grocery list* into your favorite search engine.

TIP

Coupons are a fabulous way to save money. And yes, you can find coupons for whole foods — even produce. Check online at different coupon sites (and check their legitimacy at www.cents-off.com), read through the store's weekly ad (you can usually find it near the store's entrance), and check newspapers, especially the Sunday food sections. If a store is out of a particular sale or coupon item, ask for a rain check. You should receive a notice when the product is back in stock, and the store should still honor your coupon.

Don't be afraid to ask for help when you're at the store! If you can't find a certain item, ask whether the store stocks it or whether you can have it ordered. Most grocers are happy to oblige. In fact, they may start stocking more clean foods if more shoppers request them.

Mapping out the good and bad supermarket aisles

The grocery store has been specifically designed to get you to spend as much money as possible. In fact, some companies do nothing but design store layouts and hold focus groups to make displays as enticing as possible. They even do studies on the type of music that will keep you in the store as long as possible! But you don't have to fall victim to this intelligent design; you can outwit it by planning a shopping strategy.

To make shopping easier and more effective, try the following:

>> Don't deviate from your shopping list unless you see a good sale on clean food your family likes.

>> Don't shop when you're hungry. Foods that you would normally pass up may look too good to ignore if your blood sugar level is low. So be sure to eat something healthy before heading to the store.

>> Avoid the center aisles of the grocery store. In most grocery stores, you find the clean foods (produce, meat, and dairy) at the perimeter of the store. The highly processed foods, like mixes, frozen dinners, and snack foods, are in the center aisles.

>> Look up high and down low on grocery store shelves for the best buys. Food manufacturers pay money for prominent placement on store shelves. Less processed foods are usually placed in a more inconvenient location.

>> Buy perishable foods toward the end of your shopping journey so they don't have time to warm up. Perishable foods include meats, frozen foods, dairy items, and anything else that starts out cold.

>> Try to avoid temptation at the store. If you don't buy junk food, it won't be within reach when you're hungry. Sometimes making a lifestyle change is as simple as that.

>> Be strong and resist the impulse buys that surround the checkout lanes. The checkout lanes are the final source of temptation, the place where all the candy bars, magazines, and little treats developed to tempt children lurk.

After you make it through the store, get everything home as quickly as possible. Perishable foods shouldn't be out of refrigeration longer than two hours (one hour if the temperature is above 80 degrees F), and frozen foods shouldn't have time to thaw. You may want to think about keeping an insulated cooler in the car to keep cold foods cold on the way home.

Shopping at Farmers' Markets, Food Cooperatives, and CSAs

The grocery store isn't your only shopping option when you're living an eating clean lifestyle. Because you're buying fewer processed foods, farmers' markets, food cooperatives, and Community Supported Agriculture (CSA) are ideal places to find great whole food. They offer fresh food that's often organically produced, grown right in your area, and minimally processed.

In this section, we look at what to buy and what to avoid from these providers. We discuss some questions to ask before you buy your items and the best ways to save money while getting the freshest food.

Farmers' markets

Most towns have farmers' markets; at the very least, you can find a farm stand or two just outside of town or on a street corner. Farmers' markets offer everything from seeds to baked goods. The produce, eggs, dairy products, and meat they have for sale are usually very fresh and of excellent quality. The farmers have harvested the produce that day or the day before, and many of the farmers farm organically. So you can see why farmers' markets fit perfectly into the eating clean lifestyle.

When you go to a farmers' market, follow these tips to get the best food and the best deals:

» **Bring your own containers and cash.** Sturdy reusable bags with solid handles are your best bet. Most vendors only accept cash. For the most part, prices are firm at farmers' markets, but sometimes at the end of the day, you can bargain for a better deal.

» **Ask lots of questions.** Ask how the farmers grew the food, whether they grew it organically, when they picked it, and how long it will last before you have to use it. Some farmers even tell you how to cook the product or offer recipes.

» **Have an idea of basic price ranges for these foods in the grocery store.** Saving money is a big part of shopping, so if you're paying $8 for a pint of raspberries at a farmers' market when perfectly good organic raspberries are available in the store across the street for $5, you're wasting your money.

» **Shop with the seasons.** One of the best things about farmers' markets is that the food is all local and available when nature says it's ready. You won't find strawberries in late fall, but you can find pumpkins, onions, and apples that taste fantastic.

» **Have fun and experiment.** Browse through the aisles, get to know the farmers and vendors, and relish the experience. Use this time to teach your kids about whole foods and show them why they're so good to eat.

Food cooperatives

Food cooperatives (coops) are customer-owned businesses that usually stock organic foods and specialty items. You can find hundreds of coops all around the country and the world. Education is a big focus for these organizations, and many of them offer classes that teach nutrition, basic cooking techniques, and the how-to's of eating a healthy diet.

To get the best experience out of a coop, follow these tips:

» **Consider joining the coop.** To join, you usually pay a one-time fee, but then you can have a say in how the organization is structured and which products it offers.

» **Attend classes and workshops.** Many coops have nutrition experts and even dieticians among their members. These people may be available for consultation to help get your diet on the right track.

» **Bring your own bags to save on packaging and costs.** Most of the vendors have bags you can use, but they may charge you for them. Recycle supermarket bags to be environmentally and economically conscious.

» **Ask questions.** The staff is very knowledgeable about the food offered. Many times the meats, dairy, and produce are grown and produced locally, and the staff has regular contact with the suppliers.

» **Enjoy the feeling of community.** Belonging to an organization that meshes with eating clean goals is a big bonus.

Community Supported Agriculture (CSA)

Community Supported Agriculture (CSA) is a deal consumers make directly with farmers to purchase their harvest. The farmers offer shares that consumers purchase. Then when the farmers harvest the produce, gather the eggs, and process the meat, the consumers get a basket of very fresh foods delivered every week during the growing season.

CSAs can focus on fruits and vegetables, but they can also include meats, eggs, cheeses and other dairy products, flowers, plants, and even baked goods. Depending on your particular agreement, the farmer may deliver a set basket to you, or you may be able to go to the farm and pick out items yourself. And supporting local farmers helps decrease the *carbon footprint* (amount of pollution produced) in your food budget. Read more about this in Chapter 21.

WARNING

Before you become a part of a CSA program in your area, be aware that it involves shared risk. If the farmer experiences a crop failure because of a severe hailstorm or drought, you take the loss along with the farmer. In this type of agreement, you must take a long-range view. You're investing in a local farm, reducing waste and travel costs, and investing in the future. If a crop is poor one year, odds are it will be excellent the next. As long as you understand this concept, you'll most likely have an excellent experience with a CSA in your area.

An organization called Local Harvest can help you find CSA farms in your area and can help with any problems or complaints you may have about them. Check out their website at www.localharvest.org/csa for details. As part of the local food movement, Local Harvest encourages family farms, in-season eating, and clean eating.

Chapter 10

Incorporating Organic Food into Your Eating Clean Plan

O rganic foods was the hot phrase of the 1970s. Everyone remembers the yogurt eaters, usually dressed in sandals and some kind of woven shirt, wearing their long hair held back (or not) in a headband, and muttering about free-range chicken and pesticide-free grapes.

Turns out they were right. Eating natural foods is the basis of the clean eating lifestyle. Of course, you don't have to wear clothes made of hemp and woven sandals to eat well, but whatever rocks your boat.

The market for organically grown foods has exploded over the last several decades, growing by about 20 percent a year, making it the fastest growing portion of the American food system. Close to 70 percent of all Americans buy organic food, albeit occasionally. Organic food production is better for the earth and for you, so its popularity is really no surprise.

In this chapter, we look at some facts about pesticides, herbicides, growth hormones, and antibiotics in food, and we explain how organic foods are different. We take a look at the standards the government sets for organic foods, particularly meat and produce. We go over the fifteen grocery store items you should always try to buy in organic form and then look at foods that are safe even if they aren't grown organically.

Getting the Skinny on Organic Foods

If you're old enough to remember Euell Gibbons, you likely remember his famous commercial for Grape-Nuts cereal in which he stated, "Ever eat a pine tree? Many parts are edible." Many people mocked him because they didn't understand what Mr. Gibbons was really saying. He was really just advocating a natural diet of whole, organic foods.

So what does the term *organic* mean? Organic foods are what your ancestors ate 100 percent of the time for hundreds of thousands of years; they're what your body is meant to eat. Nonorganic foods, on the other hand, have been around for only 150 years. But because people living today haven't been around for 150 years, they don't realize what a radical change organic to nonorganic truly is. No wonder organic food advocates say that what most people eat is literally making them sick!

REMEMBER

Organic foods are grown or produced without pesticides, herbicides, fungicides, artificial fertilizers, growth hormones, synthetic chemicals, antibiotics, or additives. Farmers use different methods to produce organic produce, meats, and dairy products, but none of them involve manmade chemicals.

In this section, we look at some facts about the chemicals used to grow nonorganic food, the keys to organic food production, and the rules regarding organic food labeling.

Organic produce

Farming is a tough business. It's dangerous, difficult, and doesn't create great wealth for the individual farmer. And when a farmer chooses to forgo chemicals, the job gets even more arduous. So what's different about organic farming, and why do some farmers choose to grow food organically? Many organic farmers believe that the way they produce food is better for everyone, including themselves, their families, and the environment. After all, just think about the number of chemicals a modern farmer has to handle every day: herbicides, growth hormones, pesticides, and artificial fertilizers. Reducing occupational exposure to these toxic chemicals naturally reduces the risk of disease.

But how does food produced organically compare to food produced with all the modern-day chemicals? Read the following sections to find out.

The basics of organic produce

Food grown organically is

>> Fertilized with compost or manure rather than artificial chemicals

>> Hand weeded, tilled, cultivated, or mulched instead of being sprayed with herbicides

>> Treated with traps or beneficial bugs like ladybugs to prevent insect damage instead of being sprayed with pesticides

>> Grown in soil that's enhanced by crop rotation and *green manure* (that is, cover crops like clover) rather than chemical fertilizer

>> Grown from heirloom seeds harvested naturally rather than genetically modified seeds that produce sterile plants

So what does this mean to the eating clean lifestyle? Well, the goal of the eating clean lifestyle is to eat as close to nature as possible, and you can't get much more natural than organic food. On the other hand, there's nothing clean about pesticides or weed killers. Those compounds become part of the food, and they remain on the food even after you wash or peel it.

The problems with herbicides, pesticides, and other chemicals

Here are some facts about foods produced with chemicals:

>> In the United States, farmers use more than 800 million pounds of pesticides on crops every year; that's nearly 3 pounds per citizen!

>> Pesticides remain in your body fat for years after consumption. In fact, babies are born with pesticides in their fatty tissue, passed on by their mothers!

>> The hormone disrupters (such as plasticizers, insecticides, and other agricultural chemicals) found on certain nonorganic foods, especially foods packed in plastic and berries, may contribute to obesity, cancer, and other diseases.

>> Pesticides run off farms and flow into ponds, streams, rivers, and lakes; from there, they get into your water supply.

>> Insecticides aren't species-specific, meaning that they kill any bug, including beneficial bugs that destroy harmful insects. For example, ladybirds kill aphids, which destroy plants, but insecticides kill ladybirds. The green

> lacewing larvae controls spider mites, mealybugs, and thrips that destroy crops, but insecticides kill the beneficial lacewing.
>
> ≫ Farmers often treat produce with more than one pesticide. In a recent test, scientists found residue from 14 different herbicides and pesticides on strawberries.

What do these facts mean for you and others who eat nonorganic produce? You've probably heard a lot about *inflammation*. Doctors and researchers think that inflammation in your body's cells causes disease, from cancer to heart disease to degenerative diseases, like Parkinson's and multiple sclerosis. Pesticides and herbicides promote inflammation and cause mutations in cells. These chemicals can also mimic the action of hormones like estrogen in the body, thus increasing the risk for cancer and other diseases. In other words, exposure to these chemicals is risky.

But no one knows just how risky that exposure is. One of the main problems with pesticides is that scientists don't really know how much exposure can cause health problems. However, they do know that the amount that causes a problem most likely varies from person to person and that children are more susceptible to these chemicals than adults.

Some chemicals are additive; that is, exposure to them adds up because they build up in the body. So eating one apple sprayed with an additive chemical won't hurt you, but eating hundreds of chemical-sprayed apples over the years may be harmful. In fact, some additive chemicals are called *cocarcinogens,* meaning that they don't cause cancer on their own but they do increase the rate of cancer development when they come in contact with other chemicals.

WARNING

Pesticides may also have synergistic effects, meaning that when you consume two or more pesticides, they may react with each other to cause more damage than each would on its own. So studies showing that one pesticide is safe may not be accurate in the real world when that pesticide combines with other chemicals. Considering that the total number of household pesticides alone is more than 20,000, the potential for synergistic effects is very large.

A 2010 Harvard study found that organophosphate insecticides (OP), the most common pesticides used in the United States, are very toxic, especially to children, even in tiny amounts. That study focused on the development of attention deficit disorder (ADD) and found that children who are exposed to more pesticides have double the rate of ADD. Even so, researchers don't know the exact long-term effects of pesticide and insecticide exposure.

For these reasons, looking for at least some foods grown without chemicals makes a whole lot of sense. Although organic produce isn't necessary to the eating clean lifestyle, many people make a conscious effort to seek out untreated produce.

Organic meat and dairy products

Farmers don't have to use pesticides or herbicides to raise beef, chicken, pork, and fish. But to make large factory farms more efficient and profitable, manufacturers often add chemicals to the mix. Plus, if farmers feed their animals produce grown with pesticides and herbicides, those chemicals become part of the animals, too.

Read on to find out more about the difference between regular meat and dairy products and their organic counterparts.

The basics of organic meat and dairy products

Meat and dairy products that are produced organically are

>> Not fed growth hormones, which can remain in the meat and may be linked to premature puberty in humans.

>> Grown without antibiotics, unless an outbreak of disease actually occurs in the barn or coop.

>> Grass fed instead of being fed grain by humans. (Actually, the cows feed themselves grass, as cows have done for hundreds of thousands of years.)

>> Usually free range, meaning that their farmers allow them to roam freely instead of keeping them caged in buildings, resulting in healthier animals that don't need antibiotics.

In addition, to be labeled organic, animals must spend at least one-third of the year grazing on pasture, and 30 percent of their food must come from grazing. What does this mean for you, the consumer? Grass-fed meat has a lower fat content, more omega-3 fatty acids, and more conjugated linoleic acid (CLA), a good fat. (For more details on organic labeling, skip to the later section "100 percent organic standards and labeling.")

Unfortunately, these organic methods of producing food are much more time- and labor-intensive than relying on factory farming and chemicals. As a result, these products do cost more than nonorganic foods — sometimes much more. You have to decide whether you're going to spend more money for these products.

The problems with hormones, antibiotics, and other chemicals

In contrast to grass-fed, hormone-free, organically farmed animals, many farm animals from nonorganic producers are

- » **Fed growth hormones to stimulate growth:** These chemicals remain in the animals after they're slaughtered, and then humans consume them. Scientists don't know yet whether these hormones can disrupt human hormone balance.

- » **Routinely given antibiotics:** Because the living conditions of these animals can be poor, especially on large factory farms, disease can be rampant. Farmers routinely give the animals antibiotics to prevent infections. Those antibiotics remain in the meat, milk, and eggs that humans consume and may contribute to the development of resistant bacteria (or *superbugs*, as they're sometimes called).

- » **Sometimes fed food containing animal byproducts to reduce costs:** To be blunt, this practice is a form of cannibalism. Some scientists think that it has lead to diseases like mad cow disease.

- » **Fed plastic pellets for roughage (a digestion aid) or food that contains manure or urea:** These unpalatable ingredients are, to say the least, disgusting. And they harm the animal in many ways, including making them more susceptible to disease.

- » **Contained in small pens and not allowed access to the outdoors:** Cramped growing conditions lead to stressed animals, and stress in animals can lead to disease.

- » **Fed artificial, chemically produced food instead of being allowed to graze on grass and plants, as nature intended:** This practice introduces more chemicals, including pesticides and herbicides, into the food chain.

The U.S. Department of Agriculture (USDA) and the U.S. Food and Drug Administration (FDA) do state that meat and dairy products produced with these artificial ingredients and under these unnatural conditions are safe to eat. But the studies conducted on these ingredients and conditions really don't address long-term effects, particularly the effects they have on children, whose rapid growth rate may make them more susceptible to such chemicals. Research is finding more and more evidence that raises doubt about these official USDA and FDA statements.

Despite this evidence, many beef producers dispute claims that their nonorganic practices result in unsafe food. As a matter of fact, you may remember the lawsuit Texas beef producers brought against Oprah Winfrey in the 1990s based on a state law that protects agricultural products from "defamatory remarks" (we always thought that law was silly — can a cow really have its feelings hurt?). Ms. Winfrey produced a show on mad cow disease in 1996 after an outbreak of the disease in Britain killed 10 people. The cattlemen lost that suit when the court said that "statements of opinion based on truthful, established facts are protected by the First Amendment."

Still, even if nonorganically produced meats and dairy products are safe, many people who live the clean eating lifestyle prefer to eat meats and dairy products that have not been produced with these methods. Some worry about the way the animals have been treated, others want to eat food that's as pure as possible, and others think that organic meat, eggs, milk, and cheese just taste better. Not to mention these farming methods are pretty unpalatable.

100 percent organic standards and labeling

Everyone from seed suppliers and farmers to food processors can obtain organic certification on their products. Requirements vary from country to country. In the United States, farmers and food processors must meet specific organic standards set by the USDA.

In 2002, the USDA established the National Organic Program (NOP) to help consumers find out more about the organic products on the market. The NOP standards apply to certifiers, producers, processors, and handlers. Look for a small sticker directly on the whole, single-ingredient foods you buy or a sign placed near the food that says *USDA Organic.*

TIP

Foods made with multiple ingredients, which you eat only sparingly on the clean eating diet, have different types of organic labels, so be sure to look closely at the label on any organic foods before you buy them. As with all product labeling, different terms mean different things. Here's what the most common "organic" labels mean in the United States:

>> **100 percent organic:** The food must be made with only organically produced ingredients.

>> **Organic:** The food must contain 95 percent organic ingredients.

>> **Made with organic ingredients:** The food must contain 70 to 95 percent organic ingredients.

If the product has less than 70 percent organic ingredients, the word *organic* may appear only on the ingredient list next to the particular ingredient, but the product can't display the USDA organic seal.

The use of these labels is voluntary, even though only farms that have been certified organic can place them on their foods. To receive the organic certification, an organic-certifying agent examines the farm and farm records to make sure that it conforms to the organic standard, which is a set of regulations and operating guidelines set by the USDA's NOP. When farmers or processors receive the organic certification and use that certification on the label, the certifiers must make information about how the food is grown and produced available to the public. The use of the label is voluntary. Making the information public, once the label is used, is not.

One exemption to this regulation is a farm that produces less than $5,000 worth of organic food annually: It doesn't have to become certified and may still label its foods *organic* as long as it states that it complies with NOP standards. But the farm can't use the USDA seal, and it can't sell its ingredients to a producer and call them *organic*.

WARNING

If you see other organic-sounding terms on a food label, don't assume that the food is organic. For instance, words like *all-natural* and *hormone-free* on food labels don't mean the foods they represent are organic. After all, arsenic is "natural" but you certainly wouldn't want to eat it!

Confused yet? Don't be. Unless you're a true purist, buying foods labeled *organic* is optional when you're living the eating clean lifestyle. But whether you eat organic food or not, make sure you shop at stores and markets where you trust the merchants, always wash produce before eating it, and cook all your food properly. If you follow these simple steps, the odds are you'll be just fine.

Are Organic Foods Healthier?

Are organic foods really better for you? That's the million-dollar question, isn't it? So far, study results have been mixed. Studies and reviews in popular mainstream journals (such as the *American Journal of Clinical Nutrition*) usually show that organic and nonorganic foods have no significant difference in nutritional values. But nutritional content varies from year to year and even from farm to farm, so getting exact measurements can be difficult.

On the other hand, some research does show that organic foods contain more nutrients and, thus, may be healthier than their conventionally grown counterparts:

>> Dr. Walter Crinnion published a review in the *Alternative Medicine Review* in 2010 that showed that organic foods do have a higher content of magnesium, iron, and vitamin C than conventionally grown produce. Organic foods usually also have higher levels of anthocyanins, flavonoids, and carotenoids, which are important antioxidants called phytochemicals. (For details on these compounds, see Chapters 3 and 4.)

>> Some studies on the nutritional content of organic tomatoes have shown that they do have more nutrients, especially phytochemicals, than tomatoes grown conventionally, as long as the organic tomatoes were grown on *mature* organic farms (farms that have been certified organic for at least three years). The reason that tomatoes grown on mature organic farms have more nutrients may be that the soil used to grow the tomatoes has had time to build nutrients naturally and is of higher quality than the soil on conventional farms.

» A review released in 2008 by The Organic Center looked at studies that compared matched pairs of foods — one organically grown, the other grown using pesticides and other chemicals — and analyzed their nutritional content. The term *matched pair* is important because the foods were not only the same (carrots compared to carrots), but they were grown in the same area, in the same climate, and with similar plant genetics, similar rain amounts, and the same harvest time. Here's what the researchers discovered about organic foods:

- Organically grown produce had higher levels of 8 of the 11 nutrients tested.

- Organically grown produce had higher levels of polyphenols and other antioxidants, which help protect your body against the inflammation that can cause cancer and heart disease.

- Nutrients in the organically grown produce were in a more biologically active form, meaning that the body could more readily absorb them.

- Conventionally grown produce grew bigger faster because of artificial fertilizer, giving them less time to absorb essential nutrients from the soil.

One more reason why you may want to choose organic produce is that they contain more phytochemicals, which are beneficial vitamins, minerals, and other chemicals. Plants produce phytochemicals in self-defense against pests and problems that can attack the plant while it's growing. Because conventionally grown crops are "protected" by insecticides and pesticides and don't need phytochemicals, they don't produce as many of them as their organic counterparts.

Pesticide and herbicide residue on conventionally grown produce and hormones and antibiotics in meat are present in very small quantities, and organically grown produce may still have small amounts of these chemicals due to drift from neighboring, nonorganic farms. The government says that these amounts are too tiny to make a difference in your health. But organic food advocates say that researchers haven't done enough testing on these chemicals to say conclusively that they're 100 percent safe.

For now, organic producers can't claim that their food is better for you or safer than nonorganic food. The only claim they can make is the organic sticker they put on their foods. You get to draw your own conclusions (or do your own research).

So what's the bottom line? If you transition to a clean diet and eat whole foods and avoid processed foods, you'll be eating healthier than you were before. You may consider organic foods to be the frosting on the cake because they'll most likely have a positive effect on your health, too. Even if we discount the research, intuitively, foods grown with chemicals that are literally poisons can't be as safe or wholesome as foods grown without them.

...archers haven't done extensive testing on the effects of pesticides and other chem-
...s on children (for obvious reasons — who would expose a child to these chemicals?),
...t because children's bodies are growing at such a rapid rate, these chemicals likely
...ave more of an effect on them. In fact, the folks at the Environmental Working Group
(EWG) have found that many children exceed the Environmental Protection Agency
(EPA) "safe dose" of pesticide and herbicide consumption by a factor of ten or more.

So you may choose to purchase organic foods, especially the ones we list in the section
"Avoiding the filthy fifteen," for your children. After all, just a few bites of some of these
foods can exceed the adult safe dose of organophosphate insecticides.

Whether you buy organic foods is a decision you must make for you and your family. If
you can afford to do so and if this issue is important to you, by all means, buy organic
foods. Focus on the filthy fifteen (see the section "Avoiding the filthy fifteen") and remember the foods that are still very low in chemical residue even if grown conventionally (see
the section "Identifying Some Safe Nonorganic Foods"). Then relax. Who knows, a more
relaxed attitude about food and life in general may be just the ticket to better health.

WARNING

If you have a history of disease in your family, especially cancer or diseases like
Parkinson's and multiple sclerosis, which may be triggered by chemicals, try to
buy organic foods whenever possible. Also look for safe household cleaners, garden chemicals, and pesticides. Going "all organic" can also address depression,
your emotions, GI issues, and attention deficit hyperactivity disorder (ADHD).

Making Informed Decisions about the Food You Buy

Every time you buy a product in the grocery store, you make a decision. You look
for firm fruits and vegetables with good color and no bruises. The meat you buy is
sweet smelling and firm, with little juice in the package. But do you know how to
choose produce that's low in pesticides? Some fruits and vegetables have low
pesticide residues, even when they're conventionally grown. Other fruits and vegetables are so susceptible to pesticide use that you should avoid them unless
they've been organically grown.

In this section, we look at the fifteen foods you should try to buy from organic
farms and explain why doing so is important. We discuss the dangers of imported
produce, and we look at good sources of healthy and clean protein.

Avoiding the filthy fifteen

The Environmental Working Group (EWG) has compiled a list of the most contaminated fruits and vegetables, which we call the *filthy fifteen*. (It's actually called the *dirty dozen*, but why not expand it?) According to the EWG, if you purchase these fifteen foods grown organically, you could reduce your family's exposure to pesticides and herbicides by 80 percent.

Not many people can afford to eat 100 percent organic produce and organic, naturally raised meat, seafood, and dairy products. To get the most bang for your buck, figure out which foods usually contain the most pesticide and herbicide residue and try to buy those organically grown.

REMEMBER

The fifteen foods you should try to purchase organically grown (in order from most pesticide residue to least) are

>> **Celery:** This vegetable doesn't have a skin, so you can't wash off the pesticides used on it while it's growing. A recent study found residue of 64 pesticides on celery.

>> **Peaches:** These fruits have very delicate, permeable skins, so conventional farmers treat them with many different pesticides to keep pests away from them. More than 96 percent of all tested peaches contained pesticides.

>> **Strawberries:** These delicate fruits are heavily sprayed with chemicals, especially when you buy them out of season and they're imported from other countries.

>> **Apples:** Even peeling apples doesn't remove pesticide residue. The latest tests found that apples are grown with at least 42 different pesticides.

>> **Cherries:** These delicious fruits contain chemicals even when they're grown in the United States.

>> **Bell peppers:** You can find bell peppers in so many colors today, including orange and purple, but their thin skins offer no protection against chemicals.

>> **Carrots:** Carrots grow in the soil, so they come into direct contact with fungicides, chemical fertilizers, and pesticides. Peeling them doesn't remove pesticide residue.

>> **Pears:** Although pears have slightly thicker skins than berries, farmers spray them heavily with chemicals because so many insects love them. Unfortunately, farmers have to use more and more chemicals as the insects become resistant to the pesticides.

>> **Blueberries:** Because these fruits are delicate with very thin skins, they absorb more chemicals while they're growing and you can't get rid of the chemicals by washing the berries.

>> **Nectarines:** More than 95 percent of all tested nectarines had pesticide residue.

>> **Spinach:** This leafy green vegetable can contain residue from as many as 48 pesticides.

>> **Grapes:** Imported grapes are the culprit here. This fruit's thin skin lets chemicals permeate into the fruit, and even kings, who have grapes peeled for them, aren't immune to exposure.

Noticing a trend here? If you can't remember this list of foods, just think about the skin of fruits and vegetables as a protective barrier. The thinner and more delicate the skin, the less protection against chemicals.

>> **Potatoes:** This vegetable grows directly in the soil, so it's exposed to pesticides, herbicides, and fungicides and is at high risk for contamination.

>> **Leafy greens:** Leafy greens, such as Swiss chard, butter lettuce, and parsley, are very delicate, so insects love to eat them. They're one of the most heavily sprayed and treated crops.

>> **Tomatoes:** If you've ever grown tomatoes, you know how insects love them. Farmers sometimes heavily spray them, although they may be safer than other foods on this list.

TIP

If you can't find (or afford) organically grown varieties of these fifteen fruits and vegetables, you can take several steps to make sure you and your family are getting the nutrients you need without all the pesticides and other chemicals:

>> Substitute alternative foods that are safe even if they're nonorganic (see the section "Identifying Some Safe Nonorganic Foods" for a list of safe alternatives). For instance, if you can't find organic apples, buy watermelon or bananas instead.

>> Always wash fruits and vegetables (whether they're organic or not) before you eat them. See the nearby sidebar for details on how to make your own produce wash.

>> Peel potatoes and apples, but remember that many beneficial nutrients lie just under the skin so you discard those along with the pesticides.

>> Discard the outer leaves of leafy greens.

>> Eat a wide variety of foods. Don't, for instance, consume just a few foods like strawberries, apples, and potatoes. The more different fruits and vegetables you eat, the more micronutrients you consume. And you limit your exposure to the same pesticides.

MAKING YOUR OWN PRODUCE WASH

You can buy produce washes to help remove contaminants from the food you eat, but they can be expensive. So you may want to make your own. Just follow these simple steps:

1. **Combine 1 cup of plain white vinegar, 1 cup of water, 1 tablespoon of baking soda, and 1 teaspoon of salt in a spray bottle and shake well.**

2. **Spray the mixture on fruits and veggies.**

3. **Allow the sprayed food to stand for 5 to 10 minutes.**

4. **Rinse well and eat.**

You can store this mixture for about a week before you make another batch.

You can also rinse your produce, sprinkle it with baking soda, and then gently scrub it using your fingers. Just be sure to rinse your produce well with water before you eat it.

Realizing the dangers of imported produce

Locovores, or people who try to eat food produced within a 10- or 20-mile range of where they live, have a good point. If you eat produce out of season, such as strawberries in December or sweet corn in February, odds are that the produce didn't grow in the United States.

The two main problems with imported produce are

>> **Less than 1 percent of all imported fruits and vegetables are inspected by the government when they reach U.S. shores.** In fact, in 2007 the FDA inspected only 11,000 containers out of the 33 billion pounds of imported produce.

>> **Although the United States bans many pesticides and herbicides from use, other countries continue to use them.** In other words, many U.S. manufacturers produce banned pesticides and then export them to other countries. Those countries use them on the food they grow and then ship that food right back to the United States.

TIP

To combat the dangers of imported, pesticide-infested produce, read labels carefully. Think about the amount of risk you want to take, and try to find organic foods. Or grow your own food! Just don't let the fear of pesticides stop you from eating fruits and vegetables.

Eggs with legs, grass-fed beef, and other healthy proteins

Meat, fish, dairy products, and eggs can be laden with hormones, antibiotics, pesticides, and insecticides. Consumer groups and organizations, such as the EWG, that recommend that you eat organic produce also recommend that you eat organic proteins. These products are a bit different from fruits and vegetables because the toxins are stored in the fat.

The fat in meats contains not only flavor but also pesticide and chemical residue. An animal's body processes these fat–soluble toxins in the liver, and the liver sends them to fat cells for storage to minimize harm done to the animal's body. Because it takes 16 pounds of grain or grass to produce 1 pound of beef, the chemicals on the grain or grass are concentrated in the meat's fat.

Here's what you need to look for when purchasing meat, dairy products, and eggs:

» **Meat:** Organically raised, grass-fed beef and chicken is better for you and tastes better. Everyone has heard horror stories about diseased animals being slaughtered for human consumption. But even milder offenses, like feeding these animals grains or animal byproducts, can affect their health — and yours when you eat their meat. Look for labels that state that the meat is grass fed, organic, hormone-free, and free range.

» **Dairy products:** Organically produced milk and cheese is free from synthetic growth hormones, especially rBGH (recombinant bovine growth hormone), antibiotics, and artificial ingredients. You may want to purchase these products from small, local farms to support the organic industry. Look for the organic label on the product package.

» **Fish:** How to label fish is still up for debate. Wild fish can't have the organic label because no one controls what wild fish eat. But farm-raised fish can have that label, even though they may contain higher levels of contaminants and fish farms produce water pollution and parasite outbreaks. You also have to consider the issue of mercury and other heavy metals in fish. For these reasons, most experts recommend limiting fish consumption to two or three times a week. You can choose organic or wild fish or farmed fish depending on the price and the taste. Stay tuned to this developing story.

» **Eggs:** We use the phrase *eggs with legs* to illustrate that eggs laid from chickens allowed to roam in the sunshine are better for you than eggs laid by caged hens. Studies have found that eggs that come from very large flocks (almost always caged hens) have more salmonella bacteria than eggs from free-range, small flocks. The nutrient content of free-range eggs is higher, too. Look for the terms *free range* and *cage-free,* along with the organic label.

Identifying Some Safe Nonorganic Foods

If you read the preceding section, you may be discouraged. Don't be! Now that you know what types of food to avoid, we're ready to start listing the foods you can eat with confidence, even if they aren't organically grown or raised. In this section, we look at why many fruits and vegetables can be perfectly safe to eat, with little to no chemical residue, even if they are produced with pesticides and herbicides. We also list the foods you can buy from conventional farms that are very low in pesticide residue.

Why nonorganic can be okay

Quite a few fruits and vegetables don't absorb as many chemicals while they're growing as the ones we list in the section "Avoiding the filthy fifteen." And a few crops just don't attract bugs and other pests, so farmers don't need to treat them with insecticides in the first place. You can purchase these foods, grown conventionally, with confidence that they're safe to eat.

REMEMBER

The foods we list in the next section have tougher skins or other mechanisms that keep the chemicals out of their flesh, but you must still wash all produce before you eat it. In fact, you need to wash these fruits and vegetables before you even slice into them. No conventionally grown food is completely free from chemical residue, and the bacteria and chemical residue that lie on the skin or rind will spread into the flesh when you cut into it if you don't wash it first. Wash all your produce using the homemade produce wash we describe in the sidebar "Making your own produce wash" and then peel, slice, or cut the food.

Clean foods that you can buy nonorganic

To save money and to make the shopping experience easier, you can buy these foods conventionally grown:

>> **Asparagus:** This vegetable doesn't have thick skin; insects just don't like it! By the way, you can buy thick or thin spears; they're all tender when cooked properly.

>> **Avocado:** The thick skin on the avocado protects it from pesticides. Wash it thoroughly before peeling.

>> **Bananas:** This fruit's natural container protects it against pesticide and herbicide contamination. And yes, you need to wash bananas before peeling them!

- **Broccoli:** Poor broccoli. Like children, bugs just don't like it. Rinse it well before cooking.

- **Cabbage:** Not many pests like cabbage, so farmers don't have to use a lot of pesticides to get it to grow to a good size. Rinse it well and remove the outer leaves before eating.

- **Eggplant:** This strange purple fruit has a thick skin that protects it from chemicals. Wash the skin and peel it before using.

- **Grapefruit:** Grapefruit's thick skin protects the tart and sweet fruit from chemicals.

- **Kiwi:** This strange little fruit, with the brown rough skin and bright green interior, has natural protection. Rinse before slicing and don't worry about getting rid of the seeds; they're edible.

- **Mangoes:** Mangoes are a delicious fruit with tender, sweet flesh that tastes like wild peaches. They also have thick skin that protects the fruit from chemicals. Wash before peeling.

- **Onions:** Not many insects enjoy munching on onions, so farmers don't need to treat them with pesticides and fungicides. Wash and peel them before chopping or slicing.

- **Papaya:** This sweet and juicy fruit has a thick skin that keeps pesticides and other chemicals away from the flesh.

- **Pineapple:** Do you ever wonder about the first person who contemplated eating a pineapple? It has a formidable container that encloses the sweet fruit and seals out contaminants. Of course, wash the pineapple before you slice into it.

- **Sweet corn on the cob**: The husk and silk on ears of corn protect the tender kernels from chemical exposure. Remove the husk and wash the corn before cooking it.

- **Sweet peas:** These little gems come in their own protective package. They win the price for "vegetable least likely to have pesticide contamination."

- **Watermelon and cantaloupe:** These summertime favorites have thick rinds that are pretty impervious to chemicals. Rinse well before slicing. But if you make pickled watermelon rind, look for organic varieties.

These products usually don't need multiple pesticide or herbicide applications, which reduces their (and your) exposure to those chemicals. In recent studies, many of them had no detectable pesticide residue, and most had only one type of pesticide — which is good news, since pesticide synergy can increase its toxic effects.

Chapter 11

Preparing Clean Foods

W hen you're trying to eat clean, you want the foods you work so hard to purchase to stay as clean as possible during preparation (see Chapter 9 for tips on stocking an eating clean kitchen). One way to keep your foods clean is to use the healthiest and safest cooking methods, such as steaming, poaching, and stir-frying. Cooking food changes its composition, makes some nutrients more available to your body, and makes some foods, like meats and seafood, safer to eat.

Another way to keep your foods clean is to join the *raw food movement,* which, as you may have guessed, involves eating uncooked foods. This relatively new phenomenon is based on the premise that enzymes in fruits and vegetables — which are destroyed when the food reaches temperatures of 118 degrees — are beneficial to your body and health.

In this chapter, we look at the healthiest ways to prepare clean foods, and we show you which unhealthy methods to avoid. We also discuss ways to combine foods to make their nutritional content more accessible to your body. Finally, we look at how to use leftovers to get every vitamin, mineral, and micronutrient out of them.

Understanding the Best and Worst Cooking Methods

In Paleolithic times, just plopping food on the fire was considered haute cuisine. But times have changed! When preparing clean food for you and your family, you have many different cooking methods to choose from. Like the foods you eat, some of these methods are better — that is, healthier — than others.

We're not saying that you can't ever use less healthy methods to cook your food. We simply want you to be aware of the risks inherent in each cooking method and to know how to make your food as healthy as possible.

In this section, we explain how to cook and chill foods the healthy way and how to incorporate the increasingly popular raw food diet into your eating clean lifestyle. We also tell you which cooking methods to avoid and why.

Heating before eating

Cooking food definitely has some advantages. For one, many foods are just more palatable after you expose them to heat. Cooking allows you to combine foods to get more nutrients and flavor out of every bite. In addition, cooking food does the following:

>> **Breaks down the cell structure of foods, making some foods easier to eat:** For example, whole grains and many root vegetables are easier to eat after you cook them.

>> **Makes some nutrients more available:** For example, your body gets three times more lycopene from cooked tomatoes than it does from raw tomatoes. Your intestines absorb five times more carotenoids from carrots after you cook them.

>> **Makes food safer by killing bacteria and parasites present in meats, eggs, and seafood:** Chicken and turkey flesh contain bacteria all the way through, so you have to cook these meats to 165 degrees to make sure you kill all the bacteria. Similarly, you kill the bacteria on the surface of solid cuts of beef, pork, lamb, and seafood when you sear the exterior and raise the internal temperature to 145 degrees. All ground meats should be cooked to 160 degrees.

REMEMBER

Cooking foods changes their structures. Breads rise and set, the protein in meats unravels and reforms to become firm, fats melt, starches set, and cell structures weaken. How these changes occur can change the characteristics, textures, flavors, and nutrition levels of the foods being cooked.

The following are the best cooking methods for cooking clean whole foods:

>> **Steaming:** With this method, you expose food to steam produced by simmering water or other liquids. You don't need any additional fat to steam food. The gentle heat from the steam cooks proteins and starches but doesn't damage or destroy as many vitamins as other harsher cooking methods. Because you don't expose the food to much liquid while it cooks, you preserve the water-soluble vitamins in the food.

>> **Poaching:** You cook poached foods in water that's barely simmering. This cooler cooking method helps preserve vitamins that heat would destroy or damage. Like steaming, poaching doesn't require any additional fat. This method is also good for cooking delicate foods that are naturally low in fat, like fish and eggs.

>> **Stir-frying:** This cooking method cooks food very quickly in just a small amount of fat (usually some kind of oil). Because you heat the food so quickly when stir-frying, you preserve more nutrients. You can stir-fry foods in a little bit of water or broth, too.

>> **Baking:** You can use this gentle, dry-heat cooking method for every type of food. Foods baked at lower temperatures (below 400 degrees) retain more nutrients.

>> **Using a slow cooker:** *Slow cookers* are special tabletop appliances that cook food in a ceramic container surrounded by low heat. The food in a slow cooker cooks for hours in a sealed environment, thus preserving nutrients and flavor.

Most of these cooking methods use relatively low heat compared to other methods. For instance, a professional pizza oven can reach temperatures of 800 degrees or more, and a grill can achieve temperatures of more than 600 degrees. In contrast, the healthy cooking methods we list here use much lower temperatures of 200 to 400 degrees, and lower temperatures are one of the keys to healthy cooking.

WARNING

Food cooked at high temperatures with little water can develop compounds called *advanced glycation end products* (AGEs), which form when proteins and sugars combine under high heat. AGEs are toxic to the body and have been linked to inflammation, which contributes to diseases like diabetes, kidney disease, and heart disease. Unfortunately, these compounds are what make some foods, such as the browned crust on meats and breads, taste good. Studies have found that cutting AGE intake in half can increase your lifespan.

AGEs are another reason to avoid processed foods. Many processed foods are exposed to high temperatures during their production, so they can have high AGE contents. Although crispy, browned french fries and a crusty, grilled steak may taste good, they aren't the best foods for your health.

Of course, we're not saying that you can't ever eat a browned roast or crusty bread again. Those textures and flavors are part of the enjoyment of food. But if you or members of your family are at higher risk for certain diseases, like diabetes or heart disease, try to limit your intake of these foods.

Chilling out before eating

Chilling food is primarily linked to food safety. Perishable food must be refrigerated to keep it safe. Some recipes, such as main dish salads, cold soups, and some entrees, require chilling before eating. Others, such as sorbets and desserts, require freezing before eating. Since chilling (or freezing) is just lowering the temperatures of food, it's a clean preparation method. However, you must be careful when using this preparation method because chilled food can be unsafe.

WARNING

To keep food as safe and as fresh as possible, make sure you keep your refrigerator set below 40 degrees. When the temperature range is between 40 degrees and 140 degrees, harmful bacteria can multiply and produce toxins that can remain in the food even after it has been heated and cooked. (Temperatures below 40 degrees drastically slow the growth of bacteria, and most bacteria die above 140 degrees.) So be sure to keep all perishable foods (meats, cheeses, seafood, eggs, and dairy products) out of this unsafe temperature zone. In other words, serve hot food hot and cold food cold. Don't leave perishable foods or chilled foods out of refrigeration for more than two hours, or one hour if the ambient room temperature is above 80 degrees.

Make sure to set your freezer to 0 degrees or below and keep a freezer thermometer in that appliance to check the temperature. Before you freeze foods, chill them in the refrigerator. If you add hot foods directly to the freezer, they may raise the ambient freezer temperature too much and thaw other frozen foods. If you inadvertently leave a frozen food out of the freezer for more than an hour, you can refreeze it if it still has ice crystals on it. But if the food has completely thawed, you must use it immediately or discard it.

REMEMBER

Whole foods, which are a key part of the eating clean lifestyle, are the safest foods to eat chilled. Prepared or processed foods that are chilled, such as processed meats, prepared salads, and soft cheeses, can be contaminated during processing and handling. Because chilling doesn't kill bacteria — it only suppresses its growth — these foods can be dangerous to the very young, the elderly, and people with compromised immune systems.

Forgoing cooking altogether: The clean raw food diet

Some foods really are better for you if eaten raw. After all, cooking does destroy some active compounds and nutrients, especially those that are heat sensitive.

Not a lot of recent medical literature is available on the raw food diet, which may be why some nutritionists think it lacks credibility. The studies that have been done show that cooking vegetables, in particular, destroys important nutrients while making other nutrients more available. Other studies show that eating raw vegetables helps reduce the risk of some types of cancers, especially cancers of the esophagus, stomach, mouth, and larynx.

Raw foodists eat most raw foods without doing any preparation other than cleaning and perhaps peeling them. For a few raw foods, like grains and sprouts, they soak them before eating to improve their flavor and make them easier to digest. Some raw foodists even eat raw eggs, fish, meat, milk, and cheese. But it's difficult to find high-quality foods, like sushi-grade fish, that you can eat raw without fear of contamination (which is why most proponents of the raw food diet are *vegan*, meaning they consume no animal products at all).

The safest foods to eat raw include

» **Garlic:** Raw garlic has *allylic sulfides* (potent anticarcinogenic compounds) that are destroyed when heated. Read more about these compounds and other phytochemicals in Chapter 4.

» **Fruits:** Vitamins in fruits, like vitamins C and B, are water soluble and heat sensitive. Eating fruits raw lets you absorb more of these nutrients.

» **Nuts and seeds:** Although toasting brings out the flavor of nuts, it can also create AGEs that can contribute to disease development. Toasting nuts also oxidizes some of the essential fatty acids they contain. Oxidized fatty acids can damage cells and increase the risk of heart disease.

» **Leafy greens:** You can cook these foods before eating them, but most people eat them raw for texture.

Raw foods also offer some digestive benefits. The enzymes contained in raw foods apparently aid your body's enzymes in the digestive process. Although your stomach acid denatures some food enzymes, some enzymes remain active and others reform in the intestine.

Although heat (via cooking) destroys enzymes in the food you eat, most scientists think that a healthy human body can produce enough enzymes to safely digest food. However, animal experimentation has demonstrated that animals fed a diet of entirely cooked food developed abnormal enlargements of the pancreas. Animals fed an entirely raw food diet didn't develop this abnormality.

Going completely raw sounds okay in principle, but not many people can handle a diet of mostly raw foods. Plus, the clean raw food diet limits the types of foods you can eat. Foods that you must cook before consuming include

- **Rhubarb:** You can eat this vegetable raw in small quantities, but it contains oxalic acid, which the cooking process reduces. Oxalic acid can cause joint pain and kidney stones when ingested.

- **Kidney beans and other dried legumes:** Beans contain phytohemagglutinin (PHA), which is a toxin. This substance deactivates when you cook the beans.

- **Eggplant:** Raw eggplant is very fibrous and difficult to eat and digest.

- **Meats and seafood:** Most meat and seafood products are safer if you cook them before eating. Sushi-grade fish, which is extremely fresh and high quality, can be eaten raw, but it can be difficult to find.

You certainly should include raw foods in your diet, but you don't have to completely adhere to the raw food diet to eat clean. On balance, combining raw and cooked foods in your diet is best. Hey — If the enzymes in raw foods improve digestion, why not eat them? And why not include as many different kinds of fruits and vegetables as you can to make sure that you're getting as many micronutrients as possible?

REMEMBER

If you want to try the complete raw food diet, make sure that you check with your doctor first and follow food safety precautions carefully.

Avoiding less healthy cooking methods

Some cooking methods aren't as healthy as the ones we discuss in the earlier section "Heating before eating." For example, many people enjoy grilled and deep-fried foods, but they aren't good for the body, especially when consumed on a regular basis. These methods can burn food, heat it to very high temperatures, and cook it unevenly.

Cooking methods to avoid include

- **Microwaving:** The microwave oven doesn't make foods radioactive, but it can cook them unevenly. All microwave ovens have hot spots and cold spots, with higher and lower concentrations of energy. When cooking meats, microwaves may leave some uncooked or undercooked portions. And a few disturbing experiments show observable changes in the blood of children and adults who eat a steady diet of microwaved foods.

- **Grilling:** The grill is a fun way to cook, and it can be a healthy way to prepare foods. But you should use the grill only occasionally. The very high heat of the grill can char your food, making it taste good but also developing carcinogens called *heterocyclic amines* (HCAs) on the food's surface. Plus, any fat that melts off the food, drips onto the coals, and drifts back onto the food in smoke that contains *polycyclic aromatic hydrocarbons* (PAHs), which are also carcinogenic.

>> **Deep-frying:** Fried foods absorb at least 10 percent of the oil they're cooked in, more if the oil isn't hot enough. This cooking method creates lots of AGEs — just think of browned french fries or doughnuts. Oils used in deep-frying also change and are damaged. For example, some of the oils turn into trans fats in the heating process.

>> **Roasting:** Roasting is a specific form of baking done at a higher temperature. Roasted foods are higher in fat than foods baked in dry heat; this extra fat can cause AGEs to develop.

Boiling, broiling, and pan sautéing fall in between the good and bad cooking methods. Boiling foods can leach water-soluble vitamins out of the food; in other words, all the good stuff goes right down the sink when you drain the food. Broiling can be fine as long as you don't burn or overcook the foods. Pan sautéing is also fine as long as the heat isn't too high and you use just a little bit of oil.

If you really love grilled and broiled foods, you can do the following to make these cooking methods safer:

>> Choose leaner cuts of meat so fat doesn't burn and form PAHs.

>> Place a drip pan directly under the grilling food. If the melting fat drips into a drip pan rather than onto the coals, it won't burn and turn into carcinogen-ridden smoke.

>> Marinate meats before you grill or broil them to stop the development of carcinogenic products. Marinating can also help reduce the bacteria present on meat that can cause food poisoning. The antioxidant spices and herbs in the marinade are the good guys. Rosemary and garlic are particularly effective ingredients to include in a marinade.

>> Reduce the cooking temperature so the food is less likely to burn. As a bonus, cooking meats at a lower temperature can make them more tender, too.

Combining Foods to Boost Nutrition

Combining foods for weight loss has been a principle in the diet industry for a long time. But that's not what we're talking about here. If you eat particular foods together, compounds in the foods will help your body absorb nutrients more efficiently and effectively.

Foods contain literally thousands of natural bioactive chemicals, and those compounds work better in your body when they combine with other natural chemicals. That's why eating whole foods in the eating clean plan is better for you than eating a poor diet and adding nutrients from supplements (see Chapter 2 for more on whole foods and their place in the eating clean plan).

In this section, we look at different food combinations and explain why you should try to pair them. Your body is an amazing machine. Just like a machine, it works best when the parts are all in harmony with each other. Some food combinations enhance nutrient absorption. Others enhance your immune system, and still others help your body heal.

Combining nutrients to increase their effectiveness in your body

Different foods contain different nutrients. Not only have food scientists and researchers been discovering more micronutrients in foods, but they've also figured out that certain combinations of those nutrients increase the efficacy of each individual nutrient.

Eating different foods together combines different phytonutrients for best nutrition. For optimum nutrition, include the following food combinations in your diet. (For more information about the nutrients we mention here and why they're so good for you, see Chapters 3 and 4.)

>> **Citrus fruits plus foods high in protein:** Vitamin C helps your body absorb more iron from meats and other high-protein foods.

>> **Apples plus grapes and berries:** The quercetin (a flavonoid) in apples combines with catechins in grapes and ellagic acid in berries to help reduce the formation of blood clots in your arteries and veins.

>> **Foods high in vitamin C plus iron-rich nonmeat foods:** The vitamin C changes the non-heme iron in leafy greens and whole grains, which is difficult for the body to absorb, into a form more useful to your body.

>> **Tomatoes plus cruciferous vegetables:** The combination of antioxidants in tomatoes plus broccoli, cauliflower, kale, and other cruciferous (also called brassica) veggies boosts the effectiveness of all of them.

>> **Spice mixes:** One reason curry powder is so good for you is that it contains turmeric, which can help prevent Alzheimer's disease and cancer. When combined with the compound bioperine, which is found in black pepper, your body can absorb more curcumin, the active ingredient in turmeric. Bioperine also helps increase absorption of other micronutrients.

>> **Good fats plus vegetables:** The healthy fats in avocados or butter, for instance, increase the amount of carotene and lutein your body absorbs from foods like lettuce, spinach, and carrots.

>> **Good fats plus vitamin E-rich foods:** The fat helps your body absorb this essential vitamin.

>> **Vitamin C plus protein:** Vitamin C helps your body use protein to repair damage or injury. Eating this combination is especially important after surgery or any other medical procedure.

>> **Potassium with sodium:** If you eat a high-sodium food, eat foods high in potassium (vegetables and fruits) with it. Potassium helps your kidneys secrete excess sodium.

>> **Carbs plus protein:** This combination not only helps keep you feeling satisfied longer but also helps your body repair damage.

Deciding what to eat with what

As you study the list of food combinations in the preceding section, you may notice that you already combine a lot of these foods and nutrients. You drink orange juice in the morning with your scrambled eggs, combining vitamin C with protein. You find a lot of spice combinations in many cuisines, enhancing their antioxidant properties. You cook carrots in a little bit of butter, which helps your body absorb more beta carotene and other carotenoids, and you cook tomatoes in olive oil for a pasta sauce, which increases the amount of lutein your body can use.

Here are a few ideas of yummy food-specific combinations you can add to your diet to boost your nutrition:

>> **Add berries to your morning cereal.** The vitamin C in berries helps your body absorb more protein from the cereal.

>> **Add peanut butter to whole-wheat toast.** The fat in peanut butter helps your body absorb more of the Vitamin E in the whole grains.

>> **Make pot roast with lots of carrots.** The vitamin A precursor in carrots pairs with the zinc and protein in the pot roast to make the vitamin more useful to your body.

>> **Pair tomatoes with broccoli in a stir-fry.** These foods contain powerful antioxidants that, when acting together, are even more effective.

>> **Make a mixed green salad with avocados and olive oil.** The oil helps your body absorb beta carotene and other carotenoids from the leafy greens. Carotenoids need fats to be absorbed, so fat-free salad dressings aren't the best choice.

» **Pair leafy greens with tomatoes.** The vitamin C in tomatoes helps your body absorb the iron in the greens.

» **Drop a lemon slice into your green tea.** Catechins in the green tea are more available to your body when paired with the vitamin C in lemons.

» **Drink a smoothie made from yogurt, bananas, and berries.** The carbs and protein in the bananas and yogurt help repair your body, and the vitamin C in the berries helps your body absorb more iron.

» **Eat a fruit salad.** Combining fruits like raspberries, cranberries, grapes, and apples helps all the antioxidants in these foods work better together.

» **Enjoy a salmon or tuna salad made with yogurt instead of mayonnaise.** The vitamin D added to the yogurt helps your body absorb the calcium present in the fatty fish.

» **Make a meat marinade with rosemary, garlic, and curry powder.** These foods combine to help reduce the formation of carcinogens on grilled meats.

» **Add lots of fruits and vegetables to stews and casseroles.** Combining vitamin C with protein helps your body repair damage more efficiently.

This list could go on and on! Eating a varied diet is really the best way to ensure that you get as many nutrients as possible out of each meal. Combining whole foods in new ways not only makes your diet more interesting but also makes it healthier.

Well, the news can't all be good, can it? Here are a few food pairings you should avoid:

» **Milk and tea:** The casein in milk makes the tea's antioxidants less effective.

» **Milk and chocolate:** Just like milk and tea, the casein in milk makes the chocolate's antioxidants less effective.

» **Coffee, tea, or wine and high-iron foods, like legumes, leafy greens, and whole grains:** The tannins in the beverages interfere with iron absorption.

Using Leftovers Safely and Effectively

Did you know that the average American household throws away almost $400 of food every single month? That shocking amount of waste is not only bad for your wallet; just think of all the nutrients you're throwing away!

In this section, we look at simple and safe ways to use up clean leftovers. We also show you how to safely store these foods. After all, following a clean lifestyle is pointless if you let food go to waste or if you get sick because you ate foods that weren't safe and wholesome.

Planning to use every last bit of food

Because incorporating leftovers into your weekly meal plan involves spending more time in the kitchen, you may want to consider setting aside a morning or afternoon once a week to prepare foods ahead of time. For example, you could cook a whole chicken on Sunday, eat some of it for Sunday dinner, and put the leftovers in the fridge. Then on Monday, you could make a chicken sandwich with some of the leftovers. On Tuesday, you could whip up a quick chicken and whole-wheat pasta salad, and on Wednesday, you could use the bones to make stock for a soup to have during the weekend (or freeze that stock to use in later meals). Think of whole foods as the building blocks for recipes.

Unfortunately, some families seem to be allergic to leftovers. You may have to use some creative energy to turn your leftover food into something appealing, but doing so doesn't have to be difficult. In fact, if you bring your family and some creativity into the mix, turning leftovers into delicious new meals can be a fun challenge!

Here are some ideas for transforming leftovers into yummy new meals:

>> **Change the flavor of the food.** Say you cooked a whole chicken with some lemon and garlic one day for dinner. To make chicken salad with a twist out of the leftovers, mix some yogurt with curry powder and a bit of honey or agave nectar. Cube the chicken and add it to the curry yogurt mixture along with some chopped apples for a curried chicken salad. Or add some Tex-Mex ingredients, like jalapeño chiles, black beans, and avocado, to the chicken, to make a Mexican chicken wrap.

>> **Transform the food into something completely different.** Meatloaf is a popular and budget-friendly recipe that most kids love. Transform your leftover meatloaf into a delicious pizza. Just crumble up the leftover meatloaf, and top a whole-wheat pizza crust with some pureed tomatoes, the meatloaf, fresh tomatoes, leftover vegetables, and a bit of grated cheese. Bake and devour. Turn your leftover salmon into a quiche and use your leftover veggies in a quick soup.

>> **Serve the food in a new way.** If you have some leftover vegetable soup, puree it, add some yogurt to make it creamy, and serve it inside some warm, hollowed-out whole-wheat rolls.

>> **Wait a day or two before offering the leftover food.** Serving a meal based on chicken three days in a row can get monotonous. Mix things up by serving a vegetarian meal or something based on beef in between the chicken dinners.

Don't forget to get your family's input about leftovers. If your family really likes a new recipe you make, think about ways to tweak it a bit and use the same preparation or combination of flavors to wake up leftovers.

Safely storing and using clean leftovers

The big issue with leftovers is food safety. If you store food improperly and it makes you or your family sick, it doesn't really matter how clean or healthy the food was to begin with. The most basic rule for leftovers is this: When in doubt, throw it out. Getting sick, paying a doctor, or ending up in the hospital for a serious illness is much more expensive than tossing out food that's past its prime.

To safely store and use leftovers, do the following:

» Refrigerate cooked food within two hours of serving, or one hour if that day's temperature is above 80 degrees.

» Store leftovers in the refrigerator for three to four days at the most.

» Freeze leftovers for longer storage. Make sure to wrap the food well in freezer-safe packaging, label it, and use it within a few months.

» Cover food completely while it's in the fridge or freezer. Those appliances are dry inside, and food can dry out or even absorb flavors from other foods while sitting on the shelf.

» Use the fridge to cool the food. That's its job! Transfer soups and casseroles to a shallow container so the food cools quickly and gets through the danger zone of 40 to 140 degrees F quickly (see the section "Chilling out before eating" for more details).

» Keep cooked and uncooked foods separate in the fridge and freezer. Never store uncooked meats above cooked foods or above foods that you plan to eat raw. Meat juices that drip onto cooked or raw food can contaminate it.

» Make sure that you thoroughly reheat foods before serving them again. Use a food thermometer and reheat casseroles and most other leftovers to 165 degrees. Reheat soups, stews, and gravies to a rolling boil.

» Follow basic food safety rules. Always wash your hands before food preparation, during preparation, and after cooking. Wipe down all surfaces with a soapy cloth and wash dishes in soapy water or in the dishwasher. Never put cooked food on a plate that held uncooked food.

Basically, just use common sense; keep the kitchen, fridge, freezer, and pantry clean, and your family should stay safe and healthy.

4

Adapting the Eating Clean Plan to Fit Your Life

Chapter 12

Eating Clean on the Go and in Social Situations

So you have a nice clean kitchen at home (in every sense of the word). But what do you do when you have to venture out into the big bad world? Everyone knows what lurks out there: unclean food! From fast-food burgers to the office doughnut cart to street vendors, danger and temptation lurk around every corner.

But remember that one of the precepts of the eating clean diet is that *you are in control.* You have armed yourself with the most important weapon of all: knowledge! After you figure out what clean food is and where to find it, you can eat out at the scariest greasy diner and still have a satisfying meal.

In this chapter, we take a look at restaurant menus and go over the key terms you need to look for so you know what (and what not) to order when eating out. We also examine how to pack clean lunches and snacks for when you don't want to eat out. To round out the chapter, we discuss how to stick to your eating clean diet at social gatherings and parties and what to do when you fall off the wagon. (Don't worry! Everyone does it every now and then!)

Understanding Restaurant Menus

Restaurants can be enticing, charming, and tantalizing. The aromas that waft out of the kitchen, the gentle clink of glassware, the snick of a fork on a plate, and the tinkle of ice cubes in glasses all evoke warm and cozy feelings. But restaurants can also serve some of the unhealthiest food on the planet. Just look at recent news stories about the amount of trans fats and sodium restaurants put in their foods. (Did you know the amount of sodium in a single restaurant meal can put you over an entire day's allotment?)

In this section, we look at how to read a restaurant menu and pick out the cleanest foods. We offer ways to talk to the chef and ask about different menu items and specialty orders. And we show you how the phrase "on the side" can help you stick to your clean eating lifestyle with little fuss or muss.

Getting familiar with key menu terms

A restaurant menu is designed to tempt you into ordering (and eating) as much as possible. Menus describe foods in the most mouth-watering terms. In fact, limiting yourself to one entree is hard to do! But by studying the menu before you order (and knowing what to look for), you can stay on your clean eating plan and feel just as good when you leave the restaurant as you did when you entered it.

In the past 30 years, one of the biggest changes in restaurants has been portion sizes; they're bigger today than they've ever been. A healthy 3-ounce serving of meat is about the size of a pack of cards. Nowadays, an 8-ounce steak is considered a "petite portion" in many restaurants!

TIP

One of the best ways to stay on the clean eating plan when you eat out is to automatically cut down portion sizes. Eat half of what's on your plate and take the rest home. You may also want to order from the appetizer or child's menu rather than the adult section for more reasonably sized portions.

The good

Here are some terms and descriptive phrases to look for on a restaurant menu. When you see these terms next to a meal, you know it's worth your consideration.

>> **Baked:** Baked chicken, fish, and vegetables are usually simple and prepared without sauces. But be sure to ask if the baked food you're thinking about ordering comes with any sauces. If it does, ask for the sauce on the side (see the later section "Ordering sauces on the side and substituting clean foods when possible" for details).

- » **Broiled:** Broiling foods is a fairly healthy preparation method. A simple broiled fish, seasoned with fresh herbs and spices, is a clean choice.

- » **Organic:** A restaurant that stresses that its food is organic most likely prepares the food in a clean manner and doesn't need (or want) to cover up food with sauces or heavy seasoning.

- » **Poached:** Poaching is another clean preparation method. Plus, poached foods are usually whole foods. Imagine trying to poach a burger or grilled cheese sandwich!

- » **Primavera:** This term means the dish contains lots of vegetables, usually fresh and in season.

- » **Steamed:** Steaming is one of the cleanest and healthiest ways to prepare food. These foods usually aren't processed or served with a sauce.

The bad

You need to watch out for and avoid many common restaurant terms. These terms provide definite clues about how the food is prepared and how many additional calories are packed into each dish. When browsing through a menu, look for and avoid the following terms:

- » **A la king:** This term means that a rich sauce coats the food. A la king foods usually come on a white English muffin or other white bread, which is low in fiber. The sauce is high in sodium and may contain lots of trans fats.

- » **Alfredo:** This term means the dish contains a sauce made of cream and butter, adding lots of fat and unnecessary calories.

- » **Au gratin:** Au gratin foods are topped with buttered breadcrumbs and cheese and broiled to produce a crisp crust, which produces those pesky advanced glycation end products (AGEs).

- » **Battered:** Battered food is fried! This cooking method creates AGEs and adds lots of calories (see Chapter 11 for more details).

- » **Breaded:** Breaded food is usually deep-fried or pan-fried. The breading usually consists of white bread. Fried foods can be high in trans fats, especially if the oil is used over and over again, as it is in many restaurants.

- » **Carbonara:** This term means the meal comes with a sauce of eggs, cream, and cheese, which also means the food will be high in unnecessary calories.

- » **Crispy:** This term usually means the food has been fried, often breaded or battered and then deep-fried. Fried foods are higher in AGEs and carcinogens.

- » **Fried:** This term includes pan-fried and deep-fried foods. The frying method adds calories and creates AGEs.

>> **Parmigiana:** This term usually means the food is coated in cheese and breadcrumbs and then fried. Foods prepared this way may have an entire day's worth of fat in one serving.

>> **Pickled:** Pickled foods have been treated with a high-sodium mixture and usually have preservatives and additives.

>> **Smoked:** While smoking adds wonderful flavor to food, it also adds polycyclic aromatic hydrocarbons (PAHs) and benzopyrene, two compounds that can cause cancer.

>> **Smothered:** Any food with this term next to it is usually covered in a rich gravy that's high in sodium and saturated fat.

>> **Stuffed:** Stuffed foods are usually stuffed with cheese or other high-calorie ingredients that are also higher in additives and trans fats.

When you're eating out, use common sense. Use the eating clean principles we cover in this chapter and the rest of the book to choose healthy foods from the menu. Don't be afraid to ask questions about how the food is prepared or to request special preparation methods. Often, chefs are happy to omit the MSG or salt from your order.

Asking the waiter or chef for clarification

For clean eaters, preparation methods are almost as important as the ingredients themselves. So when you're trying to eat clean while eating out, you have to become that annoying person who asks the waiter how the food is prepared. But remember that waiters are there to answer your questions. Chefs tell them about each dish on the menu, so the waiters should know what's in the food.

If your waiter doesn't know how a food is prepared, ask him to ask the chef or ask to speak to the chef yourself. After all, you're giving the restaurant your hard-earned money. You have the right to know what's in the food you're eating. But don't demand answers to your questions; be respectful of the chef and your waiter (and your fellow diners).

Before you order a meal with the following menu terms, ask your waiter or the chef for more details:

>> **Braised:** Braised food can be healthy if the chef cooks it in a low-sodium liquid. However, some braised foods are very rich, with lots of salt and fat added.

>> **Grilled:** Although grilling can be unhealthy because of the development of carcinogens, especially on seared and burned parts of the food, a simple

grilled chicken or steak, served without a sauce, can be a good option in many restaurants. Ask the chef to cook your food without grill marks, which can contain carcinogens.

>> **Sautéed:** This cooking method can be healthy if the chef doesn't use much oil. Ask that the chef leave out any sauce usually used in the food's preparation.

>> **Stewed:** This preparation method can be clean if the chef cooks the food at a low temperature without a lot of added salt, fat, or artificial ingredients.

>> **Stir-fried:** This preparation method can be healthy, as long as the chef doesn't use much oil and adds few preservatives and artificial ingredients. You can request that the chef reduce the oil used in preparation. Just be sure to request no sauce or less sauce, too.

TIP

One way to get the chef on your side is to explain that you have special dietary needs. No chef or cook wants to make a customer sick. Stressing that you just can't eat certain foods can help you get what you want — as long as you ask politely, of course!

Ordering sauces on the side and substituting clean foods when possible

Many chefs pride themselves on making the most delicious and richest food. Sauces, which usually consist of lots of salt, fat, and sugar, make food taste good. While a simple pan sauce made by adding broth or another healthy liquid to a pan is healthy, most sauces and dressings don't belong on the clean eating plan.

SALTY RESTAURANT KITCHENS

When Linda, one of the authors, was working for Pillsbury, she had to work in a restaurant kitchen to prepare some frozen foods for a client meeting. She'll never forget that day for one reason: She was shocked to see how the chefs simply poured salt into every pot sitting on a burner. She had to stop herself from intervening!

Many restaurant meals contain much more than the daily recommended intake of 2,300 milligrams of sodium. In fact, eating just one meal very high in sodium can spike your blood pressure, leading to an increased risk of heart attack or stroke. For instance, Olive Garden's Tour of Italy lasagna meal has more than 6,000 milligrams of sodium. Researchers at the Center for Science in the Public Interest found that in 17 restaurant chains, 85 out of 102 meals had more than four days' worth of sodium. Bottom line: Ask for unsalted foods when you eat out.

When you order a meal in a restaurant, you can ask for most sauces and dressings "on the side." Sauces or dressings on the side come in a little cup, so you can add as much or as little as you want to your food before you eat it. The chef should be able to accommodate this request. If he can't, he should let you know so that you can choose a different menu item.

Follow these guidelines when eating out to help you stay on track with your eating clean lifestyle:

>> **Ask that an olive oil and vinegar dressing be served on the side of any salad you order.** Sometimes you can ask for additional vegetables to be added to a salad. And choose dark greens over the ubiquitous iceberg lettuce.

>> **Ask to make sure the fruits in any fruit salad you order are fresh or frozen.** Fruit salads can be a good clean choice, as long as they're not canned in heavy syrup or served with a dressing.

>> **Ask to have more vegetables added to your meal.** For instance, if a vegetable pizza is on the menu, ask that your pizza include more vegetables than cheese.

>> **Create your own meal if a menu offers a la carte items.** For example, you may be able to combine poached fish or broiled chicken with some steamed vegetables and a fresh fruit salad.

>> **Ask that the sauce be placed on the side rather than on the food.** Because most restaurant items are prepared in bulk but finished as they're ordered, the chef should be able to handle this request.

>> **Unless the menu says *no substitutions,* try to substitute cleaner foods for less healthy choices.** For example, ask for a vegetable side dish in place of white pasta or for brown rice in place of white.

If all else fails and you have to order something that isn't clean, remember that unless you're following the eating clean plan 100 percent of the time, you can consider this meal part of the 20 or 30 percent slack you've built into your eating clean lifestyle. Every single meal doesn't have to be perfectly balanced nutritionally. Enjoy your meal, even if it does contain some processed foods! (See Chapters 1 and 2 for details on building your own eating clean plan.)

Packing Good Lunches and Snacks

Having food on hand is always a good idea when you're making a change in your eating lifestyle. It can help calm your nerves as you try to navigate this new eating plan and can help stop temptation when you face that dessert cart or hot dog stand.

In this section, we look at the basics of packing clean, healthy snacks and lunches. We list some quick things you can grab on your way out the door and show you how to plan good, clean lunches and snacks to get you through the work week.

Making clean snacks

Many clean foods, like apples and bananas, are portable, which makes them great candidates for snack time. Plus, you can make lots of simple snacks to take with you so you don't have to go hungry or choose an unhealthy filler food.

When you're planning and making snacks, try to pair protein with carbohydrates. This combination helps ensure that you provide fuel for your body and avoid the insulin spike that can occur after you eat a carb-heavy meal. The protein can be anything from yogurt to nut butter to cottage cheese to hummus to nuts. The possibilities are endless!

TIP

We offer you quite a few easy-to-make and portable recipes in Chapter 18 of this book, including choices like Sweet and Spicy Nuts and Stuffed Dates. Plus, you can find plenty of other easy options, like the ones in this list, that don't require recipes:

» **Popcorn:** Air pop some popcorn and mix it with some dried fruit, nuts, and a few dark chocolate chips for your own snack mix.

» **Mini wraps:** Put together a mini wrap sandwich, using foods that you don't have to refrigerate. Mash up an avocado with a little lemon juice and some mustard and spread it on a mini whole-wheat tortilla. Top it with lots of veggies, like shredded carrots, sliced mushrooms, and baby greens, roll it up, put it in a container, and stash it in your purse or work bag.

» **Fresh veggies:** Plain fresh veggies make a wonderful snack. You can pair carrot or celery sticks, soybeans, and pepper strips with a dip made from plain yogurt and some herbs or spices.

» **Homemade veggie chips:** Make your own veggie chips. Thinly slice carrots, sweet potatoes, beets, or radishes and toss them with olive oil. Place the veggies on a cookie sheet, sprinkle them with spices, and bake them at 400 degrees for 15 to 20 minutes until crisp.

» **Curry berries:** Mix some different types of berries in a small container. Top them with curry powder and shake the container gently to coat.

» **Peanut butter and crackers:** Pack some clean organic peanut butter along with whole-wheat crackers, preferably homemade.

» **Clean prepackaged snacks:** Some protein bars or granola bars are made from wholesome ingredients. Just be sure to read the nutrition labels on any packaged snacks before you buy them!

Make sure that you pack your snacks and lunches safely. If the snacks contain perishable foods (meats, cheeses, dairy products, and so on), store them in an insulated container along with a frozen ice pack or cold pack. Make sure the containers you use are reusable (to be kind to the earth) and seal them tightly. And remember that your snacks should be small — no more than 200 to 300 calories.

Packing clean lunches

Packing your own lunch is not only economical but also the best way to eat clean. Lunch is full of perils and potholes, including fast food, vending machines, and the doughnut or muffin you grab at the last minute because you don't have time to eat a real lunch.

The following sections provide some tips to help you pack the best lunches for you and your kids. Turn to Chapter 16 for some quick and easy (and delicious, of course!) lunchtime recipes.

Lunch for yourself

When you make your own lunch, think about what you like to eat and what fits into your schedule. A wrap sandwich made from sturdy dark-green lettuce or a whole-wheat pita bread sandwich is great for lunch on the run. Soups, either hot or cold, can be another great choice, and salads, of course, are the ultimate healthy lunch as long as you follow a few basic rules.

When making your clean lunch, be sure to follow these guidelines:

>> **Pack in as many vegetables or fruits as possible.**

>> **Make your own salad dressing and use only a small amount on your homemade salad.**

>> **Use greens that are as dark as possible on your salad or sandwich for the most nutrition.**

>> **Add a protein source, like cubed cheese, nuts, or cooked meats (such as chicken or fish), to salads, sandwiches, and soups.**

>> **Consider using unusual breads or wraps and clean condiments for sandwiches.**

   Whole-wheat or rye bread is a better choice than white, and using condiments like clean mustard or yogurt is better than using mayo or salad dressing.

>> **Combine protein with carbohydrates in your lunch for quick energy and long-lasting satisfaction.**

Add hard-cooked eggs and cheese to a green salad or pack peanut butter with celery sticks.

>> **Incorporate a lot of little snacks into your lunch.**

A few cubes of cheese, a handful of nuts, some fresh fruit and veggies, and perhaps some yogurt make a great lunch that's easy to throw together.

Lunch for the kids

Packing clean lunches for children is a whole different ballgame. The most important thing to do is to have them participate in making their lunches. If they have some choice and control, they'll be more likely to eat the good, clean lunches you've packed. (For tips on getting your kids to eat what you want them to, see Chapter 13.)

Remember that children don't have a lot of time to eat lunch at school and that the cafeteria is full of distractions. Your goal is to get your children to eat a few bites of some nutrient-dense, healthy food to keep them going throughout the rest of the school day. So make each bite count.

Here are some tips to keep in mind as you pack your kids' lunches:

>> **Pack a lot of small snacks.** If your kids love nuts and fruit, pack nuts and fruit, along with some cheese or slices of turkey or chicken. And don't forget a carton of organic juice or milk.

>> **Use bento boxes to pack lunch every day.** These cute boxes are divided into sections, so they keep food from touching other food (one key childhood gripe) and make the food more interesting.

>> **Make a *snackable* lunch yourself.** Put clean crackers, slices of cheese and meat, and a container of yogurt into a bento box and *voilà!* A clean version of the little meal kit kids love.

>> **Make kid-friendly and easy-to-eat roll-up sandwiches or wraps.** Pack all the makings of the sandwich and let your children make their own creations at lunchtime.

>> **Pack some hot soup or cold salad in a small thermos.** Soups and salads packed with lots of vegetables are the best.

>> **Create your own combinations with dips and trail mix.** Small containers of fruit, organic applesauce, plain yogurt, or homemade clean dips go great with some homemade trail mix.

FOOD ALLERGIES IN SCHOOL

One topic that has made the news recently is the increase in food allergies, especially among children. Many school districts have banned certain allergenic foods, like peanuts, to protect the kids who can have severe allergic reactions (like anaphylactic shock) to these items. Be sure to check with your school before you pack your child's lunch. Respect food allergies and comply with the rules schools have set because allergic reactions can be life-threatening. Giving up peanut butter is a small price to pay to save a child's life.

TIP

Be sure to empty and clean your kids' lunchboxes every day as soon as they get home from school. Bacteria can multiply quickly in just a little bit of food spilled inside a lunchbox or thermos. Wash the box and thermos with hot, soapy water and dry them thoroughly before you fill them the next day.

Avoiding unhealthy lunches and snacks

When you pack your lunches and snacks, try to avoid processed foods. Yes, we know this little tidbit seems super obvious, but we have to say it anyway.

Although a protein or granola bar may seem like an easy solution to the snack question, you must read the label first. Many snack bars are high in sugar and preservatives, and trans fats are common in almost all packaged bars. If you're making a sandwich for lunch, those deli meats you turned to in the past are now off the list because they're highly processed and high in sodium, preservatives, and additives.

TIP

When you're packing up food for the day, think whole foods. Whole fruits and vegetables are the easiest foods to pack for lunches and snacks. They come in their own containers, they're packed with nutrients, they don't need refrigeration, and they taste great.

If you choose to pack perishable foods, be sure that your lunchbox is well insulated and that the cold or frozen packs you add will stay cold for the hours when the box is sitting next to your desk. You may want to run a test on your lunchbox on the weekend. Put food in the box along with the cold pack. After four or five hours, use an instant-read thermometer to check the temperature of the perishable food. If it's above 40 degrees, enough bacteria could grow to make you sick. Either refrigerate your lunchbox or pack nonperishable foods.

You know you're not going to pack nacho cheese chips or bakery cookies in your lunchbox. But you need to remember safety as you pack your lunch and snacks, too.

- **Don't pack hot meats, like baked chicken, fish, pork, or beef.** An insulated lunchbox is designed to keep foods cool, not to cool them down to a safe temperature. Make sure you thoroughly cook and thoroughly chill all meats before you pack them in your lunchbox.

- **Don't pack frozen foods, like yogurt pops.** They'll melt, even when you pack them with a frozen gel pack.

- **Consider packing only nonperishable foods.** Good, clean, nonperishable foods include peanut butter or other nut butters, vegetables, nuts, fresh and dried fruits, and crackers.

- **Throw away any leftover food that's perishable.** That insulated lunchbox doesn't rechill food. So don't be tempted to save perishable food for your snack later on in the day.

Dealing with Dinner Invitations the Clean (and Polite) Way

Dinner invitations are one of the real joys in life. You get to see family and friends and enjoy great conversation while someone else does the cooking. But what happens when you're eating clean and you receive a dinner invitation from someone who uses processed foods?

You have several options in this situation. You can let your hostess know that you're on a special diet and ask about the menu. You can offer to bring something that you can eat. Or you can abandon the diet for one night and chalk this meal up to the 20 percent side of your 80/20 plan (that is, your plan to follow the eating clean lifestyle 80 percent of the time; see Chapters 1 and 2 for details).

In the following sections, we provide some tips for how to deal with a party invitation that doesn't ask for food preferences, and we offer you some clean potluck solutions. Above all, remember that dinners and parties are social situations during which every guest needs to make some compromises for them to be successful.

Knowing what to do when the invitation doesn't ask about food preferences

Considering the guests' dietary needs as well as their likes and dislikes is an important part of planning a party. If you're giving the party, ask all your invitees whether they can't or won't eat certain foods and whether they have any special favorites or foods they really don't enjoy. Then try to plan the menu around these preferences, keeping it within your budget, cooking skills, and taste.

So many people are on special diets these days (gluten-free, sugar-free, vegan, vegetarian, and allergy diets, just to name a few) that making a special request for a dish you can eat isn't out of the ordinary. The key is in handling your special request politely.

If you're invited to a party and the host or hostess doesn't ask about food preferences, you have several options for what to do next:

>> **Mention that you're on a new eating plan and ask if you can bring anything**. If the hostess acquiesces, bring a dish that you have tried and know you can make and enjoy.

>> **Ask if you can do anything to help.** Asking how you can help may lead to a discussion about what she plans to serve. If you don't think you can eat anything on the menu and your hostess says not to bring anything, eat something before you go to the dinner.

>> **Eat a small meal before you go so you can pass on foods you don't want to eat.** Combine protein, such as a small portion of cooked chicken, with some carbs and healthy fat, such as a toasted English muffin spread with some organic butter. This type of combination will satisfy you for a couple of hours.

>> **If all else fails, take small portions of the foods at the dinner and eat just a bit of them.** That way, you don't starve, you don't insult your hosts, and you keep the party pleasant. After all, everyone's personal diet choices are his own business.

WARNING

However you decide to handle the dinner invitation, here's what you definitely shouldn't do after you arrive:

>> **Don't make a big deal out of the fact that you can't eat certain foods on the menu.** The people issuing the invitation are opening their home to you. You go to these gatherings for social interaction and companionship, not just to eat.

>> **Don't comment on the foods that are unhealthy or made with processed ingredients.** The host and hostess have worked hard on this party, and their offerings came from the heart. If you see something you can't or won't eat, just pass by it quietly. Announcing "I can't eat that" and explaining why in detail is rude.

>> **Don't preach about your diet choices and lifestyle.** If you bring a dish to the party, hand it over without much comment. If people ask you about the food or ask for the recipe, then share your clean eating plan with them and tell them about your new lifestyle if they seem interested. But don't be a proselytizer; people don't like being preached to about their diet choices!

If you feel that you have to decline a particular party invitation, perhaps because the party is based around a barbecue or is a celebration of desserts, be polite about it. Thank the hostess for the invitation and tell her how touched you are that she thought of you. You may want to send a bottle of wine or some flowers before the event to express your appreciation.

Considering some clean potluck solutions

Potlucks are a great choice for entertaining. Not only are they a fun way to share your favorite dishes, but they're easier on the hosts and their pocketbook. If you offer (or are asked) to bring something to a potluck party, you can choose to bring something clean or throw caution to the winds and make your most indulgent and decadent recipe. If you're lucky, the decadent dish and the clean dish will be one and the same! (Check out Chapters 15 through 18 for some delicious clean recipes.)

TIP

If you're giving a potluck dinner, you can assign courses to your guests or even offer recipes. However you divide the duties, make sure all your guests can tell what each recipe is and what's in it. A great way to make a potluck party a more congenial event is to ask your guests to bring recipe cards along with their dishes. These recipe cards can start conversations as well as alert people to foods and ingredients that they may not want to or cannot eat.

If you're invited to a potluck dinner, be sure to make a dish you feel comfortable making. You may want to bring a dish based on a popular recipe that you've "cleaned up" just to demonstrate your wonderful new eating lifestyle. In fact, because the clean variations taste better than the versions made with processed foods, you may win a few converts to the eating clean lifestyle!

When you're trying to decide what to take to a potluck dinner, consider these good, clean choices:

>> **Casseroles:** Casseroles are a great way to stretch meat (especially organic meats) and combine two courses into one. Make sauces from scratch (avoiding the usual creams and cheeses, of course), use lots of vegetables, and add herbs and spices for seasoning rather than lots of salt.

>> **Appetizers:** A clean dip made with organic yogurt and fresh herbs paired with baby vegetables is a welcome addition to any meal. Even kids love dipping tiny veggies into a savory dip.

>> **Desserts:** Making clean desserts not only ensures that you have something to eat but also pleases other guests who are trying to watch their intake of fat and artificial ingredients.

>> **Soups:** You can make clean, indulgent soups by pureeing vegetables and using that mixture in lieu of heavy cream.

>> **Salads:** Salads can range from a baby spinach salad with homemade dressing to a main dish pasta salad (whole-grain pasta, please!) packed with vegetables and cooked chicken. In fact, you can essentially bring your very own salad bar to a potluck to give everyone a choice.

Picking at Party Food

Parties in general can be hazardous to the clean eating lifestyle. But by using a few simple tricks, you can ensure that what you eat stays as close to your clean eating plan as possible.

In the following sections, we look at how to build a plate from a buffet to make it healthy, and we describe some ways to politely say no when you come across someone at the party who wants to sabotage your diet efforts (every party has one!).

Eating healthy at parties: It's possible!

When you're at a party, whether it's a cocktail party with appetizers, a buffet where you can build your own plate, or a sit-down dinner where they bring the meal to you, remember that you're in control. After you master the tricks we present in this section, you'll be able to eat as cleanly as possible, even when faced with processed, salty, unclean foods.

First of all, pace yourself. Remember that your brain takes 20 minutes to realize that you've had enough to eat (see Chapter 5 for details). Eat slowly and savor every bite.

Next, watch your alcohol intake. While one glass of red wine is actually good for you, the negatives increase and the positives decrease with every additional glass. Alcohol kills brain cells, and it leads to poor judgment and decision making.

After you master these first two tricks, use the following tips to eat as healthy as possible at parties:

>> **If you have a choice, choose a smaller plate.** Having a reasonable amount of food on a small plate looks like more than a little bit of food on a big plate. Remember: You eat with your eyes first.

>> **Divide your plate into four sections and designate each section for a particular type of food.** Pile veggies and fruits into two of the sections. Then put protein in the third quarter. Allocate the fourth quarter for the indulgent treats, like garlic bread, scalloped potatoes, and fried foods. This method allows you to follow the 80/20 rule (actually, it's the 75/25 rule, but that's pretty close!). (See Chapters 1 and 2 for more on the 80/20 rule.)

>> **Choose colorful foods.** Don't build a beige or brown plate. Keep in mind that the more colorful the food, the more vitamins, minerals, phytochemicals, fiber, and antioxidants it contains.

>> **Look for the plainest foods.** Any food that's smothered in a sauce or covered with cheese or buttered breadcrumbs probably isn't a clean food. Broiled chicken, sautéed vegetables, a simple fruit salad, whole-wheat bread, and more fruit for dessert are usually your best choices.

>> **Drink lots of water and other plain beverages like tea.** These liquids help fill you up and cut back on the time you spend eating.

>> **Make conversation, not the food, the focus of your night.** A party's main focus is to get together with others, not eat. Keep this fact in mind and enjoy yourself.

If you've been eating clean for some time, you probably notice something interesting when you attend parties and other social get-togethers: You naturally gravitate toward the healthier foods. In time, processed foods and foods made with unhealthy ingredients start to taste, well, kind of strange. Plus, if you enjoy feeling light and clean after eating clean foods, just the sluggish feeling of being overstuffed after you eat too many processed foods will help you get back on track before the next party.

Explaining your diet when you have to

Every crowd has at least one person who chooses to focus on what you're eating (or not eating). This person may be genuinely interested in learning more about you, or maybe basic human nature gets the better of him and he just has to find out why you're behaving a bit differently. Occasionally, malice may play a role. Whatever the reason behind this inquisition, too many questions can become too intrusive fast.

As you deal with people who question your diet and lifestyle, remember that you're in control. Here are a few things you can do when someone persistently questions your motives or tries to press food on you:

>> Explain that you're on a new eating plan. Your explanation can be as brief or as detailed as you want it to be.

>> Claim a food allergy if the food pusher won't give up.

>> Master the art of the graceful exit. Claim that you want to talk to someone who just came in, or use the time-honored excuse of needing to use the restroom.

>> Turn the question around and ask the person why he's eating what's on his plate. Stick to your guns and your plan and don't let yourself be coerced into eating something you don't want to eat.

Getting Your Mojo Back: What to Do When You Fall off the Plan

If there's one certainty in life (besides death and taxes), it's that you're going to fall off the clean eating plan at some point. Nobody's perfect, so go ahead and accept this fact now. By realizing that you will fall, you make the process of getting back on track a whole lot easier.

When you fall off the plan, follow these steps to pick up the pieces and get back on track:

1. **Forgive yourself.**

   You're only human, and taking a few detours from the eating clean plan isn't the end of the world.

2. **Regroup and try to think about why you went off the plan.**

   You always have a reason, and just maybe it was a good one!

3. **Learn from your mistakes.**

   The next time you get the feeling that tripped you up, or something bad happens and you feel like binging on junk food, try other remedies to help you feel better. Drink some water, go on a walk, call a friend, or read a book.

4. **Be determined to start again.**

   After all, you're not back at square one. One or two (or three or four) missteps don't cancel out all your hard work. Hopefully you enjoyed your misstep. What's the point of breaking the rules every now and then if you don't have fun while doing it? Try to relax!

Chapter 13

Getting Your Family on the Bandwagon

Getting your family to cooperate in a new endeavor is never easy, especially when that endeavor involves changing the daily diet. But don't give up yet! We're here to help make your family's transition to clean eating smooth and relatively painless.

Starting your children on the clean eating path is easier when they're very young. Kids learn by example (as anyone who's ever accidentally let a swear word slip out knows), so their eating habits start with you. The first step toward a new family diet begins when you make the change. Of course, the whole process will be easier if your spouse is on board, too, but you can be the pioneer all by yourself if necessary. The older kids get, the more resistant they are to change, but change is still possible.

Participation is the other key to a healthy diet. Kids want to learn. In fact, this yearning for knowledge is one reason babies fight naps; they know they'll miss something while they're sleeping. So make buying, preparing, and eating a clean diet a fun and educational adventure. Your family will benefit for life.

Even if your kids turn green at the thought of green vegetables or your spouse thinks salads are for rabbits, you can change their minds (and their eating habits) by using the tips and tricks we provide in this chapter.

Transitioning from Twinkies to Turnips

If you're reading this book, you're most likely the person responsible for feeding your family. As such, you wield a lot of power! Now that you're determined to feed your family a more nutritious diet, you're ready to start implementing the necessary changes.

In the following sections, we look at how to make changes and plan your family diet makeover with as little fuss as possible. Because transitioning your family to an eating clean diet is such a personal process, we look at plans to make changes gradually or quickly (your choice!).

As with all makeovers, seeing big changes takes time. So you need to develop a plan to switch your family to the eating clean lifestyle. You can start slowly or blast right in. Either way, start by talking to your kids (and spouse) about food and healthy lifestyles; then get them involved in planning and preparing your new food. (See the section "Inviting Participation" for details.)

REMEMBER

Realize that transitioning your family to an eating clean lifestyle is going to be more work than calling in a pizza order or piling everyone into the car for a trip to a fast-food joint. But the payoff is tremendous. A healthy family that stays healthy for life is the best reward for any parent. Make small changes, be persistent, try new recipes, and don't give up! Eventually, even the most stubborn family members will improve their eating habits.

Making changes the slow way

When you make small, gradual changes, seeing results takes a little while. But if your family is very resistant to the idea of a diet change, small and gradual is the way to go. While sneaking good foods into your family's diet isn't the ideal way to improve their eating habits for life, some subterfuge may be necessary. But as your eating habits gradually change, your family will most likely start to enjoy the healthier food you prepare.

For a gradual makeover, pick one or two changes a week. Get rid of the most unhealthy foods first and substitute slightly healthier choices. After you make these changes, you can gradually add clean, whole foods and switch to unprocessed foods until your family's diet is where you want it to be. Just remember that habits take a few weeks to become ingrained and success breeds success. So don't give up along the way!

For the slow-road makeover, take things one week at a time. The changes you make don't have to be in any particular order, but you can use the game plan in Table 13-1 to help you get started.

TABLE 13-1 Gradual Transition to the Eating Clean Lifestyle

Week	Change to Make	Tips for Implementing the Change
Week one	Substitute a homemade meal for one fast-food meal.	Make hamburgers at home, offer baked french fries, and serve some fresh fruit with a dipping sauce for dessert. Gradually increase this switch until fast food is only an occasional treat. (See Part 5 for a whole collection of clean meal and dessert recipes.)
Week two	Stop buying soda pop.	In its place, make lemonade, iced tea, or fruit juices. If your family members love the carbonation of soft drinks, add seltzer water or ginger ale to your homemade beverages. For a fun twist, freeze some of the lemonade or tea into ice cubes to add to your cold drinks.
Week three	Switch from refined grains to foods with some whole wheat.	Choose pasta with added fiber or the kind that's made from whole grain but looks like regular pasta. In place of white bread, pick a sandwich bread that has some whole wheat but still tastes mild. Try making muffins or pancakes with whole-wheat pastry flour rather than all-purpose flour. Every week, add more whole grains and use fewer refined grains until most of your grain choices are clean.
Week four	Instead of buying flavored chips and salty snacks, look for baked snacks that are low in sodium.	Make your own clean snacks, like baked pita chips seasoned with curry powder or cumin or nut and dried fruit mixes. The trick is to make these healthy clean choices available and within reach. (See Chapter 18 for some yummy clean snack recipes.)
Week five	Add one or two fresh fruits to your everyday menu.	Mix a chopped apple into pancake batter, or add some sliced strawberries to a green salad. Mix pears with onion, jalapeños, and lime juice for a fresh salsa to serve with grilled pork chops.
Week six	Add one or two vegetables to your everyday menu.	Toss a chopped red bell pepper or diced zucchini into a green salad. Stir some cooked and pureed cauliflower into mashed potatoes or add chopped and steamed cauliflower to macaroni and cheese. Add some green beans to your favorite chicken soup recipe or stir parsnips into a beef stew.
Week seven	Stop buying canned products and frozen prepared meals.	Use your slow cooker to make healthy soups, pasta sauce, casseroles, and chilies. Freeze your leftovers in individual containers that you can later reheat for a quick lunch or snack.
Week eight	If you're still serving fried foods, start making the change to baked, steamed, and poached preparations.	Marinate boneless, skinless chicken in lemon juice and herbs and bake it until it's juicy and tender instead of frying it. Poach some salmon in the slow cooker with fennel and squash. Make some muffins with whole grains and fruit instead of buying doughnuts or pastries.

(continued)

TABLE 13-1 *(continued)*

Week	Change to Make	Tips for Implementing the Change
Week nine	Make over some of your favorite recipes using clean foods.	If your family loves Mexican food, substitute canned refried beans with your own pinto beans that you mash with pureed onions and garlic. Use ground turkey or chicken rather than ground beef for burritos. Choose whole-grain tortillas in place of plain flour or corn tortillas. Finally, reduce the amount of cheese you use in your Mexican recipes.
Week ten	Focus on portion sizes.	Most Americans don't realize that a serving of meat should be only the size of a deck of cards or that a serving of chopped fruit or ice cream is only ½ cup. Until you're used to choosing the correct amount of each food, measure it out.

REMEMBER

By week ten, many of these habits will likely be second nature. Go back over the list again, making more drastic changes, like eliminating fast food altogether or switching to 100 percent whole-grain breads and pastas. Continue making changes by phasing out foods that aren't clean and adding more that are. If you're ready to move to the fast-track way at this point, check out the next section.

Making changes the fast way

If you want to see more change in less time, the fast-track way to an eating clean lifestyle may be a better fit for you and your family. Getting good results, like clearer skin or more energy, fast can be powerful motivation to continue with drastic change. This method is for people who embrace change and who want to take control of their health fast. For some people, making a drastic change is easier to do since it immediately removes all tempting unclean foods from their diet.

REMEMBER

Make sure that your family is basically healthy before you make any drastic changes. Talk to your family doctor about eating clean and tell her about your new lifestyle. Then dive in!

The changes to ingrained habits you have to make during the fast-track transition to an eating clean lifestyle can be jarring and difficult, but the payoff can be tremendous. Take a look at Table 13-2 to see what these quick changes include.

WARNING

If you go from eating one to two servings of fruits and vegetables a day to eating five to seven, your digestive tract may rebel, causing you to suffer from gas, bloating, and digestive upset. If you experience such discomfort, cut back on the produce and add another serving every few days.

For recipes and more ideas about your new diet, check out Part 5 of this book.

TABLE 13-2   **Fast Transition to the Eating Clean Lifestyle**

Week	Change to Make	Tips for Implementing the Change
Week one	Get rid of all soft drinks, packaged salty snacks, and junk food.	Instead of buying diet soda, potato chips, crackers, tortilla chips, packaged cream puffs, packaged cookies, bakery cakes, and ice cream desserts, make your own snacks, like the Sweet and Spicy Nuts from Chapter 18, using fresh fruits and vegetables, nuts, seeds, and whole grains.
Week two	Give away canned foods and processed foods to your local food bank.	Instead of buying canned meats, beans, fruit, cake and pudding mixes, canned soups, pasta sauces, broth, sweetened cereals, jams, granola bars, and snack mixes, buy only organic produce, meat, and dairy products (if you use them).
Week three	Switch to whole-grain foods.	Only purchase whole grains, like brown rice, quinoa, spelt, wheat grains, and steel-cut oatmeal, and avoid refined flour or grains. Get rid of all sugar and sugary foods. Use stevia, organic honey, or agave syrup to sweeten foods. Don't switch to artificial sweeteners, as they're heavily processed.
Week four	Make everything you eat from scratch.	Pack your fridge full of good clean foods and only fill your pantry with items like whole grains, nuts, dried fruit, seeds, tea, and spices. Don't fry foods; instead, choose cooking methods like poaching, steaming, and slow cooking.
Week five	Think about getting rid of all dairy products and all wheat products, especially if anyone in your family has allergies.	Stop buying dairy products and get rid of all your wheat flour and grains — everything except corn and rice. Many Americans are lactose intolerant and feel better when they don't consume any dairy products. Many people are gluten intolerant or have celiac disease, which makes eating wheat difficult. Add supplements to your diet, like multivitamins, cod liver oil, fish oil, and vitamins D, C, and B complex.

Helping your family make the transition

No one — your family included — can make the transition from an unhealthy lifestyle to a clean lifestyle without a little help. And you must be patient! Making the switch may take some coaxing, and it'll definitely take some time. But with the tips we offer in this section, you'll be able to get even reluctant family members on board the clean eating plan.

TIP

To help your family, especially your kids, make the switch to a clean eating plan, consider these tips:

>> **Make sure that your child sees you enjoying a good variety of foods, especially fruits and vegetables.** Children learn by imitating, and you can set a good example by enjoying healthy foods right in front of them.

>> **Remember that kids naturally eat smaller portions than adults.** When you add a new food to your repertoire, let your children try a very small amount. Just a fraction of a teaspoon is a start. Eventually, they'll learn to enjoy foods that promote health.

>> **Set realistic goals.** Don't expect miracles overnight, and realize that you and your family will have lapses. Don't give up when you have one of these lapses. Just pick up where you left off and celebrate success with a trip to the zoo or a day at the beach. Don't forget to pack healthy snacks to take with you!

>> **Don't force foods or make your children sit at the table until they eat all their food.** If you do, you'll probably end up with some very picky eaters. Never present food as a punishment. Instead, concentrate on positive reinforcement and conversation about healthy foods.

>> **Make food fun.** Most children like finger foods, so cut fruits and veggies into smaller pieces. Offering a dip for raw produce is another way to tempt children into trying something new. Or cut vegetables into fun shapes with tiny cookie cutters.

>> **Make sure the new food looks appealing.** People eat with their eyes first, so a honeydew melon cut into balls or fun shapes with a cookie cutter and zucchini cut into long ribbons with a vegetable peeler may tempt your family into trying a bite.

>> **Kids need to feel like they have some control.** When you're planning a meal, ask your children whether they'd like to have carrots or peas. Or ask them whether they'd like to have grilled chicken or broiled salmon. Your kids appreciate having input in food decisions and knowing that you respect their opinions.

>> **Don't reward with dessert.** You're trying to get your family to enjoy and appreciate healthy food for its own sake. A reward of dessert or something sweet only reinforces bad eating habits.

What about the other adults in the family? If your spouse or significant other has bad eating habits, you may need to sit down and have a conversation about food, nutrition, and health. Being proactive is important. You don't want to face an angioplasty or diagnosis of diabetes before you make changes in your family's eating habits.

Enjoying the benefits of clean eating

After your family has been eating well for a few weeks, they'll start noticing positive changes in their mood, energy level, and appearance. Teenagers' skin will most likely improve, their hair will have more gloss, and they may start to shine a little brighter in academics, sports, and team activities. Lucky for you, all these benefits help reinforce your clean eating message! In fact, these benefits may be all the reinforcement they need.

REMEMBER

Be sure to make the dinner table a pleasant place to be. Initiate conversations with your children and significant other. Don't spend this precious time criticizing or discussing serious problems. Instead, talk about your day, good things that have happened lately, and the food you're eating.

If you're eating alone, make the eating experience pleasurable and beautiful. Use nice china, crystal goblets, candles, and music. Yes, just for you! The food you're eating is going to improve your life, so you might as well make the experience as wonderful as possible.

Getting worthwhile results from small changes

You may remember a television show called *Honey, We're Killing the Kids* that focused on a family's bad eating habits. The nutritionist in the show immediately threw out all the junk food, processed food, and sugary foods in the house, which was a good thing. But then the family's diet plans went straight to prunes, kale, squid, and whole-wheat pasta instead of making incremental changes or switching to more appealing clean foods. In fact, the families on the show were interviewed after the shows aired, and many of them had gone back to their unhealthy eating habits.

TIP

Making drastic, fast-track changes to your diet can backfire. And you can find plenty more appealing clean choices than kale and prunes. Instead of making such huge changes, which can trigger protests, hunger strikes, and the temptation to sneak candy and snack foods, start slowly. If your family is really picky, begin by adding some good foods that are naturally sweet.

Here are some small changes you can make to get your family started on the eating clean program:

>> **Instead of eliminating dessert, throw out the chocolate-covered ice cream bars and buy frozen yogurt or 100 percent juice bars.** These better-for-you desserts usually have less fat and more vitamins and fiber. And they're sweet enough to keep everyone happy.

- » **Start out with sweet fruits and veggies, such as baby carrots and strawberries, rather than sour or bitter produce, like grapefruit or broccoli.** Most kids love bananas. So cut them into chunks, roll them in yogurt and chopped nuts, and freeze them for healthy popsicles. Blanch some sugar snap peas and serve them with guacamole made with cherry tomatoes. Choose baby carrots rather than kale or romaine lettuce at first.

- » **Don't introduce more than one new food at a meal.** The sight and aromas of new foods can easily overwhelm kids. So add sugar snap peas one day and cantaloupe wedges the next.

- » **Talk about the new food as you introduce it.** Describe the taste and texture to your family; then serve it. Face it, if someone offered you something totally unfamiliar, wouldn't you want a description and some reassurance before you put it in your mouth?

- » **Let your children touch and smell the food before they taste it.** In fact, let them gradually work up to touching and smelling the new food during the times when you introduce it. Don't expect them to taste the new food the first time or even the tenth!

TIP

Most children have a repertoire of 20 to 30 foods that they enjoy, especially if they're picky eaters. Unfortunately, those foods usually include candy, chips, soda, and other foods that just aren't good for their health. If you add one new food every week or so, in a year, your children could be enjoying 50 or more new foods, and they'll be well on their way to a lifelong habit of healthy eating.

Avoiding Stumbling Blocks

Every adult has dealt with a child who just doesn't want to eat healthy foods. But did you know that biological reasons can actually explain why kids really don't like some foods like Brussels sprouts and celery and really do like foods like chocolate and soda pop? It's true!

In this section, we look at why many people love sweet foods and why some people do just about anything to avoid bitter foods. Like most things hardwired into the body's systems, you (and your family) can relearn food preferences over time and with some practice and diligence.

Combating your innate sweet tooth

First of all, everybody is born with a sweet tooth. Breast milk, the best food for infants, is naturally sweet. So babies are biologically designed to crave and enjoy sweets. In fact, researchers have found that if you place sugar in an infant's mouth, she will relax and smile. And according to research published in the journal *Physiological Genomics*, some people are born with a gene variation called GLUT 2 that predisposes them to crave sugar. No wonder so many people would rather eat a chocolate candy bar than some steamed broccoli!

REMEMBER

Sweet foods aren't all bad. In fact, they help your body produce instant energy. Back when humans were foraging for food, foods high in sugar produced enough energy for humans to keep working and reproducing to keep the species alive. That preference for sweet foods also helped early humans pick out fruits that were ripe and, thus, had the highest nutritional value.

Now that most of the industrialized world has basically an unlimited supply of food, the human sweet-tooth preference can backfire. The major problem today is that people take in too many calories with not enough nutrients. To combat this issue, sweet-food fans need to get as much nutrition as possible out of each calorie.

Another reason why many people give in to their sweet tooth is that sweet foods increase the production of a group of brain chemicals called *endorphins*, including *serotonin*, which leads to a feeling of euphoria and helps suppress pain. Yes, by eating sweet foods, you literally get a sugar high!

TIP

One way to fight this natural, built-in craving is to start adding other endorphin-creating activities, like exercise, laughter, and meditation, into your life.

Different people have different numbers of sweet-detecting taste buds on their tongues. People with more sweet taste buds can taste sweet flavors more intensely, or at a lower concentration than others. That's why some people think that sugary cereal is too sweet, while others enjoy it by the bowlful. (Check out the section "Changing food preferences: It's not easy but it can be done" for tips on how to change your sweet-tooth-inspired food preferences.)

Dealing with your natural dislike of bitter foods

On the other end of the taste bud spectrum, people are biologically programmed to dislike bitter foods. Scientists have long suspected that bitter taste buds evolved to protect early humans against toxic plants, which usually have a very bitter taste. In a 2006 issue of *Current Biology*, a research paper confirmed that suspicion. In general, people are divided into three groups: those who are very sensitive to bitter tastes (called *supertasters*), those who have intermediate sensitivity, and those who are insensitive. See the next section for tips on how to change your (and your family's) food preferences.

Changing food preferences: It's not easy but it can be done

No matter how picky your children are, their eating habits will improve over time with some effort. The trick is to be consistent, to offer choices so your children feel like they have some control, and to stick with it.

Don't be discouraged if your kids refuse to try a food the first time they see it. It may take up to 20 to 30 separate introductions to a particular food before they trust it enough to take a bite. Of course, some kids will never learn to enjoy some of the more bitter foods like broccoli rabe or kale. Your child may also have a lower number of sweet taste buds and more sensitive bitter taste buds, leading him to gulp down sugary foods and refuse bitter foods. That's okay! Broccoli rabe and Brussels sprouts aren't an integral part of a healthy diet.

Emotions also play a part in food preferences thanks to a process called *conditioning.* Kids may associate some foods with unpleasant experiences. If, for example, they were offered broccoli at a birthday party where a child was sick at the table, they may automatically reject that food because of the association. If your children have negative feelings toward certain foods, wait a few weeks or months before trying to add those foods to their diet. On the other hand, kids automatically associate some foods with pleasant experiences. Birthday cake and chocolates for Valentine's Day are just two examples.

REMEMBER

As you move along in your clean eating plan, try to gradually add more bitter and, conversely, less sweet, foods to your family's diet. You can change food preferences over time. For example, to move from sweet to less sweet foods, gradually shift from offering sugar snap peas to snow peas to green beans to edamame to broccoli. Repeated exposure to different flavors trains your brain to accept new tastes. The trick is to keep adding new foods to your table. As long as your family sees you enjoying healthy foods, and as they see the available food change over time, they'll start eating more healthy foods with enjoyment.

Inviting Participation

One of the best ways to get your family to try new foods is to have them participate in meal preparation. We don't mean just stirring a pot or two or cleaning up after dinner. We're talking about growing food, buying it, planning meals, and cooking.

In the following sections, we look at some ways to get your family interested in food preparation — hunting and gathering, if you will. The key is to make the whole process — from growing to preparing — enjoyable.

Grow it!

Now we're not saying that you have to turn your backyard into a miniature farm, as the characters in the British comedy series *Good Neighbors* did. Just a few pots on your kitchen windowsill or on the deck in your backyard or a few square feet in the garden can provide you with fresh fruits and veggies that will taste better and be better for you than anything you can buy at the store.

With just a little effort, you can grow

- » Herbs or lettuce on the windowsill
- » Tomatoes, runner beans, and bell peppers in pots
- » Strawberries in planters
- » Apple and pear trees in the backyard

TIP

Focus on growing foods that are part of your family's favorite recipes. For example, a *pizza garden* can include tomatoes, basil, green onions, and bell peppers. A *salad garden* can include all kinds of different types of lettuce, and a *snack garden* can consist of sprouts, sugar snap peas, grape tomatoes, and sunflowers.

Assign some gardening tasks to your children, or give them each a pot or a few square feet of land that they can watch over. Start by growing foods that are ready to eat quickly, like sprouts or fast-growing lettuce so they get some immediate reward. Giving your kids simple tasks like pulling weeds and watering plants can help them feel involved. And nothing's better than picking some sweet peas or cherry tomatoes right off the vine and enjoying the sweet, fresh taste.

REMEMBER

Research shows that when kids participate in gardening, they become more interested in trying the food they grow, their science test scores increase, and their social and life skills improve. Bet you didn't know you could grow smarter children along with basil and parsley!

In fact, many school districts around the country are starting youth gardens on school grounds. Growing food can provide many life lessons, including learning about soil composition, sustainable ecosystems, wildlife, weather and the seasons, nutrition, and botany. Bring up this topic at a school board meeting or ask your child's teacher about incorporating a garden into her lesson plans.

Plan it!

Before you can buy food and prepare it, you need to come up with a plan for what you want to buy and cook. Why not get your family involved in the planning? Teaching kids how to plan meals and make shopping lists gives them skills they'll use for life. You can have each child plan one meal for the week, incorporating some of her favorite foods, and then have her help you figure out which foods you need to purchase to make that meal. If planning a meal seems like too much, you may want to begin by asking your child to plan snacks instead. Offer a few choices to get the ball rolling, and take her suggestions and ideas seriously.

TIP

Each planning session can turn into a painless lesson. Explain to your child that for the most energy during the day, a meal needs to include a good variety of different whole foods. If she wants pizza, suggest vegetable toppings rather than pepperoni and a crust made with whole-wheat flour rather than white flour. Or if she loves baked chicken, choose a recipe that includes vegetables or fruit to add flavor and nutrition. Explain that her plate should be as colorful as possible so that it's healthy, nice to look at, and delicious to eat.

Enlist your child's imagination when planning meals. If she prefers processed fish sticks, tell her that this time you're going to buy fresh fish and make your own fish sticks. Use condiments like ketchup or mustard to make faces on the fish sticks and serve them with a flavorful dipping sauce.

REMEMBER

Planning sessions are a good opportunity to teach kids about minimizing waste and using leftovers. For that baked chicken, use up leftovers in chicken sandwiches made with homemade bread or a chicken salad made with apples and grapes.

Buy it!

Taking children grocery shopping can be a challenging experience, but it can also be a great learning opportunity. If children help choose the celery that's the brightest green color or the crispest lettuce or the most colorful bell peppers, they'll be more likely to eat it.

To make the grocery store experience more enjoyable, set down a few rules before you leave home. Give each of your kids a list of things to put in the shopping cart, and make a game out of the outing. Try these activities:

>> Give each child one or two coupons and have them match up the coupon to the product on the shelves. Of course, only clip coupons for minimally processed foods, and choose foods that are as natural as possible to stick to your clean eating plan.

>> Turn the experience into a scavenger hunt. Ask your kids to find milk with the red cow on the package or a bunch of bananas with exactly six bananas.

>> Make a game out of the produce aisle by having the kids bag fruits and vegetables and then guess how much each bag will weigh.

>> Have your kids keep a running total of the food cost. Give them a small calculator and tell them the price of each item or let them check the prices themselves.

>> Look for unusual fruits and vegetables and ask the kids what they might taste like or how you could prepare them. Try something new at each shopping trip.

>> Teach your kids to read labels by making a game out of finding bread with whole-wheat flour as the first ingredient or pasta sauce with fewer than seven ingredients.

After a successful shopping experience, be sure to create some sort of reward. Take everybody to the park or to the bookstore for a new book. Because you're teaching your kids to eat for health as well as enjoyment, rewarding them with food isn't a great idea. Teach them to reward themselves with more intangible things like exercise or a game.

TIP

Because you want to feed your family the freshest food at the best prices, think about visiting farmers' markets. These outdoor markets are fascinating. Not only do you get to see food in its natural state, but you can learn a lot from the vendors. Ask them how they grow the food, how long the food takes to grow, and what the vendors' favorite ways to prepare it are. Strolling through the aisles of a farmers' market can be a wonderful way to interest your kids in the journey from farm field to table.

Cook it!

Every child should learn how to cook. You can find simple kitchen tasks that are appropriate for children of any age. If you aren't sure about your own cooking skills, take some time to read cookbooks that can help you improve, like the latest edition of *Cooking Basics For Dummies* by Bryan Miller, Marie Rama, and Eve Adamson (Wiley).

REMEMBER

When you get kids involved in the kitchen, teach them basic safety information, like always washing their hands before and after a cooking or preparation session, separating cooked and uncooked foods, being careful with knives and hot surfaces like the oven and stovetop, and cooking food to the correct doneness. Start by reading through the recipe, collecting all the ingredients and utensils, and making sure you understand how the recipe comes together. Then make the food and clean up while it's cooking.

Age-appropriate tasks help your family get involved in food preparation in a safe way. Be sure to pair tasks with your kids' fine motor skills. For example:

>> Preschool children can roll lemons and limes before juicing, count out slices of bread, wash fruits, sift flour, shake jars, peel oranges and hard-cooked eggs, put muffin liners into muffin tins, and use cookie cutters.

>> Middle school children can peel fruits and vegetables, break eggs (and wash their hands afterward!), read over a recipe and plan how to proceed, beat batters, and even do some supervised cooking with a wok or skillet.

>> Teenagers can prepare a whole meal after you teach them basic cooking and kitchen safety.

If your children just aren't interested in preparing a meal, start piquing their curiosity with some fun kitchen activities. Show them how to make a volcano using vinegar and baking soda or make modeling clay with cornstarch. Look for child-size kitchen tools to pique their interest. What child can resist a tiny rolling pin or miniature muffin tins?

After they see how fun cooking and baking can be, you can enlist their help to make Clean Edamame Guacamole and Kale Chips with Spanish Salsa or other fun recipes from Part 5. The kitchen can be a fascinating place. And when kids learn how to cook healthy foods, they gain a skill for life that will improve their health and well-being. Besides, cooking as a family is fun!

Chapter 14

Meeting Special Dietary Considerations

Special diets seem to be making their way into mainstream culture. Everybody knows somebody who's allergic to something or who can't eat one type of food or another. Food allergies, gluten sensitivity, and issues with meat and other animal products are three of the most common reasons why people practice special diets.

The good news is that even if you have someone with a food allergy or some strong food preferences in your family, you can still eat a clean diet. In fact, the clean diet is probably the best way to accommodate these needs and preferences!

In this chapter, we look at what food allergies are, why their numbers seem to be increasing, and how you can plan your meals to avoid allergenic foods. We also delve deeper into gluten sensitivity and look at the protein in wheat, barley, and similar products that can produce serious medical symptoms in people who are allergic or sensitive to it. We finish up by considering how vegetarian and vegan diets fit into the eating clean plan.

Food Allergies and Sensitivities

If you've ever faced a food allergy — whether you're the one with the allergy or someone in your family has it — you probably feel, well, picked on. After all, you now have a list of foods that are off your menu forever. Luckily, avoiding processed foods makes staying away from allergenic foods easier. An apple, for example, contains only apple — not 25 other ingredients that may or may not contain the food you're allergic to.

Doctors estimate that only 2 to 6 percent of the population actually has a true food allergy with development of antibodies specific to that food. The two major ways used to diagnose food allergies are blood tests and elimination diets. A small group of physicians, the American Academy of Environmental Medicine, also uses very precise skin tests called *dilution-titration* and *provocative neutralization*. Although "scratch tests" are relatively accurate for inhalant allergies, doctors generally consider them an inaccurate test for food allergies.

In this section, we look at what food allergies really are, how the body reacts to the food in question, and how to tell the difference between an allergy and a sensitivity. Then we list the main allergenic foods and give you tips on how to avoid them.

Understanding food allergies

A food allergy can develop at any point during your life. You can develop an allergy when you're 99 years old or never experience one at all. Doctors don't know what triggers an allergy, but they do know what happens when one develops.

Getting to know your immune system

A food allergy occurs when your immune system decides that one or more foods are attacking your body, and, as a result, it fights back. Your immune system is incredibly complex, comprised of lymph nodes, bone marrow, white blood cells (T-cells, b-cells, and many others), the spleen, the thymus gland, and tonsils. Its purpose is to protect you against bacteria, viruses, and any other substance your body perceives as foreign. The immune system usually works pretty well, keeping you healthy and free from disease. But sometimes it overreacts, causing allergies to develop.

Note: Food allergies can run in families, so genetics may play some part in development of this condition. Some studies also suggest that exposing fetuses to certain foods in utero can generate allergies. Pediatricians advise parents to introduce potentially allergenic foods to babies and toddlers gradually, in stages, so that if an allergy exists they can identify it early and eliminate the particular food from the child's diet.

REMEMBER

When you have an allergy to a food and you eat it, your body reacts to the protein (or sometimes other molecules) in the food. People rarely have an allergic reaction to a food the first time they eat it. But sometimes people who are allergic to one type of food experience cross-reactivity to unrelated allergens the first time they eat or are exposed to that other allergen. For instance, people who are allergic to grass could have an immediate allergic reaction to potatoes, melons, tomatoes, watermelons, oranges, cherries, or peanuts. Or someone with a peanut allergy could have an immediate reaction to legumes, wheat, corn, plantains, or melons.

If your body decides a food is a foreign substance, it will create one of the following two types of antibodies in your blood:

>> **IgE antibodies:** These antibodies are associated with immediate allergic reactivity. The next time you eat an IgE-provoking food, the IgE antibodies, which are attached to mast cells in your mouth, esophagus, stomach, and skin, will release histamines and other chemicals into your bloodstream to "protect" you against the invader, causing a rapid allergic reaction.

>> **IgG antibodies:** These antibodies are associated with more delayed allergic reactions, which are usually more subtle and harder to connect directly with the food that provoked them.

WHEN ALLERGIES TURN DEADLY

Although only a very small percentage of food allergens can be life-threatening, some people are so allergic to certain foods that they can die after simply kissing someone who has eaten it or touching that particular food. Everyone has heard of children with very severe peanut allergies. These severe reactions cause a systemic cascade in the immune system, overwhelming the body with histamines, which can cause a sharp drop in blood pressure, a narrowing of the airways, and anaphylactic shock. If not treated immediately, anaphylactic shock is deadly.

If you're severely allergic to one or more substances, always carry a medical ID along with an epinephrine pen or kit. This pen contains a measured dose of adrenaline (also known as epinephrine) in a syringe. If you have a severe allergic reaction to a substance, you inject yourself with this pen to stop the symptoms. There are different sizes of the pens for children and adults. Treatment for a severe allergic reaction doesn't stop with this injection; it just buys you time. You must still go to an emergency room for further treatment.

Sometimes food allergies simply go away, or resolve. Scientists don't understand why this happens. Many children can literally outgrow allergies to eggs, soy, wheat, and milk. In fact, as many as 85 percent of children with allergies to those foods will outgrow them. Unfortunately, allergies to fish, shellfish, and nuts are usually life-long and can be very serious.

Identifying food allergy symptoms

Symptoms of an immediate food allergy (one caused by IgE antibodies) may include, from least to most serious

>> Rash or hives

>> Tingling in the mouth

>> Abdominal pain

>> Dizziness or fainting

>> Difficulty swallowing

>> Nausea or vomiting

>> Difficulty breathing or wheezing

>> Stomach pain

>> Diarrhea

>> Chest pain

>> Swelling of the mouth or tongue

>> Drop in blood pressure

>> Anaphylactic shock

A visit to the doctor is in order if you or anyone in your family has experienced any of these symptoms after eating a specific food. Your doctor can run tests to positively identify the allergenic food and prescribe an EpiPen, which administers epinephrine, a chemical that stops the allergic reaction. She can also refer you to a nutritionist who can help you identify all the places where the allergenic foods can hide (such as eggs in salad dressings or peanuts in cookies).

REMEMBER

The vast majority of food allergies are not life-threatening, but they certainly are unpleasant. Although some symptoms are easy to connect with their offending foods, others are much more difficult to identify and require help from a physician skilled and knowledgeable in food allergy diagnosis and treatment. These physicians are often not the same as those skilled and knowledgeable in treating inhalant allergies.

Dr. James C. Breneman, former chair of the Food Allergy Committee of the American College of Allergy, says that food allergies, particularly nonimmediate, delayed-response-type food allergies, can be partially or completely responsible for the following symptoms:

» Arthritis

» Chronic lower back pain

» Eczema

» Itching

» Asthma

» Recurrent infections of throat, sinuses, lungs, and bladder

» Bedwetting

» Canker sores

» Gallbladder attacks

» Migraine headaches

Dr. Wright (one of the authors of this book) has followed Dr. Breneman's recommendations about the connection between food allergies and seemingly nonrelated symptoms since 1981 and has observed that you can prevent nearly 100 percent of gallbladder pain attacks, as well as nearly 100 percent of all bedwetting incidents, by carefully identifying and then eliminating specific food allergies.

Living with food allergies

If you've been diagnosed with a food allergy, you must be vigilant about what you do and do not eat. Fortunately, changing to the eating clean lifestyle can make avoiding particular foods much easier. Because common allergens, including gluten, MSG, nuts, and soy can appear in everything from salad dressing to candy bars, you automatically eliminate some allergens from your diet by sticking to whole foods. So eat whole, unprocessed foods and a healthy mix of clean meats, fruits, vegetables, and whole grains and you may get control of your allergies as well as a healthier body.

REMEMBER

Read labels carefully on the processed foods you do buy and figure out what names your particular allergen can hide behind. For people with severe allergies, eating a roll that was baked in a factory that uses eggs or soy in another product can be enough to trigger a reaction. For this reason, the FDA requires manufacturers to list the top-eight food allergens in "plain language" (in other words, no pseudonyms) on food labels. (If you're wondering which allergens make the top-eight list, check out the section "Avoiding key allergens.")

Be careful of cross-contamination! For someone with a severe allergy, eating a cookie that you removed from the cookie sheet with a spatula that touched a nut can be enough to trigger a reaction. If someone in your family has a severe allergy, keep your home and kitchen completely free of the offending food. For more information, see *Food Allergies For Dummies*, by Robert Wood (Wiley).

Decoding food sensitivity or intolerance

Food sensitivities and food intolerances are an entirely different matter. Some sensitivities are not intolerances. Areas of the body besides the gut and immune system can react to foods in an allergic fashion. For example, your nervous system can be sensitive to certain foods, causing you to have a seizure when you eat them. Many more people have food sensitivities than have true food allergies.

People can be intolerant to or sensitive to a variety of different foods and food ingredients. The most common ones are

- » Lactose
- » Gluten
- » Fructose
- » Yeast
- » Additives and preservatives
- » MSG

A *food allergy* is a biological response to a perceived attack on your body. A *food intolerance* usually means someone doesn't have the enzymes to digest a particular food. And a *sensitivity* is any type of negative response to a food, such as flushing or a rapid heartbeat. Diagnosing a food sensitivity or intolerance can be very difficult, because the reaction to the food can be delayed by hours or days, while the body's reaction to a true food allergy usually happens within minutes. Plus, food sensitivity or intolerance sometimes depends on the amount of food you consume. For instance, some people aren't sensitive to a certain food unless they consume a large quantity.

Symptoms of food sensitivity or intolerance include

>> Nausea

>> Vomiting

>> Diarrhea

>> Heartburn

>> Irritability

>> Cramping

>> Headaches

HOW FOOD MANUFACTURERS HIDE ALLERGENS

Unfortunately, some of the less common allergens can hide behind different names on food labels. People who are allergic or sensitive to MSG, for instance, must read labels and watch out for dozens of terms ranging from *autolyzed yeast* to *calcium caseinate* to *soy protein*.

Allergens can hide in other places in processed foods, too. For example, food manufacturers can use peanuts or peanut protein in curry paste or pudding mixes, and eggs can hide in salmon pate or pasta shells.

The easiest way to protect yourself against hidden allergens (and to keep you healthy at the same time) is to eat clean, whole foods and make your own curry pastes, pudding, salad dressings, and snack foods.

If you or a family member is experiencing any of these symptoms, you and your doctor can try to pinpoint which foods are behind them by doing one of the following:

>> **Elimination diet:** In this diet, you eliminate most foods from your diet and consume very basic, bland foods in their place for a certain period of time — usually one or two weeks. Then you add foods back into your diet, one at a time, and monitor the symptoms closely.

   If you decide to try an elimination diet, be sure to do so only under the care of a physician or nutritionist.

>> **Breath test:** If your body is unable to digest lactose, for instance, your doctor may have you take a breath test to verify that lactose is the problem. After eating a food containing the suspected ingredient (lactose, in this case), you breathe into a bag at certain intervals. The doctor then tests the air in the bag for the presence of hydrogen. Human breath usually contains very little hydrogen, but your body produces more hydrogen gases when bacteria in your GI tract cause undigested lactose to ferment. This test can also be used to test for lactose or sorbitol malabsorption.

As with food allergies, the only way to control a food intolerance is to avoid the offending food. Lucky for you, the eating clean lifestyle makes managing food intolerances much easier. After all, eating whole foods and avoiding processed foods help you keep hidden ingredients out of your diet so you can feel better and be healthier.

Avoiding key allergens

Although people can be allergic to or intolerant of many different kinds of food, nine foods cover 90 percent of all food allergies. Avoiding the foods you're allergic to is key. Watch out for cross-contamination and be vigilant. With practice, you'll get good at recognizing the presence of these foods in products.

Here are the nine main allergens, along with clean alternatives you can substitute for them in recipes and daily life:

>> **Cow's milk and other dairy products:** A cow's milk allergy appears only in the first year of life. Infants who are nursed until they start eating regular food are most vulnerable to this allergy. Children may outgrow a milk allergy. People with lactose intolerance aren't allergic to milk; they can't digest lactose, the sugar in milk, which means they can't eat any dairy products made with cow's milk.

   Why not nurse your infant for as long as you can? It's basic "clean eating" for babies! If you don't or can't nurse your infant, or if your child is allergic to cow's milk, look for organic formulas, and be sure to prepare them with clean, safe water. These formulas should not contain processed refined sugars, synthetic preservatives, palm oil, or carrageenan — read labels carefully. If you're eating clean, your infant can, too!

>> **Peanuts:** Peanut allergies can be life-threatening, and the tiniest amount of nut or nut dust can trigger a severe reaction. The protein in peanuts is very complex, which is why the reaction to it is so severe. If you don't outgrow this allergy, the reaction can become more severe over time.

Substitute other types of nuts as long as you know you're not allergic to them. In baking recipes, coconut or oatmeal make good substitutes for peanuts, and soy nuts provide a similar crunch and texture.

>> **Tree nuts:** Tree nuts include pecans, walnuts, Brazil nuts, and macadamia nuts, among others. Manufacturers use them in many foods you may not think contain nuts, like cereals, salad dressings, sauces, and ice cream. Although tree nut allergies can be quite severe, many of them aren't life-threatening.

Substitute toasted oatmeal or toasted breadcrumbs for chopped nuts in recipes.

>> **Eggs:** People usually outgrow allergies to eggs, but they can be lifelong and very serious. If you have an egg allergy, you must avoid anything made with eggs or egg protein, so watch out for terms on food labels like *albumin* and *egg protein.*

You can find some good egg substitutes in the store that mimic the function of eggs in baked goods. You can also combine 1 tablespoon of ground flaxseed with 3 tablespoons of water, beat the mixture well, and substitute it for one egg.

>> **Fish:** Fish allergies include allergies to cod, haddock, salmon, tuna, halibut, and other freshwater and saltwater fish. If you or someone in your family has a fish allergy, be careful with products like salad dressing, Worcestershire sauce, gelatin, and omega-3 supplements, which may contain fish products or extracts.

Substitute chicken or pork for fish in recipes.

>> **Shellfish:** An allergy to shellfish can be an allergy to mollusks, including oysters and clams, or to crustaceans, including shrimp, crayfish, lobsters, and crabs. Avoid all shellfish and watch out for products like glucosamine, which can be made from the shells of crustaceans. Also avoid snails, squid, and scallops.

Or just substitute chicken or pork for shellfish in recipes.

>> **Wheat:** If you suffer allergy-type symptoms after eating wheat, you may have a true wheat allergy, or you may have celiac disease or non-celiac gluten-gliadin intolerance (check out the section "Gluten Sensitivity and Celiac Disease" for details). Food labels can hide many forms of wheat, using terms like *farina, modified food starch,* or *bran,* so be aware of the complete list of terms to avoid. You can find these terms on the Internet on sites such as www.glutenfreefoodslist.net and www.projectallergy.com.

Substitute gluten-free mixes, flours, and other products for wheat-containing products.

>> **Corn:** Corn allergies can be mild or severe, and many people with corn allergies show cross-reactions to other grains as well. People with corn allergies may react to corn pollen, cornstarch, or grass pollen. So avoid foods like corn tortillas, margarine, corn oil, corn syrup, cornmeal, grits, hominy, and many breakfast cereals.

Substitute tapioca or arrowroot for cornstarch in recipes, and be sure to read labels carefully. You can find corn products in everything from peanut butter to fish sticks to cheese spreads.

>> **Soy:** Soy allergies can be difficult to accommodate because you find soy byproducts in many processed foods. Plus, a protein in soybeans can cause a cross-reaction in people with peanut allergies. Read labels and get familiar with the list of terms used to identify soy in processed foods (go to www.projectallergy.com for a list of these terms). Avoid edamame, tofu, tempeh, miso, and soy nuts.

You can substitute peas, green beans, or lima beans for edamame in recipes. Use sour cream in place of soft tofu.

Following the clean eating plan can help you avoid these allergens, but keep in mind that you may need to be more strict about staying on the plan. While many people employ an 80 percent clean, 20 percent not clean strategy for their eating clean plan, you may find that your compliance needs to approach 100 percent. Regardless, relying on fresh, unprocessed, whole foods is an excellent way to control allergies and intolerances.

REMEMBER

After you're diagnosed with an allergy and get familiar with the foods you need to avoid, you'll discover that adapting recipes to work with the foods you can eat is fairly easy to do. For instance, you can use quinoa in place of couscous in a salad recipe, substitute chicken thighs for salmon, or use almond milk or rice milk in place of cow's milk. As long as the food you use as a substitute is clean and fresh and a reasonable replacement for the allergenic food, most recipes work out just fine.

GMO FOODS AND ALLERGIES

In 1996, some manufacturers started putting DNA from certain foods into the seeds of soy, corn, cottonseed, and canola plants; the results are called *genetically modified foods* (or GMO foods). Specifically, manufacturers modified soybeans with a gene from a Brazil nut. Predictably, people allergic to tree nuts had reactions to those soybeans.

GMO foods may also be creating new proteins that many people could be allergic to. But no one will know for sure until people become sick.

Try to avoid GMO foods if you have allergies, and avoid them even if you don't!

Gluten Sensitivity and Celiac Disease

Celiac disease and non-celiac gluten sensitivity are both part of a special category of food allergies. A gluten allergy doesn't result in breathing problems or shock (like some severe food allergies do), but it can cause long-term damage to the body if left uncontrolled. People who are sensitive to gluten react to *gluten*, a protein found in wheat, rye, barley, and oats.

Celiac disease is a genetic disorder that develops into a chronic illness in which gluten damages the villi in the intestines, leading to poor absorption of nutrients and serious illness caused by vitamin deficiencies. *Non-celiac gluten sensitivity* is a response to the glutenin and gliadin proteins that make up gluten, and it's also associated with significant nutrient malabsorption.

In this section, we look at the differences between non-celiac gluten sensitivity and celiac disease, and we show you how to handle these conditions with the eating clean diet plan.

Identifying gluten sensitivity

Both non-celiac gluten sensitivity and celiac disease cause poor absorption of many essential nutrients, including essential amino acids, minerals, folate, and fat-soluble vitamins, including vitamin D. Celiac disease and a sensitivity to gluten can also lead to depression, chronic illnesses, or serious diseases like osteoporosis and cancer. (In fact, men who develop osteoporosis at a relatively young age often have non-celiac gluten sensitivity.)

In addition to malabsorption and other chronic illnesses, non-celiac gluten sensitivity may also cause the following symptoms:

- Mouth sores
- Chronic indigestion
- Intestinal gas
- Bloating and cramping
- Ulcers
- Chronic diarrhea
- Chronic constipation
- Muscle weakness
- Chronic fatigue
- Bone or joint pain
- Skin rashes

Symptoms of celiac disease may include:

- Chronic diarrhea
- Abdominal pain
- Weakness
- Smelly, fatty stools
- Bone or joint pain
- Osteoporosis
- Weight fluctuation
- Thyroiditis
- Osteoporosis
- Bone or joint pain
- Unexplained anemia

There's considerable overlap in symptoms of these two problems with gluten, but not total identity. Unfortunately, many of these symptoms can also be symptoms of other diseases or medical conditions, so be sure to see a doctor skilled and knowledgeable in the diagnosis of food allergies and sensitivities if you suspect a gluten sensitivity.

Doctors confirm a diagnosis of celiac disease with blood tests to measure the presence of antibodies against gluten and an intestinal biopsy to examine the intestinal wall. The diagnosis of non-celiac gluten sensitivity is best made with the anti-gliadin secretory IgA antibody test, done with a stool specimen.

Unfortunately, gluten sensitivity can be difficult to diagnose. A low or low-normal level of *triglycerides*, commonly measured blood fats, is often a sign of non-celiac gluten sensitivity. But the elimination diet can be the most inexpensive and efficient way to pinpoint gluten sensitivity. Eliminate gluten from your diet, and if you feel better, it's probably the problem.

REMEMBER

People who test negative for celiac disease can still be sensitive to gluten. After you and your doctor rule out other diseases, and if you feel better eliminating gluten from your diet, continue on that path. Also keep in mind that you can have non-celiac gluten sensitivity with no gastro-intestinal symptoms at all; just look at the previous list of symptoms for proof!

SHOULD YOU AVOID GLUTEN EVEN IF YOU AREN'T SENSITIVE?

So should people who aren't gluten sensitive or who don't have celiac disease avoid gluten? Some nutritionists think so. Interestingly enough, human beings don't need to consume any gluten-containing foods to be healthy.

If you aren't experiencing symptoms of gluten sensitivity or celiac disease, you can try a short experiment: Eliminate gluten from your diet for a period of two to three weeks and see how you feel. If you feel much better without gluten in your diet, then try to avoid it.

Dr. Christiane Northrup says that many women over the age of 40 should avoid gluten because it can be difficult to digest. People who suffer from fibromyalgia, certain skin conditions like dermatitis herpetiformis, asthma, rheumatoid arthritis, or irritable bowel syndrome (IBS) may also want to avoid gluten because gluten can aggravate those conditions. Talk to your doctor or a nutritionist about this issue to decide whether you should adopt the gluten-free lifestyle.

If you think you have a gluten sensitivity but all your tests are negative, try eliminating gluten from your diet anyway. Go on a gluten-free diet for a few weeks; then add gluten back in. If your symptoms reoccur, you may want to kick gluten to the curb.

Developing a gluten-free diet and lifestyle

If you or a member of your family has been diagnosed with celiac disease or non-celiac gluten sensitivity, removing gluten from your diet is very important. After all, "cheating" on this diet can permanently damage your intestines, which can lead to osteoporosis, depression and other mental illnesses, cancer, and other diseases associated with malnutrition (see the preceding section for details).

Setting up a gluten-free kitchen is an important first step in managing gluten sensitivity or celiac disease. Empty and thoroughly clean your kitchen and everything in it, including bread machines, toasters, cutting boards, and all utensils that may have been in contact with wheat, barley, rye, or oats. Even a tiny crumb can cause a reaction in someone with a severe case of celiac disease or gluten sensitivity.

Throw away any foods that contain gluten or that you suspect may have gluten. Then go shopping for safe foods, keeping a list of forbidden ingredients close at hand. Remember that gluten can hide in many different products, including prescription drugs, grated cheese, soy sauce, beer, and whiskey.

TIP

If you have to avoid gluten, you can include processed foods in a clean eating plan to make it work for you. Gluten-free baking mixes, gluten-free flour mixes, pasta made from rice, and other gluten-free products contain unusual ingredients like xanthan gum, which helps add structure to baked goods. But that and other additives like guar gum and gelatin are natural products so they still fit into your clean eating lifestyle. If you crave bread but can't eat gluten, use a gluten-free substitute instead of depriving yourself or eating wheat products.

If you have to buy processed foods for someone with celiac disease or non-celiac gluten sensitivity, be sure to avoid foods with the following label terms and ingredients:

- » **Barley:** This grain can hide in ingredient lists under the terms *malt, flavorings, coloring, flavor enhancers, hydrolyzed plant protein,* or *hydrolyzed vegetable protein.* Rice is a good substitute.

- » **Bran:** Bran is the outer covering of a cereal grain. It can come from corn and rice, as well as wheat, rye, and oats. Make sure the bran in any food's ingredient list comes only from corn or rice before you buy it.

- » **Bulgur:** Bulgur is simply wheat grains that have been processed or crushed so that they cook quickly. Use quinoa or rice as a substitute.

- » **Cereal:** Avoid any cereal product made from wheat, oats, barley, rye, triticale, or spelt. Look for cereals made from rice, corn, millet, quinoa, sorghum, wild rice, and teff.

>> **Couscous:** This pasta is made from steamed and cooked wheat. You see it most often as a side dish or in salads. Substitute millet or quinoa for couscous in recipes.

>> **Dinkle:** Dinkle is another name for spelt, which is a form of wheat.

>> **Farina:** People often cook and serve this cereal as a hot cereal or a side dish similar to polenta. For a substitute, use cooked cornmeal.

>> **Flour:** If you see this general term on a label, contact the manufacturer to find out which type of flour is in the product. However, we recommend avoiding these products even if you know the flour doesn't contain gluten, simply because manufacturers can change formulations without giving any notice.

>> **Food starch:** This ingredient can come from wheat, potatoes, rice, or corn. The term is too unspecific to be safe; avoid products with food starch in them.

>> **Graham flours:** This term is just another name for wheat flours. Substitute gluten-free flour mixes.

>> **Hulls:** Again, this word is too broad. Hulls from which grain? Unless the food's label specifically says *gluten-free,* assume that the hulls contain gluten and avoid it.

>> **Kamut:** A member of the wheat family, this ancient grain is very large. Some people who are gluten sensitive can eat this grain, but try it only under a doctor's or nutritionist's supervision. Substitute quinoa for this ingredient in recipes.

>> **Malt:** This ingredient is made from dried sprouted grain, usually wheat; It's used in brewing and as a food additive.

>> **Matzo:** Unleavened bread is usually made from wheat, so although it's unleavened (without yeast or baking powder), it isn't suitable for a gluten-free diet.

>> **Modified food starch:** Used as a thickener, stabilizer, and emulsifier, this ingredient appears in many foods. It's usually corn based, which is acceptable, but it may be made with wheat. Check with the manufacturer to make sure. (If the product is made in the United States, it must have a wheat ingredient disclaimer on the label.)

>> **Oats, oat bran, gum, or fiber:** Oat products don't contain gluten naturally, but cross-contamination is a real concern. Add oats to your diet carefully, and be sure to use only those products that have been grown and processed in a gluten-free environment or dedicated mill. See the nearby sidebar for more on oats.

>> **Rye:** Rye is one of the big three grains to avoid in a gluten-free diet because it contains gluten.

>> **Seitan:** This vegetarian protein substitute (which is often called *wheat meat*) is made from gluten, so people with gluten sensitivity and celiac disease need to avoid it.

>> **Spelt:** Although spelt is a non-wheat flour, it does contain gluten, although at a lower concentration than wheat. It's on the unsafe list for people with celiac disease and gluten sensitivity.

>> **Triticale:** This grain is a cross between rye and wheat, two of the main grains you must avoid on a gluten-free diet.

>> **Udon:** This Japanese noodle is made from wheat. Substitute rice noodles or other gluten-free noodle products.

>> **Wheat:** Obviously, you must avoid this one!

Because the eating clean plan focuses on eating lots of fruits and vegetables, clean meats, and grains like rice and corn, it's a fairly simple way to accommodate a gluten-free diet. Plus, you automatically eliminate a lot of potential problem foods because one main element of the eating clean plan is avoiding processed foods.

TIP

For more information about avoiding gluten, check out *Living Gluten-Free For Dummies* by Danna Korn, *Gluten-Free Baking For Dummies* by Dr. Jean Layton and Linda Larsen, and *Celiac Disease For Dummies* by Ian Blumer and Sheila Crowe (Wiley).

WHAT ABOUT OATS?

Oats are frequently grouped with the grains to avoid if you're gluten sensitive or have celiac disease. But oats themselves don't contain gluten, so why do people group them with wheat, barley, and rye? Farmers often grow oats in fields right next to wheat, barley, and rye, so cross-contamination is the big issue. Plus, manufacturers often process oats in the same plant as the other gluten-containing grains. Just a tiny amount of gluten can cause a severe reaction in some patients.

If you shop carefully, you may be able to find oats that are grown and processed with no exposure to wheat, barley, or rye. Look for oats in containers marked by the Gluten-Free Certification Organization as being gluten-free. Just be careful when you first decide to add oats to your diet and consume oats in moderation. Not all celiacs can consume uncontaminated oats.

Vegetarian Diets

People who avoid eating animal products are loosely classified as *vegetarians.* Although the eating clean plan includes clean meats and other animal products, you can easily adapt it to fit your vegetarian lifestyle.

In this section, we look at the different classifications within the vegetarian lifestyle and explain how you can accommodate each one with the clean eating plan.

REMEMBER

Because animal products are the best source of complete protein, getting enough protein is the main concern of any vegetarian diet. Combining foods and eating a varied diet are the best ways to get enough protein if you want to avoid eating animal products.

Understanding the levels of vegetarian diets

When someone claims to be a vegetarian, most people assume the person doesn't eat red meat, fish, poultry, pork, or eggs. But vegetarianism has different levels, all defined by what their proponents will and will not eat.

Here's a list of the main levels of vegetarianism, from most relaxed to most dedicated:

>> **Flexitarian:** These vegetarians sometimes eat a vegetarian diet and sometimes eat meat. They may pick a day or two out of the week to eat only vegetarian products.

>> **Pollo vegetarian:** Although you may find it difficult to believe, people in this group add chicken to their "vegetarian" diet. Because they don't eat red meat, they consider themselves vegetarians.

>> **Pescatarian:** Fish lovers add fish to their vegetarian diets. They eat salmon, halibut, cod, and other white fish, along with shellfish like shrimp and clams. Many vegetarians add fish to their diets to capitalize on the healthy benefits in omega-3 fatty acids.

>> **Ovo-lacto vegetarian:** This category includes people who eat eggs (ovo) and dairy products (lacto). Milk, cheese, yogurt, sour cream, and egg products are on this diet's list of foods okay to eat. This variation has some variations of its own: Some people add only eggs to their vegetarian diet, while others add only milk products.

>> **Vegan:** Vegans are the truest vegetarians; they don't eat any food produced by animals or made using animals.

>> **Raw vegan:** Like vegans, people in this category consume only plant-based foods, but, to take it a step further, they don't heat any of their foods above 115 degrees for nutritional reasons. This diet is also called the *raw food diet* or the *macrobiotic diet.*

>> **Fruitarian:** People in this group don't eat anything based on killing. So they eat the products of plants, such as fruit, nuts, and seeds, but they don't eat anything that harms or kills a plant, let alone an animal.

Accommodating these different vegetarian diets is easy to do with the clean eating plan. You just have to make sure that someone following one of these diets eats a wide variety of food (as wide as the plan allows) and considers adding a vitamin supplement to the diet. Protein, vitamin B12, and sometimes iron are the main nutrients you need to worry about in vegetarian diets, more so as the diet becomes "stricter." Vitamin B12 can be more difficult than protein and iron to incorporate into clean vegetarian diets, so vegetarians often have to take supplements to get this nutrient.

Combining foods for complete proteins

The main challenge for vegetarians — since most of them eat plenty of fruits and vegetables — is getting enough protein in their daily diet. Although nutritionists used to recommend eating protein at every meal, they now know that vegetarians can balance protein intake over a whole day. So you don't have to combine proteins at every meal to get a good amount of *complete protein* (that is, all the essential amino acids human beings need).

Most healthy adults need about 50 grams of complete protein every day. Pregnant and nursing women and people with chronic health problems may need more. Because only animal products (with a few exceptions) contain complete proteins, vegetarians must combine protein sources in combinations called *complementary proteins.* Of course, vegetarians who eat eggs, milk, or fish don't have to worry about getting enough protein.

Eating a variety of protein sources is key. The best protein sources for vegetarians include the following:

>> **Grains:** Only amaranth, quinoa (which is really a seed!), buckwheat, and spirulina (which is an algae) contain all the essential amino acids your body needs. Use these hearty foods as hot cereal, in casseroles, and in side dishes. Although these foods provide complete proteins, they don't score 100 percent on the Protein Digestibility Corrected Amino Acid Score (PDCAAS; see Chapter 3 for details).

>> **Soy protein:** Soy protein has all the essential amino acids and scores 100 percent on the PDCAAS scale. You can add soy flour, soybeans, and other products, including tofu, to your clean vegetarian diet.

>> **Legumes with grains:** This protein combination pairs legumes, which are missing the amino acids methionine, cystine, and tryptophan, with brown rice or wheat, which are rich in those amino acids. Other good combinations include beans with tortillas, hummus with bread, or garbanzo beans (also called chickpeas) with brown rice.

>> **Legumes with nuts:** Combining legumes, which include black beans, kidney beans, garbanzo beans, cannellini beans, and brown beans, with nuts like pecans, peanuts, walnuts, hazelnuts, and almonds provides complete protein.

>> **Legumes with seeds:** Combining seeds, including sesame seeds, sunflower seeds, pumpkin seeds, chia, and flaxseed, with legumes provides complete protein. Hummus, which is a combination of garbanzo beans and sesame seeds, is a great way to combine these foods in a vegetarian diet.

>> **Seitan and meat substitutes:** These protein sources are processed, so you may want to include them sparingly in your clean diet. But because they provide 100 percent of all the essential amino acids, they're acceptable on the eating clean plan.

Vegetarians also need to make sure they get enough calcium, iron, and vitamin B12. (The main sources for these nutrients are dairy products and red meat.) Good vegetarian sources of calcium include dark leafy greens, broccoli, almonds, rice milk, and fortified juices. Good sources of iron include lentils, soy, spinach, dark leafy greens, and garbanzo beans. One brand of nutritional yeast, Red Star T-6635+, contains active vitamin B12. Other vegetarian sources of vitamin B12 include fortified cereals and soy products, but read the labels carefully. Often, supplemental vitamin B12 is the easiest and most reliable source.

LIMITING AMINO ACIDS

The amino acid that's in short supply in any grain, legume, nut, or seed is called a *limiting amino acid*. Your body needs nine amino acids that it can't make on its own. On a vegetarian diet, legumes, grains, nuts, and seeds have all the amino acids you need, but each food is missing one or more of them.

Think of your body as a bike repair shop. If the shop doesn't get enough handlebars (one type of protein), it can make only a limited number of bicycles. But if a new supplier delivers lots of handlebars, the shop can produce many bikes. The same thing is true with vegetarian diets and limiting amino acids.

The Vegan Lifestyle

Veganism is the purest form of vegetarianism. People following this diet eat no animal products at all. In fact, some even avoid honey produced by bees, and many don't wear leather, silk, wool, or fur. Like vegetarians, vegans must eat a varied diet to get a good amount of nutrients.

In this section, we look at what nutrient–related challenges vegans face, why protein is key, and how the eating clean plan can make getting essential nutrients easier even when you're avoiding animal products.

Getting plenty of nutrients on the clean vegan diet

Most vegans already avoid processed foods because manufacturers use animal products like butter, eggs, and protein extracts to make many of them. But if you decide to go the vegan way, make sure you eat a rich variety of dark leafy greens, fruits, vegetables, nuts, seeds, legumes, and grains to get all the nutrients you need. A good multivitamin can help fill in any missing nutrients; you may also want to add specific supplements to your diet.

For best health, vegans need to focus on getting the following nutrients:

>> **Calcium:** To get enough calcium, eat a lot of dark-green vegetables, soy or rice milk that has been fortified with extra calcium, and tofu made with calcium sulfate. You may also add a calcium supplement to make sure you're consuming enough of this bone-strengthening mineral.

>> **Vitamin D:** The vegan diet doesn't include many vitamin D-rich foods. You can find fortified orange juice and rice and soy milk, but the best source of vitamin D is sunshine. Expose your skin to the sun at least a few minutes per day until the first sign of pinkness, but don't use sunscreen during this time because sunscreen limits your skin's ability to make this essential vitamin. At the point of pinkness, cover up or apply a sunscreen. You can also add a vitamin D supplement to your diet.

>> **Iron:** You can obtain iron by eating kidney beans and other legumes, blackstrap molasses, dark leafy greens like Swiss chard, kale, beet greens, soybeans, and fruits like grapes and watermelon.

>> **Vitamin B12:** The recommended daily allowance (RDA) for this vitamin is quite low, but vegans need to be sure they get enough of it. The nutritional

yeast we discuss in the section "Combining foods for complete proteins" as well as some fortified soy milks and cereals are good sources, but you may need to add a supplement to your diet.

Remembering that protein is key

Getting enough protein is the key to maintaining a balanced vegan diet. You need to combine proteins in the vegan diet the same way you do in the vegetarian diet (see the section "Combining foods for complete proteins"). Also include tofu, textured vegetable protein (TVP), and protein powder in your recipes. Remember that your body stores protein and draws upon those stores when needed, so you don't have to eat complete proteins at every single meal.

Eating a wide variety of clean vegetables, which provide good amounts of protein (albeit not the complete form), is a great way to get protein when you're living a vegan lifestyle. Here are some of the best vegetable protein sources:

» Avocados contain 3 grams of protein per serving.

» Russet potatoes, eaten with the skin, have 4 grams of protein per serving.

» Broccoli has about 3 grams of protein per serving.

» Spinach has 2 grams of protein per serving.

So enjoy the vegan lifestyle on your clean eating plan. Remember the rule of clean eating: Combine protein with carbohydrates to satisfy your appetite. Hummus, peanut butter, soy, and vegetable combinations are all delicious when you eat them with whole grains.

5
Morning to Evening Recipes

IN THIS PART . . .

Get delicious and satisfying breakfast recipes.

Learn about clean lunches for eating on the go.

Find tasty and healthy recipes for dinner.

Get some great snack and dessert ideas to satisfy the munchies.

Chapter 15

Waking Up to Great Food: Satisfying Breakfast Recipes

Everybody knows that eating a good breakfast is the best way to start the day. But do you know why? In this chapter, we take a look at why eating a healthy and balanced breakfast meal is so important. Then to help you start your day off right, we include 12 clean recipes that are easy, delicious, and satisfying.

When you make these recipes, you have a few choices for the type of ingredients you use. You can go the 100 percent organic route, you can use some convenience foods, like bottled salsa and grated cheese, or you can use whatever ingredients you have on hand.

If you're thinking a clean, homemade breakfast sounds great but you seldom have time to cook in the morning, don't skip this chapter yet! You can make many of the recipes we include here ahead of time and then just heat them in the toaster oven or on the stovetop. If you do freeze or refrigerate these recipes, remember to wrap them well and label everything. In the morning, the last thing you want to do is try to decipher what's in your freezer!

Understanding the Importance of Breakfast

During the day, how long can you go without getting hungry? Six hours is usually the maximum time between meals. So just think about how much your body needs breakfast, after eight hours of sleep!

Breakfast provides the fuel for the rest of your day. Studies show that people who eat breakfast perform better at all tasks, have more energy throughout the day, and tend to weigh less than those who skip this important meal. Eating first thing in the morning also lowers your liver's production of bad LDL cholesterol.

One of the neatest things about being a grown-up is that you get to decide what you want to eat. If you don't like traditional breakfast foods like eggs or cereal, don't eat them. Instead, eat what you like! A pasta salad with lots of chicken and fruit makes an excellent breakfast, especially if you make it with whole-wheat pasta, organic chicken, a yogurt-based dressing, and organic fruit. You can also make a breakfast pizza using homemade whole-wheat crust, scrambled eggs or tofu, sautéed veggies, and good artisan cheese.

REMEMBER

Whatever you decide to have for breakfast, keep the following guidelines in mind to get the most out of the meal:

>> **Combine protein with carbohydrates and good fats.** Your brain needs carbohydrates for fuel. Protein and fats help keep you feeling satisfied longer.

>> **Try to eat whole fruits rather than fruit juices.** If your family has a history of obesity or diabetes, avoiding fruit juices is even more important. If you like to drink your breakfast, make a smoothie with whole fruits.

>> **Turn your favorite breakfast into a clean meal.** For example, if you love frosted crisp cereal, make Baked Oatmeal instead. If you like those processed breakfast bowls found in the frozen food aisle (yes, the ones full of sodium and preservatives), try making the Wild Rice Egg Roll Ups instead.

Starting Your Day the Right Way with Some Tasty Breakfast Recipes

When you make the recipes in this chapter, follow the directions carefully. But don't be afraid to substitute some of your favorite ingredients for others, especially in the nonbaking recipes. For instance, you can add a couple of jalapeño chilies to the Avocado Toast with Scrambled Eggs or your favorite veggies to the Chicken and Spinach Mini Quiches. Whenever you make a change in the recipe, just be sure to write it down. Forgetting the little changes you make here and there is easy to do, and you don't want to lose your delicious, new creations!

REMEMBER

If you want to use organic ingredients for these recipes, that's great. But know that organic foods aren't necessary to the clean eating plan. Check out Chapter 10 for a list of the fifteen foods you should always try to buy organic and a list of the foods that are just fine grown conventionally.

STAY AWAY FROM DAIRY PRODUCTS WITH rBGH

Many people like to drink milk in the morning. Or they serve milk to their children. Although doctors skilled and knowledgeable in nutritional medicine frequently recommend avoiding cow's milk and dairy products for optimal health, dairy products can be a healthy choice for some people. Just be careful not to drink too much milk. The Harvard Physicians' and Nurses' Studies found that increased quantities of cow's milk are associated with increased risk of prostate cancer and increased risk of osteoporosis.

The hormones and antibiotics in milk can also be problematic. Bovine growth hormone, or rBGH (also called *recombinant bovine growth hormone*), first made the news a few years ago. Many countries around the world have banned the use of rBGH simply because it gets into the milk and dairy products that humans consume. Farmers use rBGH to artificially increase milk production, but it can also damage the cow's udders and cause disease.

If you do choose to consume milk and other dairy products, buy organic milk harvested from grass-fed cows. And look for the phrase *produced without rBGH* on the label.

Cantaloupe Banana Smoothies

PREP TIME: 10 MIN | **YIELD: 4 SERVINGS**

INGREDIENTS

2 cups peeled, cubed cantaloupe

1 banana, peeled, cut into chunks, and frozen

½ cup orange juice

1 tablespoon lemon juice

1 cup yogurt

1 tablespoon flaxseed

1 teaspoon vanilla extract

DIRECTIONS

1 Combine the cantaloupe, banana, orange juice, and lemon juice in a blender or food processor. Cover and blend on high until the fruits are well mixed.

2 Add the yogurt, flaxseed, and vanilla. Cover and blend on high until the mixture is smooth. Divide the smoothie evenly into four glasses and serve immediately.

PER SERVING: Calories 121 (From Fat 28); Fat 3g (Saturated 1g); Cholesterol 8mg; Sodium 36mg; Carbohydrate 21g (Dietary Fiber 2g); Protein 4g.

VARY It! You can switch up this simple recipe in many ways. For example, use honeydew melon in place of the cantaloupe or add a peeled, sliced peach or pear to the mix. Or add a handful of frozen spinach or kale for even more nutrients.

Wild Rice Egg Roll-Ups

| PREP TIME: 15 MIN | COOK TIME: 35–45 MIN | YIELD: 6 SERVINGS |

INGREDIENTS

½ cup wild rice, rinsed

5 cups water

8 eggs

1 tablespoon olive oil

1 onion, minced

⅓ cup golden raisins

½ cup minced celery

2 tablespoons minced green onions

2 teaspoons curry powder

¼ teaspoon turmeric

½ cup lowfat Greek yogurt

Six 6-inch whole-wheat tortillas

DIRECTIONS

1 Place the wild rice in a medium saucepan; add 1½ cups of water. Bring the rice and water mixture to a boil over high heat. Cover the pan, reduce the heat to low, and simmer for 35 to 45 minutes, or until the rice is tender. Drain well and set aside.

2 Place the eggs in a 2-quart saucepan and cover them with water. Bring the eggs and water to a boil over high heat; boil for 1 minute.

3 Cover the pan of eggs and remove it from heat. Let it stand for 12 minutes.

4 Uncover the pan, place it in the sink, and run cold water over the eggs until they're cold to the touch. Tap the eggs against the side of the pan under the water; let them stand for 5 minutes. Peel the eggs.

5 In a large saucepan, combine the olive oil and minced onion. Cook the oil and onion over medium heat, stirring frequently, until the onion is tender; remove from heat.

6 Chop the hard-boiled eggs and add them to the oil and onion mixture along with the wild rice, raisins, celery, and green onions. Stir in the curry powder, turmeric, and yogurt.

7 Place the tortillas on your work surface. Scoop an equal amount of the egg mixture onto each tortilla. Roll up each tortilla and serve immediately.

PER SERVING: Calories 301 (From Fat 91); Fat 10g (Saturated 3g); Cholesterol 285mg; Sodium 271mg; Carbohydrate 43g (Dietary Fiber 4g); Protein 16g.

TIP: You can make the egg filling for these roll ups ahead of time. Just refrigerate it and reheat it in a saucepan when you're ready to eat it. Or if you prefer, serve it cold.

Baked Oatmeal

PREP TIME: 15 MIN	COOK TIME: 40–50 MIN	YIELD: 8 SERVINGS

INGREDIENTS

2 cups old-fashioned rolled oats

½ teaspoon baking powder

¼ teaspoon cinnamon

⅛ teaspoon cardamom

1 cup cooked farro or barley

1⅔ cups plain almond milk

2 eggs

¼ cup maple syrup

2 tablespoons melted butter

2 teaspoons vanilla extract

DIRECTIONS

1 Preheat oven to 350 degrees. Grease a 9-inch square baking dish with butter.

2 In large bowl, combine the oats, baking powder, cinnamon, and cardamom, and mix well. Set aside.

3 In a medium bowl, combine the cooked farro or barley, almond milk, eggs, maple syrup, butter, and vanilla, and mix until combined. Stir into the oat mixture and transfer to the prepared baking dish.

4 Bake for 40 to 50 minutes or until a food thermometer registers 160 degrees.

PER SERVING: Calories 162 (From Fat 44); Fat 5g (Saturated 2g); Cholesterol 8mg; Sodium 47mg; Carbohydrate 26g (Dietary Fiber 3g); Protein 4g.

TIP: To get 1 cup of cooked barley, combine ⅓ cup barley and ¾ cup water in a saucepan. Simmer for 40 to 50 minutes or until tender, then drain, if necessary. For the farro, combine ½ cup farro with 1 cup water; simmer for 30 to 35 minutes or until tender.

Toasted Oat and Barley Hot Cereal

PREP TIME: 15 MIN, PLUS STANDING TIME | COOK TIME: ABOUT 5 HR | YIELD: 12 SERVINGS

INGREDIENTS

1 cup steel-cut oats

1 cup uncooked pearl barley, rinsed

1 apple, peeled and chopped

½ cup chopped dates

⅓ cup dried cranberries

1 teaspoon ground cinnamon

¼ teaspoon ground cardamom

1 tablespoon pure maple syrup

6 cups water

DIRECTIONS

1 Place the oats in a medium saucepan over medium heat. Toast the oats, stirring frequently, until the oats are fragrant and start to turn a light golden brown. Remove the saucepan from heat.

2 In a 3-quart slow cooker, combine the toasted oats, barley, apple, dates, and cranberries. Sprinkle the mixture with the cinnamon and cardamom and drizzle the maple syrup over everything.

3 Add the water to the mixture and stir gently. Set the slow cooker to hold for 2 hours. Then set it to cook on low for 5 hours.

4 Stir the mixture and serve warm with more maple syrup or honey to drizzle on top (if desired). Each serving consists of 1 cup of cereal.

PER SERVING: Calories 150 (From Fat 11); Fat 1g (Saturated 0g); Cholesterol 0mg; Sodium 2mg; Carbohydrate 33g (Dietary Fiber 5g); Protein 4g.

NOTE: Oatmeal and barley are whole grains, which provide lots of fiber, B vitamins, and protein. Steel-cut oats are less processed than rolled oats and can stand up to slow-cooker cooking.

Avocado Toast with Scrambled Egg

PREP TIME: 15 MIN | COOK TIME: 15 MIN | YIELD: 4 SERVINGS

INGREDIENTS

2 avocados

2 tablespoons lemon juice

5 eggs

2 tablespoons plain almond milk

1 tablespoon butter

⅛ teaspoon salt

⅛ teaspoon pepper

4 slices whole-grain bread or Whole Grain and Nut Bread (see recipe later in this chapter)

1 cup cherry tomatoes, chopped

2 tablespoons minced fresh parsley

⅓ cup crumbled goat cheese

DIRECTIONS

1 Peel the avocados, remove the pits, and place in a medium bowl. Add the lemon juice and mash with a fork until the avocado is slightly chunky. Set aside.

2 In another medium bowl, beat the eggs with the almond milk in a medium bowl. In a small skillet, melt the butter.

3 Add the eggs to the skillet and sprinkle with the salt and pepper. Cook over medium-low heat until the eggs are set but still moist.

4 While the eggs are cooking, toast the bread slices until light golden brown; set aside.

5 Then, in a small bowl, combine the cherry tomatoes, parsley, and goat cheese and mix gently.

6 Spread the avocado mixture on the toast and top with the egg. Top with the tomato mixture and serve immediately.

PER SERVING: Calories 328 (From Fat 200); Fat 22g (Saturated 7g); Cholesterol 17mg; Sodium 307mg; Carbohydrate 23g (Dietary Fiber 9g); Protein 13g.

Chicken Pear Sausages

PREP TIME: 15 MIN, PLUS FREEZING TIME | COOK TIME: ABOUT 30 MIN | YIELD: 20 SERVINGS

INGREDIENTS

1 pound boneless, skinless chicken breast

½ pound boneless, skinless chicken thighs

2 ice cubes

1 large onion, minced

2 cloves garlic, minced

1 tablespoon plus 2 tablespoons olive oil

2 Bosc pears, peeled and diced

1 tablespoon lemon juice

2 tablespoons fresh thyme leaves, minced

½ teaspoon sea salt

¼ teaspoon white pepper

1 tablespoon butter

DIRECTIONS

1 Cube the chicken and place it in the freezer for 15 minutes.

2 Remove the chicken from the freezer and place it in a food processor; add the ice cubes. Cover and pulse until the chicken is medium grind (chunky but not finely minced). Cover and refrigerate.

3 In a large skillet, cook the onion and garlic with 1 tablespoon of olive oil over medium heat until the onion and garlic are tender, about 6 to 7 minutes. Stir frequently. Add the pears and lemon juice; cook for 1 minute longer. Place the mixture in a large bowl to cool.

4 Add the ground chicken, thyme, sea salt, and white pepper to the onion mixture. Mix gently with your hands until the mixture is combined well. Form the mixture into 20 patties that are about ½ inch thick.

5 Heat the butter and 2 tablespoons of olive oil in a large skillet and add half of the sausage patties. Cook, turning once, until a meat thermometer registers 165 degrees, about 8 to 11 minutes. Move the patties to a covered dish to keep warm. Cook the remaining sausage patties. Serve immediately.

PER SERVING: Calories 38 (From Fat 15); Fat 2g (Saturated 0g); Cholesterol 11mg; Sodium 68mg; Carbohydrate 2g (Dietary Fiber 0g); Protein 4g.

TIP: You can freeze the uncooked sausage patties in a tightly wrapped container for up to four months. When you're ready to cook them, let the patties thaw overnight in the refrigerator. Sauté them in a little olive oil for 6 to 8 minutes on each side, turning once, until the temperature registers 165 degrees.

Cranberry Nut Muffins

PREP TIME: 15 MIN | **COOK TIME: 18–23 MIN** | **YIELD: 12 SERVINGS**

INGREDIENTS

1¾ cups whole-wheat flour

1 cup old-fashioned rolled oats

⅓ cup maple sugar flakes

1½ teaspoons baking powder

½ teaspoon baking soda

¼ teaspoon sea salt

2 eggs

⅓ cup plain almond milk

2 tablespoons butter, melted

⅓ cup applesauce

2 tablespoons honey

2 teaspoons vanilla extract

1 medium banana, peeled and mashed

1½ cups fresh or frozen (unthawed) cranberries, coarsely chopped

½ cup chopped pecans

DIRECTIONS

1 Preheat the oven to 375 degrees. Line a 12-cup muffin pan with paper liners or grease the pan with butter; set aside.

2 In a large bowl, combine the whole-wheat flour, oats, maple sugar flakes, baking powder, baking soda, and sea salt; mix well and set aside.

3 In a small bowl, combine the eggs, almond milk, melted butter, applesauce, honey, vanilla, and banana; mix well.

4 Stir the egg mixture into the flour mixture just until combined. Fold in the cranberries and pecans. Spoon the batter into the prepared muffin pan.

5 Bake for 15 to 20 minutes, or until the muffins are set and lightly browned. Remove the muffins from the pan and cool them on a wire rack before serving.

PER SERVING: Calories 185 (From Fat 55); Fat 6g (Saturated 2g); Cholesterol 5mg; Sodium 173mg; Carbohydrate 26g (Dietary Fiber 4g); Protein 5g.

Whole Grain and Nut Bread

PREP TIME: 15 MIN	COOK TIME: 45 MIN	YIELD: 8 SERVINGS

INGREDIENTS

2 cups whole-wheat flour

½ cup plus 1 tablespoon bread flour

⅓ cup finely chopped walnuts

¼ cup rye flour

1¼ teaspoons dry yeast

¼ teaspoon salt

1½ cups warm water

1 tablespoon olive oil

DIRECTIONS

1 In a large bowl, combine the whole-wheat flour, ½ cup bread flour, walnuts, rye flour, yeast, and salt.

2 Add the warm water to the flour mixture and stir well, just until the flour disappears. Brush the top of the dough with the olive oil.

3 Cover the bowl with plastic wrap, then a kitchen towel, and let rise at room temperature for 12 to 18 hours.

4 Sprinkle the dough with 1 tablespoon bread flour and gently knead the dough right in the bowl a few times, and then form it into a rough round loaf. Place on a 14-inch long sheet of parchment paper. Cover the dough with an upside-down large bowl and let rise at room temperature for 2 hours.

5 Preheat the oven to 425 degrees. Place a 5- to 6-quart covered cast-iron Dutch oven in the oven and heat for 20 minutes.

6 Cut an X in the top of the dough using a sharp knife or razor blade. Carefully remove the lid of the Dutch oven and lower the bread, still on the parchment paper, into the hot Dutch oven. Cover.

7 Put the Dutch oven into the preheated oven and bake, covered, for 25 minutes. Then remove the cover and bake the bread for 20 to 25 minutes longer, until a thermometer registers 210 degrees and the bread is dark golden brown. Remove the bread from the Dutch oven using the parchment paper sling, and cool on a wire rack.

PER SERVING: Calories 193 (From Fat 51); Fat 6g (Saturated 1g); Cholesterol 0mg; Sodium 75mg; Carbohydrate 31g (Dietary Fiber 5g); Protein 6g.

Matcha Chia Smoothies

PREP TIME: 10 MIN | **YIELD: 2 SERVINGS**

INGREDIENTS

1 cup apple juice

2 tablespoons white chia seeds

3 kiwifruit, seeds removed, peeled, and chopped

1 frozen banana, cut into chunks

1 tablespoon matcha powder

1 cup plain almond or soy milk

DIRECTIONS

1 In a small bowl, combine the apple juice and chia seeds and refrigerate, covered, overnight.

2 Place the mixture in a blender.

3 Add all the remaining ingredients and blend until smooth.

4 Serve immediately.

PER SERVING: Calories 280 (From Fat 59); Fat 7g (Saturated 1g); Cholesterol 0mg; Sodium 10mg; Carbohydrate 54g (Dietary Fiber 12g); Protein 5g.

TIP: Matcha is a type of Japanese green tea. The powder dissolves quickly in water and can be used in many recipes. It's packed with antioxidants, including catechins, and actually contains more of these cancer-fighting compounds than blueberries or pomegranates do.

Fruit Compote

INGREDIENTS

1 cup water

2 tablespoons honey

2 cinnamon sticks

3 apples, peeled and chopped

3 pears, peeled and chopped

8 dried apricots, chopped

8 dates, chopped

½ cup dried cranberries

⅛ teaspoon sea salt

DIRECTIONS

1 In a 2-quart saucepan, combine the water, honey, cinnamon sticks, apples, pears, and dried apricots. Bring the mixture to a simmer over medium heat. Cook, stirring occasionally, until the apples and pears are softened, about 8 to 10 minutes.

2 Use a slotted spoon to remove the fruit from the pan and place it in a medium bowl. Stir the dates, dried cranberries, and sea salt into the fruit mixture.

3 Remove the cinnamon sticks from the liquid and discard them. Return the liquid to a boil and heat until the liquid is reduced to ⅓ cup. Pour the liquid over the fruit. Cool, stirring occasionally.

4 For each serving, serve 1 cup of the fruit compote over yogurt or cottage cheese or on top of hot or cold cereal.

PER SERVING: Calories 304 (From Fat 5); Fat 1g (Saturated 0g); Cholesterol 0mg; Sodium 101mg; Carbohydrate 81g (Dietary Fiber 8g); Protein 1g.

VARY IT! This easy recipe is also delicious with waffles or pancakes or as a topping on French toast.

NOTE: Cover any leftover fruit compote and store it in the refrigerator for up to 3 days.

Chicken and Spinach Mini Quiches

| PREP TIME: 15 MIN | COOK TIME: 30–35 MIN | YIELD: 6 SERVINGS |

INGREDIENTS

1 tablespoon olive oil

1 small onion, diced

1 boneless, skinless chicken breast, cut into small pieces

1 cup baby spinach leaves, chopped

4 eggs

⅓ cup lowfat Greek or regular yogurt

½ teaspoon dried thyme leaves

⅛ teaspoon pepper

3 tablespoons flour

1 cup shredded Muenster or Monterey Jack cheese

DIRECTIONS

1 Preheat the oven to 350 degrees. Grease a 12-cup muffin pan with a bit of butter and set aside.

2 In a small saucepan, heat the olive oil over medium heat. Add the onion; cook and stir for 2 minutes. Add the chicken; cook and stir for 3 to 5 minutes or until the chicken is no longer pink. Add the spinach; cook for 2 to 3 minutes, or until the spinach has wilted and the chicken is thoroughly cooked. Remove the pan from the heat and drain if necessary.

3 In a medium bowl, combine the eggs, yogurt, thyme, and pepper; mix well. Stir the flour and cheese into the egg mixture. Add the cooked chicken mixture to the egg and cheese mixture and stir gently.

4 Spoon into the prepared muffin pan. Bake the quiches for 23 to 28 minutes, or until they are set and light golden brown.

5 Let the quiches cool for 3 minutes; then run a knife around the edge of each quiche to loosen it from the pan. Remove the quiches from the pan and serve warm.

PER SERVING: Calories 188 (From Fat 82); Fat 9g (Saturated 4g); Cholesterol 43mg; Sodium 197mg; Carbohydrate 8g (Dietary Fiber 3g); Protein 18g.

Whole-Grain Waffles

| PREP TIME: 15 MIN | COOK TIME: ABOUT 15–20 MIN | YIELD: 8 SERVINGS |

INGREDIENTS

1 cup rolled oats

2 cups whole-wheat flour

⅓ cup oat bran

2 teaspoons baking powder

1 teaspoon baking soda

½ teaspoon sea salt

1 cup cottage cheese

½ cup soy or almond milk

2 tablespoons orange juice

2 eggs

3 egg whites

2 tablespoons honey

2 tablespoons olive oil

DIRECTIONS

1 Place the oats in a food processor or blender. Cover and blend until the oats are finely ground. Place them in a large mixing bowl.

2 Stir in the whole-wheat flour, oat bran, baking powder, baking soda, and sea salt. Mix the dry ingredients with a wire whisk to blend.

3 In a medium bowl, combine the cottage cheese, soy milk, orange juice, eggs, egg whites, honey, and olive oil; mix until smooth.

4 Add the wet ingredients to the dry ingredients and mix just until combined; the batter will be lumpy.

5 Preheat a waffle iron according to the manufacturer's instructions. Brush the iron lightly with a little olive oil.

6 Add ½ cup of batter to the waffle iron, close the iron, and cook until the steaming stops. The amount of time depends on your waffle iron. Open the iron and remove the waffle. Repeat this step with the rest of the batter. Serve each waffle with butter, syrup, or honey.

PER SERVING: Calories 252 (From Fat 68); Fat 8g (Saturated 2g); Cholesterol 57mg; Sodium 537mg; Carbohydrate 37g (Dietary Fiber 6g); Protein 13g.

Chapter 16

Refueling Your Body with Some Smart Lunches

A h, lunch. Remember the three-martini lunch made famous by the movie *Wall Street*? Not surprisingly, that particular "meal" isn't clean. Lunch is a time to take a break from the workday and refuel your body, so put the martini back on the shelf and grab a salad (or pita or soup or sandwich . . . you get the idea).

Even if you're following the plan of eating every three to four hours, lunch is still an important meal. It fuels your body for the afternoon and keeps everything running after breakfast and your midmorning snack.

When you follow the eating clean plan, lunch from the hot dog stand isn't necessarily a thing of the past. You can treat yourself occasionally to a less-than-clean food. But the majority of your lunches should be healthy. Don't worry; they can be delicious, too. In this chapter, we look at what makes a healthy lunch, and we walk you through some quick and easy lunch recipes, including Clean Cobb Salad, Roasted Veggie Hummus Pitas, and Salmon Avocado Summer Rolls.

Making Smart Lunch Choices

When you're eating clean, packing your lunch is the easiest way to make sure you get in all the nutrients and energy you need to get through the rest of the day. After all, most lunch places, especially those that serve food quickly, don't offer very healthy meal choices. Packing your own lunch not only saves you money but also helps you feel secure as you embark on a new lifestyle. If you have clean food packed and ready to eat, you won't be tempted by the vending machine or the local fast-food joint.

Okay, so you're ready to pack your own clean lunch . . . now what? Despite what you may think, cleaning up the traditional lunch foods is relatively easy to do. For example, you can transform a high-sodium, high-preservative soup and sandwich meal into a good, clean choice by making your own soup or buying organic soup packed in a BPA-free can. Clean up a chicken sandwich by using whole-grain bread, cooking your own chicken, using Greek yogurt as a spread in place of mayonnaise, and adding lots of veggies.

To get the most out of your lunches, be sure to do the following:

>> **Make time to eat lunch — even in the middle of a busy workday.** Your body and brain need fuel to function well. You can eat at your desk, but try to take fifteen or twenty minutes to get outside for a change of scenery.

>> **Enjoy your food.** Try not to gulp down your meal. Chew each bite thoroughly and concentrate on the flavors and textures of the clean food.

>> **Combine proteins with carbohydrates and good fats to keep your body fueled for the rest of your day.** For example, you can make a simple sandwich full of fuel for the day by using whole-grain bread, adding a clean protein like organic cheese, and mixing in dark greens and vegetables.

KEEPING YOUR LUNCH SAFE

Follow these food safety rules when you're packing your lunch:

- If the food is perishable, be sure to pack a frozen gel pack and use an insulated bag to keep the food temperature at 40 degrees or below.

- Make sure that you keep hot foods, like soup, above 140 degrees. When packing hot soup, first rinse a thermos with boiling water to heat it and then add the hot soup. Seal the thermos tightly and place it in an insulated bag to keep it hot until you're ready to eat it.

Healthy Lunch Recipes

The best part about the lunch recipes we include here is that you can change them up to include your favorite foods. So if you love chicken, feel free to add some cooked chicken to the Clean Cobb Salad, or if you're not a big kale fan, use romaine lettuce or Napa cabbage in place of the kale in the Chicken Kale Wraps with Vietnamese Dipping Sauce.

REMEMBER

If you want to use organic ingredients for these recipes, go for it. But know that organic foods aren't necessary to the clean eating plan. Check out Chapter 10 for a list of the fifteen foods you should always try to buy organic and a list of the foods that are just fine grown conventionally.

AVOID TRANS FATS AT LUNCH

Many people choose to eat fast food at lunch, and they end up consuming a lot of trans fats. Most snack foods and many processed foods contain trans fats. Manufacturers create these fats in the lab by adding hydrogen to liquid oils to make them solid at room temperature. Trans fats cause inflammation in your body by blocking anti-inflammatory enzymes and become part of your cell walls, making them "flabby." This negatively affects every part of your body.

Trans fats have a half-life of 51 days. (You're probably used to hearing about half-life in terms of radioactive substances, but other substances have half-lives, too.) In the case of trans fats, a half-life of 51 days means that half of the trans fats you eat stay in your body for seven weeks.

Unfortunately, labels on processed foods can be deceiving about trans fats. If the food has less than 0.5 grams per serving, the manufacturer can legally claim "zero trans fats" on the label. But if that food has 0.49 grams of trans fats per serving and you eat three servings of that food, you've consumed almost 1.5 grams of trans fats! So basically what we're saying is this: Stay away from anything that has *hydrogenated* on the label.

Luckily, the U.S. Food and Drug Administration (FDA) has ordered food manufacturers to stop using trans fats in foods by 2018. But some companies will be able to petition the FDA for a special permit to use this substance. So keep reading labels and avoid this type of fat.

Clean Cobb Salad

PREP TIME: 15 MIN, PLUS STANDING TIME | **YIELD: 4 SERVINGS**

INGREDIENTS

½ cup lowfat Greek or regular yogurt

2 tablespoons sour cream

2 tablespoons buttermilk or soy milk

1 tablespoon lemon juice

1 tablespoon mustard

1 tablespoon minced flat-leaf parsley

1 clove garlic, minced or grated

2 tablespoons minced dill fronds

2 tablespoons minced chives

⅛ teaspoon black pepper

6 eggs

Water

4 cups torn romaine lettuce

2 cups baby spinach

2 ripe red tomatoes, cut into wedges

2 stalks celery, sliced

1 can cannellini beans, rinsed and drained

2 avocados, peeled and sliced

½ cup sliced almonds

½ cup crumbled blue cheese (optional)

DIRECTIONS

1 In a small bowl, combine the yogurt, sour cream, buttermilk, lemon juice, mustard, parsley, garlic, dill, chives, and pepper; mix well. Cover and refrigerate.

2 Place the whole eggs in a 2-quart saucepan; cover them with cold water. Bring the water to a boil over high heat; boil for 1 minute. Then cover the pan, remove it from heat, and let the eggs stand for 12 minutes.

3 Drain the eggs and place them back into the pan; place the pan with the eggs in the sink. Run cold water into the pan until the eggs are cool to the touch. Carefully crack the eggs under the water and let them stand for 5 minutes. Then peel the eggs and cut them into wedges.

4 On each of four plates (or in four containers), arrange the romaine lettuce, spinach, eggs, tomatoes, celery, and beans. Drizzle the salad with the dressing you made in Step 1.

5 Top with the avocados, almonds, and blue cheese (if desired) and serve immediately.

PER SERVING: Calories 451 (From Fat 263); Fat 29g (Saturated 7g); Cholesterol 324mg; Sodium 353mg; Carbohydrate 31g (Dietary Fiber 15g); Protein 23g.

TIP: To make this salad ahead of time, omit the avocados. Pack the dressing, almonds, and blue cheese separately. When you're ready to eat, drizzle the dressing over the salad and top it with almonds and blue cheese.

Slow Cooker Thai Chicken Soup

PREP TIME: 15 MIN | **COOK TIME: 7 HR** | **YIELD: 6 SERVINGS**

INGREDIENTS

1 onion, chopped

3 cloves garlic, minced

2 large carrots, sliced

2 lemongrass stalks, cleaned and bent in half

2 tablespoons peeled, minced fresh ginger root

1 jalapeño pepper, minced

4 cups low-sodium chicken broth

2 pounds boneless, skinless chicken thighs

1 tablespoon curry powder

1 teaspoon turmeric

One 14-ounce can coconut milk

2 tablespoons lime juice

1 teaspoon miso paste

⅓ cup chopped fresh cilantro

2 tablespoons minced fresh basil leaves

DIRECTIONS

1 In a 4- to 5-quart slow cooker, combine the onion, garlic, carrots, lemongrass, ginger root, and jalapeño pepper. Add the chicken broth and stir.

2 Place the chicken thighs on the vegetables. Sprinkle with curry powder and turmeric.

3 Cover the slow cooker and cook on low for 7 to 8 hours or until the chicken registers 165 degrees and is fully cooked. Remove the chicken from the slow cooker and let stand for 10 minutes, then shred. Return the chicken to the slow cooker. Remove the lemongrass from the slow cooker and discard.

4 In a medium bowl, combine the coconut milk, lime juice, and miso paste and stir with a wire whisk until blended. Stir into the slow cooker.

5 Cover and cook on low for another 20 to 30 minutes or until the soup is hot. Garnish with the cilantro and basil and serve.

PER SERVING: Calories 226 (From Fat 160); Fat 18g (Saturated 15g); Cholesterol 11mg; Sodium 126mg; Carbohydrate 12g (Dietary Fiber 1g); Protein 8g.

Clean Gazpacho

PREP TIME: 20 MIN, PLUS CHILLING TIME | YIELD: 6 SERVINGS

INGREDIENTS

4 large beefsteak tomatoes, chopped

1 cup cherry tomatoes, chopped

1 large cucumber, peeled, seeded, and chopped

1 small red onion, peeled and chopped

1 clove garlic, minced or grated

2 cups tomato juice

2 tablespoons lemon juice

2 tablespoons orange juice

2 tablespoons olive oil

¼ teaspoon sea salt

⅛ teaspoon white pepper

½ teaspoon dried tarragon

½ teaspoon dried oregano

¼ cup chopped flat-leaf parsley

DIRECTIONS

1 Place half of the tomatoes and cucumber in a blender. Add the onion, garlic, and tomato juice. Blend until smooth.

2 Pour the blended mixture into a bowl and stir in the remaining chopped tomatoes and cucumber, lemon juice, orange juice, olive oil, sea salt, white pepper, tarragon, and oregano. Taste for seasoning and add more salt, pepper, tarragon, or oregano (if desired).

3 Cover and chill for 2 to 3 hours before serving. Garnish with parsley and serve 1 cup per serving.

PER SERVING: Calories 99 (From Fat 46); Fat 5g (Saturated 1g); Cholesterol 0mg; Sodium 399mg; Carbohydrate 13g (Dietary Fiber 3g); Protein 2g.

TIP: We recommend pairing this recipe with the Chicken Lettuce Wraps we tell you how to make later in this chapter for an excellent lunch. Or you can add chopped, cooked chicken, shrimp, or salmon to the soup just before serving.

Chicken Kale Wraps with Vietnamese Dipping Sauce

| PREP TIME: 15 MIN | COOK TIME: 2 HR | YIELD: 4 SERVINGS |

INGREDIENTS

2 jalapeño peppers, seeds removed if desired, minced

1 clove garlic, minced

2 tablespoons honey

½ cup chicken broth

2 tablespoons lime juice

1 teaspoon miso paste

2 tablespoons olive oil

5 boneless, skinless chicken thighs, chopped

1 onion, finely chopped

2 cloves garlic, minced

1 tablespoon minced fresh ginger root

½ cup shredded carrots

1 tablespoon rice wine vinegar

2 tablespoons chopped fresh cilantro

10 kale leaves, thick stems cut out

DIRECTIONS

1 For dipping sauce, in a small bowl, combine the jalapeño peppers, garlic, 1 tablespoon of honey, chicken broth, lime juice, and miso paste. Blend well using a wire whisk; set aside.

2 In a large skillet, heat the olive oil over medium heat for 2 minutes. Add the chicken, onion, garlic, and ginger root; cook and stir for 4 to 6 minutes or until the chicken is thoroughly cooked. Remove from the heat.

3 Stir in the carrot, rice wine vinegar, the remaining 1 tablespoon of honey, and cilantro; cover and place in the refrigerator while you prepare the kale.

4 Rinse the kale leaves well. Place each leaf on the work surface and cut out the thick stem in a V shape. Discard the stem.

5 Bring a large pot of water to a boil, and prepare a large bowl with ice water. Drop the kale leaves into the water and cook for 2 to 3 minutes or until the kale is just tender. Immediately put the kale into a bowl of ice water. Let stand for 1 minute, then remove the kale and dry it on kitchen towels.

6 To serve, roll up the chicken mixture in the kale leaves and serve with the dipping sauce.

PER SERVING: Calories 260 (From Fat 97); Fat 11 (Saturated 2g); Cholesterol 72mg; Sodium 255mg; Carbohydrate 22g (Dietary Fiber 2g); Protein 20g.

Fruity Coleslaw

PREP TIME: 15 MIN | YIELD: 8 SERVINGS

INGREDIENTS

⅔ cup lowfat Greek or regular yogurt

2 tablespoons olive oil

3 tablespoons apple cider vinegar

2 tablespoons lemon juice

2 tablespoons raw honey, or ¼ teaspoon stevia

½ teaspoon sea salt

¼ teaspoon black pepper

1 teaspoon dried thyme

3 cups shredded red cabbage

3 cups shredded green cabbage

3 stalks celery, sliced

2 Granny Smith apples, chopped

2 cups red grapes

½ cup dried cherries

1 cup pistachios or pecan pieces

DIRECTIONS

1 In a large bowl, combine the yogurt, olive oil, vinegar, lemon juice, honey, sea salt, pepper, and thyme; mix well.

2 Stir in the cabbage, celery, apples, grapes, dried cherries, and pistachios until everything is coated with the dressing mix from Step 1. Serve immediately or cover and refrigerate for 2 to 3 hours before serving. Serve 1 cup per serving.

PER SERVING: Calories 244 (From Fat 105); Fat 12g (Saturated 2g); Cholesterol 1mg; Sodium 179mg; Carbohydrate 33g (Dietary Fiber 5g); Protein 7g.

TIP: Use this coleslaw as a condiment on chicken or beef sandwiches or stir in some leftover cooked salmon for a quick and healthy lunch.

Roasted Veggie Hummus Pitas

PREP TIME: 20 MIN | **COOK TIME: 10–12 MIN** | **YIELD: 6 SERVINGS**

INGREDIENTS

2 yellow summer squash, cut into 1½-inch pieces

2 cups button mushrooms, cut in half

1 red bell pepper, sliced

1 green bell pepper, sliced

1 large onion, chopped

1 tablespoon olive oil

1 tablespoon plus 3 tablespoons lemon juice

⅛ teaspoon black pepper

½ teaspoon plus ¼ teaspoon sea salt

1 cup canned chickpeas, rinsed and drained

2 cloves garlic, minced

⅓ cup lowfat Greek or regular yogurt

¼ cup sesame seeds

1 teaspoon ground cumin

⅛ teaspoon red pepper flakes

6 whole-wheat pita breads, split

6 leaves romaine lettuce

DIRECTIONS

1 Preheat the oven to 400 degrees.

2 Arrange the squash, mushrooms, bell peppers, and onion on a cookie sheet. Drizzle the veggies with the olive oil and 1 tablespoon of lemon juice and sprinkle with the black pepper and ½ teaspoon of sea salt. Roast, uncovered, until the veggies are tender, about 10 to 12 minutes, stirring once during roasting.

3 Combine the chickpeas, garlic, yogurt, sesame seeds, 3 tablespoons of lemon juice, cumin, ¼ teaspoon of sea salt, and red pepper flakes in a blender or food processor. Blend until smooth.

4 Combine the roasted vegetables with the chickpea mixture. Line each pita bread with a lettuce leaf, add ⅙ of the vegetable mixture, and serve immediately.

PER SERVING: Calories 314 (From Fat 69); Fat 8g (Saturated 1g); Cholesterol 1mg; Sodium 668mg; Carbohydrate 54g (Dietary Fiber 10g); Protein 13g.

TIP: If you want to pack these pitas for lunch, pack the vegetable mixture, the lettuce, and the pita breads separately. Assemble the sandwich just before eating.

Fruity Chicken Pasta Salad

**PREP TIME: 15 MIN, PLUS REFRIGERATING TIME
YIELD: 6 SERVINGS**

COOK TIME: ABOUT 10 MIN

INGREDIENTS

½ cup lowfat Greek or regular yogurt

¼ cup lowfat sour cream

3 tablespoons buttermilk or almond milk

2 tablespoons apple cider vinegar

2 tablespoons mustard

2 tablespoons raw honey, or ¼ teaspoon stevia

1 teaspoon dried thyme

½ teaspoon sea salt

⅛ teaspoon white pepper

10 cups water

4 cups whole-wheat penne or farfalle pasta

3 cups cooked chicken, cut into 1-inch pieces

3 stalks celery, sliced

2 cups red grapes

1 cup blueberries

2 cups cubed cantaloupe

½ cup walnut pieces

DIRECTIONS

1 In a large bowl, combine the yogurt, sour cream, buttermilk, vinegar, mustard, honey, thyme, sea salt, and white pepper; mix well to blend.

2 In a 4-quart saucepan, bring the water to a boil. Add the pasta; cook according to package directions until the pasta is just tender. Drain well and add the pasta to the bowl with the dressing you made in Step 1.

3 Stir in the chicken and celery until they're well coated. Gently add the grapes, blueberries, cantaloupe, and walnuts. Stir gently. Cover and refrigerate for 2 to 3 hours before serving. Serve 1½ cups per serving.

PER SERVING: Calories 492 (From Fat 129); Fat 14g (Saturated 3g); Cholesterol 68mg; Sodium 439mg; Carbohydrate 67g (Dietary Fiber 8g); Protein 31g.

Salmon Avocado Summer Rolls

PREP TIME: 20 MIN	COOK TIME: 10 MIN	YIELD: 4 SERVINGS

INGREDIENTS

1 tablespoon olive oil

One 8-ounce skinless wild salmon filet, cubed

2 cloves garlic, minced

1 tablespoon minced or grated fresh ginger root

⅔ cup mung bean sprouts

3 tablespoons thinly sliced green onion

2 tablespoons lime juice

2 tablespoons low-sodium tamari sauce

⅓ cup julienned carrots

8 brown rice paper spring roll wrappers

1 cup thinly sliced Napa cabbage

2 avocados, peeled and chopped

DIRECTIONS

1 In a medium skillet, heat the olive oil over medium heat for 2 minutes. Add the salmon, garlic, and ginger root. Stir-fry this mixture for 1 to 2 minutes or until the salmon is barely cooked.

2 Add the bean sprouts; stir-fry for another 2 to 3 minutes or until the salmon is cooked as desired. Transfer the salmon mixture to a medium bowl and stir in the onion, lime juice, tamari sauce, and carrots.

3 Place about 2 cups of very warm water in a 9-inch pie plate. Put one rice paper wrapper in the water and let stand for 10 to 15 seconds or until the wrapper is soft. Place the wrapper on the counter.

4 Top the wrapper with ⅛ of the salmon mixture, then ⅛ of the cabbage and avocado. Fold in the ends of the wrapper, and roll up. The wrapper will stick to itself as you roll.

5 Repeat this procedure 7 more times with the remaining ingredients and serve immediately.

PER SERVING: Calories 487 (From Fat 169); Fat 19g (Saturated 3g); Cholesterol 37mg; Sodium 773mg; Carbohydrate 57g (Dietary Fiber 10g); Protein 25g.

NOTE: Sprouting seeds and beans can help your body absorb more nutrients in the beans that are usually bound by phytic acid, and they're a good source of vitamin C. But raw bean sprouts have been linked to quite a few food poisoning outbreaks in the past few years, so always cook sprouts before you eat them.

Black Rice Veggie Salad

PREP TIME: 25 MIN | **COOK TIME: 35 MIN** | **YIELD: 4 SERVINGS**

INGREDIENTS

1 cup black rice

2½ cups vegetable broth

2 tablespoons lemon juice

1 tablespoon honey

1 tablespoon Dijon mustard

3 tablespoons olive oil

Pinch sea salt

Pinch pepper

1 red bell pepper, chopped

1 yellow bell pepper, chopped

1 cup whole sugar snap peas

3 celery stalks, sliced

2 green onions, thinly sliced

DIRECTIONS

1 In a medium saucepan, combine the black rice and vegetable broth. Bring to a boil over high heat; then reduce the heat to low and simmer, covered, until the rice is tender, about 30 to 40 minutes. Drain the rice if necessary and set aside.

2 In a large bowl, combine the lemon juice, honey, mustard, olive oil, salt, and pepper and mix well. Stir in the warm rice until coated.

3 Stir in the bell peppers, sugar snap peas, celery, and green onions to mix. Cover and chill for 1 to 2 hours to blend the flavors before serving.

PER SERVING: Calories 328 (From Fat 122); Fat 14g (Saturated 2g); Cholesterol 0mg; Sodium 582mg; Carbohydrate 48g (Dietary Fiber 5g); Protein 8g.

TIP: Black rice is available online and in some large grocery stores. It's really black, and very high in anthocyanins, one of the antioxidants important to good health. In fact, black rice has one of the highest levels of this compound found in any food. It is also called "forbidden rice," and was only available to Chinese royalty in ancient times. If you can't find it, you can substitute wild rice.

Bok Choy Seafood Soup

PREP TIME: 15 MIN | **COOK TIME: 2 HR** | **YIELD: 4 SERVINGS**

INGREDIENTS

One 8-ounce package brown rice noodles, broken in half

2 tablespoons olive oil

2 shallots, peeled and minced

1 tablespoon minced fresh ginger root

One 8-ounce package shiitake or button mushrooms, sliced

4 cups coarsely chopped baby bok choy

One 32-ounce box vegetable broth

2 cups water

One 6-ounce wild salmon filet, cut into cubes

1 yellow summer squash, chopped

½ pound Oregon pink shrimp or Pacific spot prawns

1 tablespoon lime juice

DIRECTIONS

1 In a large bowl, place the noodles and pour warm water over them; let stand for 10 to 15 minutes or soften them according to the package directions.

2 In a large saucepan, heat the olive oil over medium heat. Add the shallots, ginger root, and mushrooms and sauté for 3 to 4 minutes or until fragrant. Stir in the bok choy and simmer for another 2 minutes.

3 Add the vegetable broth and water and bring to a simmer. Stir in the salmon filet and simmer for 2 minutes.

4 Add the squash and shrimp and simmer for 3 to 5 minutes or until the shrimp curl and turn pink. Drain the rice noodles and add to the soup along with the lime juice. Simmer for 1 minute and serve immediately. If not serving immediately, add the noodles and lime juice at the last minute.

PER SERVING: Calories 342 (From Fat 104); Fat 12g (Saturated 2g); Cholesterol 110mg; Sodium 687mg; Carbohydrate 36g (Dietary Fiber 3g); Protein 25g.

TIP: If you can't find Pacific spot prawns or Oregon pink shrimp, choose wild shrimp from the United States or Argentina. Most other imported types of shrimp are very high in bacteria.

Fruit and Grains Salad

| PREP TIME: 20 MIN | COOK TIME: ABOUT 2 HR | YIELD: 6 SERVINGS |

INGREDIENTS

⅓ cup olive oil

2 tablespoons honey, or
¼ teaspoon stevia

¼ cup orange juice

2 tablespoons lemon juice

2 tablespoons Dijon mustard

¼ teaspoon sea salt

⅛ teaspoon black pepper

1 cup wheat berries, sorted and rinsed

3 cups plus 1½ cups plus 2 cups cold water

½ cup quinoa, rinsed well

¾ cup barley

2 apples, chopped

1½ cups cubed pineapple

2 stalks celery, sliced

½ cup dried cranberries or cherries

½ cup unsalted pistachios

DIRECTIONS

1 In a large bowl, combine the olive oil, honey, orange juice, lemon juice, mustard, sea salt, and pepper; mix with a wire whisk. Refrigerate.

2 In a 2-quart saucepan, combine the wheat berries and 3 cups of cold water. Bring the water to a boil over high heat; then cover the pan, reduce the heat, and simmer for about 55 minutes, or until the wheat berries are tender but still chewy. Drain well and add to the salad dressing you made in Step 1. Refrigerate.

3 In a 2-quart saucepan, combine the quinoa with 1½ cups of cold water. Bring the water to a boil over high heat; then cover the pan, reduce the heat, and simmer for about 25 minutes, or until the quinoa is tender but not mushy. Drain well and add to the wheat berry mixture. Refrigerate.

4 In a 2-quart saucepan, combine the barley with 2 cups of cold water. Bring the water to a boil over high heat; then cover the pan, reduce the heat, and simmer for about 40 minutes, or until the barley is tender but still chewy. Drain well if necessary and add to the wheat berry/quinoa mixture. Refrigerate.

5 Add the apples, pineapple, celery, dried cranberries, and pistachios to the grain salad. Stir gently to coat. Serve immediately or cover and chill for 1 to 2 hours before serving. Serve 1½ cups per serving.

PER SERVING: Calories 521 (From Fat 177); Fat 20g (Saturated 3g); Cholesterol 0mg; Sodium 247mg; Carbohydrate 82g (Dietary Fiber 13g); Protein 11g.

Salmon Salad Sandwich with Peach Salsa

PREP TIME: 25 MIN, PLUS REFRIGERATING TIME YIELD: 6 SERVINGS	COOK TIME: 5–8 MIN

INGREDIENTS

3 large fresh peaches, peeled, pits removed, and chopped

1 small red onion, diced

3 green onions, sliced

1 jalapeño chile, minced (optional)

1 clove garlic, grated

1 tablespoon lemon juice

1 tablespoon chopped fresh mint

½ teaspoon plus ¼ teaspoon sea salt

⅛ teaspoon cayenne pepper

Three 8-ounce salmon fillets

1 cup cold water

½ cup lowfat Greek or regular yogurt

¼ cup silken tofu

2 tablespoons orange juice

⅛ teaspoon white pepper

1 cup blueberries

2 stalks celery, sliced

12 slices whole-grain bread

6 leaves romaine lettuce

DIRECTIONS

1 In a medium bowl, combine the peaches, red onion, green onions, jalapeño chile (if desired), garlic, lemon juice, mint, ½ teaspoon of sea salt, and cayenne pepper. Stir gently to mix; then cover and refrigerate.

2 Place the salmon fillets in a large shallow saucepan. Add 1 cup of cold water and bring to a boil over medium heat. Reduce heat to low, cover the pan, and simmer for 5 to 8 minutes, or until the salmon flakes when tested with a fork. Remove the salmon from the pan and let it cool for 30 minutes.

3 In a large bowl, combine the yogurt, tofu, orange juice, ¼ teaspoon of sea salt, and white pepper; blend well.

4 Flake the salmon, removing the skin. Add the salmon, blueberries, and celery to the yogurt mixture and blend well. Cover and refrigerate for 2 to 3 hours to blend flavors.

5 When you're ready to eat, place the bread on your work surface. Top 6 slices of the bread with 1 piece of lettuce and ⅔ cup of the salmon mixture. Top each sandwich with some of the peach salsa you made in Step 1 and a second bread slice and serve.

PER SERVING: Calories 356 (From Fat 67); Fat 8g (Saturated 2g); Cholesterol 66mg; Sodium 651mg; Carbohydrate 40g (Dietary Fiber 7g); Protein 34g.

Chapter 17

Sprucing Up Supper Time with Some Delicious Dinner Recipes

D innertime can be an experience full of strife and conflict, or it can be a way to reinforce your family's ties and end the day on a high note. Not surprisingly, to create a healthy family, both physically and mentally, you need to strive to create the second type of dinnertime. Instead of allowing arguments to dominate your dinner table, encourage reflection, nutrition, and companionship — even if your kids (and spouse) don't want to eat what you've put on the table.

As kids, you probably remember being forced to sit at the table staring down cold Brussels sprouts. At the time, the "clean plate club" was an important part of mealtime, and parents were told to force their children to eat what was good for them. Well, those days are gone, but you still have to get some nutritious food into your kids (and spouse).

In this chapter, we offer some tips for how to create a calm and happy dinner atmosphere, and we show you some great recipes that even picky eaters will want to try — eventually.

Making Dinnertime a Pleasant Time with a Few Simple Tricks

Encouraging family involvement in planning meals, shopping, and preparing food helps make dinnertime a more enjoyable experience for the whole family. The following list offers some tips to help you get started. (See Chapter 13 for more tips on how to get your family tuned in to the clean eating lifestyle.)

>> **Build a colorful — not a full — plate.** This is probably the most important dinner planning tip you need to know. Dinner is a great time to get in some of the fruits and vegetables you didn't eat during the day. So try to incorporate a few different fruits and veggies as well as some protein and healthy fat sources to get the most nutrition — and color — into your meals.

>> **Think about restricting some topics of conversation.** Dinner isn't the time to get into lectures (about grades, behavior, eating habits, and so on); it's a time to get closer to your family.

>> **Think about which topics you want to encourage at the dinner table.** Healthy conversation topics can include the food you're eating, the culture it came from, the high and low points of everyone's day, and plans for the evening and the rest of the week. After a while, pleasant conversation will become more organic and natural in your family, and you can feel good that you're setting and promoting a positive lifestyle choice for your kids.

>> **Have fun with dinnertime.** Think about creating theme nights (Mexican Fiesta or Trip to India, for example), or set an inviting table with a nice tablecloth, the good china and crystal, flowers, and candles. When you make an effort to make dinnertime a fun experience, your kids will want to join in.

The recipes in this chapter are mainly just cooking recipes; that is, they adapt well to (relatively small) changes. So use your family's favorite ingredients and flavors to create healthy and delicious dinners from the basic recipes we include here. For instance, if your family isn't big on bison, substitute venison or beef in the Tex-Mex Bison Chili, or if your kids think of shrimp as a yummy treat, use shrimp in the Clean Salmon and Fettuccine with Kale Pesto.

REMEMBER

If you want to use organic ingredients for these recipes, go for it. But know that organic foods aren't necessary to the clean eating plan. Check out Chapter 10 for a list of the fifteen foods you should always try to buy organic and a list of the foods that are just fine grown conventionally.

Slow Cooker Barley Stew

PREP TIME: 15 MIN | **COOK TIME: 7–9 HR** | **YIELD: 6–8 SERVINGS**

INGREDIENTS

1 cup uncooked pearl barley

½ cup dried brown lentils

1 large onion, chopped

3 cloves garlic, minced

3 carrots, sliced

1 cup sliced button mushrooms

1 cup sliced cremini mushrooms

8 cups vegetable broth

2 bay leaves

½ teaspoon sea salt

¼ teaspoon black pepper

1 teaspoon dried basil

1 teaspoon dried thyme

2 tablespoons lemon juice

DIRECTIONS

1 Rinse the barley in a colander until the water runs clear. Place the barley and lentils in a 4-quart slow cooker. Add the onion, garlic, carrots, mushrooms, vegetable broth, bay leaves, sea salt, pepper, basil, and thyme and stir gently.

2 Cover and cook on low for 7 to 9 hours, or until the lentils and barley are tender.

3 Remove the bay leaves. Stir in the lemon juice, add more seasonings to taste, and serve warm with toasted whole-grain bread.

PER SERVING: Calories 248 (From Fat 13); Fat 1g (Saturated 0g); Cholesterol 0mg; Sodium 837mg; Carbohydrate 50g (Dietary Fiber 12g); Protein 10g.

VARY IT! You can add any of your favorite vegetables to make this recipe your own.

Turkey with Caramelized Onion Apple Pecan Stuffing

PREP TIME: 8 HR 25 MIN | **COOK TIME: 5 HR** | **YIELD: 12 SERVINGS**

INGREDIENTS

8 slices whole wheat bread, cubed

2 unpeeled apples, chopped

2 tablespoons lemon juice

1 cup small whole pecans

½ cup dried tart cherries

3 tablespoons butter

3 tablespoons olive oil

2 onions, chopped

2 eggs, beaten

¼ cup cold water

1 teaspoon sea salt

½ teaspoon pepper

One 12-pound turkey, giblets removed

2 tablespoons butter

1 teaspoon dried thyme leaves

1 teaspoon dried basil leaves

1 cup low sodium chicken broth

DIRECTIONS

1 Let the bread stand, uncovered, overnight to dry. In the morning, toss the bread with the apples, lemon juice, pecans, and cherries, and set aside.

2 In a medium skillet, melt the butter and 1 tablespoon of the olive oil over medium heat. Add the onions; cook and stir until tender. Reduce the heat to low and cook, stirring frequently, until the onions are dark brown. Do not let the onions burn.

3 Add the onions to the bread mixture along with the eggs and cold water. Season to taste with sea salt and pepper. Stuff this mixture loosely inside the turkey's body cavity and neck cavity. Sew the cavities shut with kitchen twine. (Any remaining stuffing mixture can be baked in a separate casserole for 55 to 65 minutes at 325 degrees or until a meat thermometer registers 165 degrees.)

4 Preheat the oven to 325 degrees. Place the turkey in a roasting pan. Rub the turkey with 2 tablespoons butter and sprinkle with the thyme and basil. Drizzle with the remaining 2 tablespoons olive oil. Add the chicken broth to the bottom of the roasting pan.

5 Roast the turkey for 4 to 5 hours for a 12-pound turkey, until a meat thermometer registers 170 degrees. The stuffing inside the turkey should be 165 degrees. If the stuffing is not at 165 degrees, return the turkey to the oven and cook for another 15 to 25 minutes until it reaches that temperature.

6 Let the turkey stand at room temperature for 20 minutes. Cut and remove the kitchen twine, and then scoop the stuffing out of the turkey into a serving bowl. Carve the turkey and serve.

PER SERVING: Calories 488 (From Fat 137); Fat 15g (Saturated 4g); Cholesterol 206mg; Sodium 468mg; Carbohydrate 20g (Dietary Fiber 3g); Protein 65g.

TIP: If you cut the stuffing recipe in half, you can use it to stuff and roast a couple of 4-pound chickens. Put the stuffing into the chicken cavities. Roast at 375 degrees for 60 to 70 minutes, or until a meat thermometer inserted into the thigh registers 170 degrees. Remove the stuffing, carve the bird, and eat!

Chicken Chestnut Meatballs in Orange Sauce

PREP TIME: 25 MIN	COOK TIME: 25 MIN	YIELD: 6 SERVINGS

INGREDIENTS

3 tablespoons olive oil

4 green onions, minced

One 5-ounce bag roasted peeled chestnuts

1 egg, beaten

½ teaspoon sea salt

⅛ teaspoon white pepper

½ teaspoon grated orange zest

1½ pounds ground chicken, white and dark meat

2 tablespoons butter

1 cup orange juice

½ cup chicken stock

2 tablespoons lemon juice

2 teaspoons arrowroot powder

DIRECTIONS

1 In a large skillet, heat 1 tablespoon of the olive oil over medium heat. Add the green onions; cook and stir until tender, about 2 to 3 minutes. Remove the onions from the skillet and place in a large bowl; set aside the skillet and do not clean.

2 Add the chestnuts to the green onions in the bowl and mash with a fork until fairly smooth. Beat in the egg, sea salt, pepper, and orange zest. Add the ground chicken and mix with your hands until combined.

3 Form the mixture into 1-inch meatballs. Place on a cookie sheet, cover, and refrigerate for 1 hour until the meatballs become firmer.

4 When ready to eat, heat the butter and the remaining 2 tablespoons of olive oil in the same large skillet. Add the meatballs in two batches; cook just until browned, stirring occasionally, about 5 to 7 minutes, and remove.

5 Add the orange juice, chicken stock, lemon juice, and arrowroot powder to the skillet and bring to a simmer, stirring with a wire whisk. Return the meatballs to the skillet and simmer, stirring occasionally and gently with a wooden spoon, until the meatballs register 165 degrees on a meat thermometer and the sauce is thickened, about 8 to 12 minutes longer. Serve immediately over hot, cooked brown rice.

PER SERVING: Calories 349 (From Fat 194); Fat 22g (Saturated 6g); Cholesterol 143mg; Sodium 353mg; Carbohydrate 17g (Dietary Fiber 1g); Protein 22g.

Tex-Mex Bison Chili

PREP TIME: 25 MIN, PLUS STANDING TIME | COOK TIME: ABOUT 1 HR 15 MIN | YIELD: 6 SERVINGS

INGREDIENTS

3 cups dried kidney beans

9 cups plus 9 cups water

1 pound ground bison

1 large onion, chopped

3 cloves garlic, minced

1 jalapeño chile, minced

1 red bell pepper, chopped

1 green bell pepper, chopped

3 stalks celery, sliced

3 large red ripe tomatoes, chopped

One 8-ounce can tomato sauce

2 tablespoons tomato paste

5 cups beef broth

2 tablespoons chili powder

1 teaspoon cocoa powder

1 teaspoon dried oregano

1 teaspoon ground cumin

1 teaspoon sea salt

¼ teaspoon black pepper

⅛ teaspoon red pepper flakes

¾ cup sour cream

¾ cup guacamole

¾ cup salsa

24 whole-grain tortilla chips

DIRECTIONS

1 Sort over the kidney beans to find small stones or rocks and discard them; rinse and drain the beans and place them in a large pot. Add 9 cups of water to the beans, cover them, and let them stand overnight.

2 Drain the beans, rinse them well, and add 9 cups of fresh water. Bring the water and beans to a boil over high heat; reduce the heat to low, cover, and cook until the beans are tender but still firm, about 35 minutes. Drain if necessary and set aside.

3 In a large skillet, cook the bison, breaking up the meat with a fork, for 2 minutes. Add the onion, garlic, and jalapeño chile; cook and stir until the bison is cooked, about 4 to 5 minutes.

4 Add the bell peppers and celery; cook and stir for 3 minutes. Add the tomatoes, tomato sauce, tomato paste, beef broth, and beans; stir to combine.

5 Add the chili powder, cocoa powder, oregano, cumin, sea salt, black pepper, and red pepper flakes. Bring the mixture to a boil over medium heat. Reduce the heat to low and simmer for 20 to 30 minutes, stirring occasionally, until the chili has thickened.

6 Serve with 2 tablespoons of sour cream, guacamole, and salsa and 4 whole-grain tortilla chips per serving.

PER SERVING: Calories 498 (From Fat 101); Fat 11g (Saturated 4g); Cholesterol 40mg; Sodium 1,441mg; Carbohydrate 67g (Dietary Fiber 19g); Protein 36g.

VARY IT! You can substitute 90 percent lean ground beef or ground venison for the bison if you prefer.

Butternut Mac and Cheese

PREP TIME: 25 MIN | COOK TIME: 1 HR | YIELD: 6 SERVINGS

INGREDIENTS

1 small butternut squash

2 tablespoons butter

1 onion, chopped

2 cloves garlic, minced

2 cups vegetable broth

2 cups almond milk

2 cups finely chopped cauliflower

2½ cups whole wheat or gluten-free pasta

1 cup shredded cheddar cheese

1 cup shredded Monterey jack cheese

½ cup grated Parmesan cheese

DIRECTIONS

1 Peel the squash, remove the seeds, cut into cubes, and set aside.

2 In a large saucepan, melt the butter over medium heat. Add the onion and garlic; cook and stir until tender, about 5 minutes. Stir in the squash; cook and stir for another 6 to 7 minutes or until the squash starts to brown.

3 Add the broth and almond milk to the saucepan and bring to a simmer. Lower the heat and simmer for about 20 to 25 minutes or until the squash is tender.

4 While the squash mixture is simmering, bring another large pot of water to a boil. Add the cauliflower and simmer for 5 minutes; remove the cauliflower with a large strainer. Add the pasta to the water and cook until almost al dente, according to package directions; drain and toss with the cauliflower.

5 When the squash is tender, mash right in the cooking liquid using a potato masher or immersion blender, or puree the squash, liquid, and vegetables in a blender until smooth. Stir in the cheddar cheese, Monterey Jack cheese, and ¼ cup of the Parmesan cheese. Then add the cauliflower and pasta.

6 Preheat the oven to 375 degrees. Transfer the mixture to a 3-quart baking dish and top with the remaining ¼ cup of Parmesan cheese. Bake for 20 to 25 minutes, until the casserole is bubbling.

PER SERVING: Calories 349 (From Fat 175); Fat 19g (Saturated 12g); Cholesterol 54mg; Sodium 547mg; Carbohydrate 29g (Dietary Fiber 5g); Protein 18g.

TIP: Cauliflower is an excellent substitute for pasta. Most people won't be able to tell it's in the dish. This cruciferous vegetable adds great nutrition to this classic recipe.

Arctic Char with Green Almond Sauce

PREP TIME: 10 MIN | **COOK TIME: 6 MIN** | **YIELD: 6 SERVINGS**

INGREDIENTS

1 cup watercress leaves, rinsed

½ cup blanched almonds

¼ cup flat leaf parsley

1 clove garlic, minced

3 green onions, chopped

1 jalapeño pepper, seeds removed, chopped

½ cup olive oil

2 tablespoons lemon juice

¼ teaspoon sea salt

⅛ teaspoon white pepper

2 tablespoons butter

Six 6-ounce wild-caught Arctic char filets

DIRECTIONS

1 In a blender or food processor, combine the watercress, almonds, parsley, garlic, green onions, and jalapeño pepper, and blend or process until finely chopped. Add the olive oil, lemon juice, sea salt, and white pepper, and blend or process until a sauce forms.

2 In a large skillet, heat the butter over medium heat. Add the filets and cook, turning carefully once, until the fish just flakes when tested with a fork, about 3 minutes per side.

3 Place the fish on a serving platter and cover with about half of the sauce. Serve immediately with the remaining sauce on the side.

PER SERVING: Calories 578 (From Fat 258); Fat 29g (Saturated 12g); Cholesterol 58mg; Sodium 236mg; Carbohydrate 3g (Dietary Fiber 1g); Protein 39g.

TIP: Arctic char is an excellent choice for sustainable seafood. This fish is also high in omega-3 fatty acids and is a great source of protein.

Ribollita

INGREDIENTS

2 cups cubed whole-wheat bread

2 tablespoons olive oil, plus a little extra for drizzling

1 large onion, chopped

4 cloves garlic, minced

½ teaspoon sea salt

⅛ teaspoon white pepper

1 teaspoon dried thyme leaves

2 cups sliced mushrooms

3 carrots, sliced

3 stalks celery, chopped

⅓ cup chopped celery leaves

One 32-ounce box vegetable stock

2 cups water

6 plum tomatoes, seeded and chopped

Two 14-ounce can cannellini beans, rinsed and drained

3 cups chopped kale

¾ cup grated Parmesan cheese

DIRECTIONS

1 Preheat the oven to 200 degrees. Spread the bread cubes on a baking sheet and bake for 8 to 10 minutes or until dry to the touch. Remove from the oven and set aside.

2 In a large soup pot, heat 2 tablespoons of the olive oil over medium heat for 2 minutes. Add the onion and garlic and sprinkle with sea salt and pepper. Sauté for 4 to 5 minutes or until vegetables are tender. Sprinkle with the thyme leaves.

3 Add the mushrooms, carrots, and celery; sauté for another 3 minutes, stirring frequently. Then add the celery leaves, vegetable stock, water, plum tomatoes, and beans, and stir.

4 Bring to a simmer, then reduce the heat to low, cover, and let simmer for 15 to 20 minutes or until the vegetables are tender. Stir in the kale and simmer for another 5 minutes or until the kale is wilted.

5 Stir in the bread cubes and simmer for another 5 to 10 minutes or until the bread has thickened the soup. Serve with the Parmesan cheese and drizzle each serving with some olive oil.

PER SERVING: Calories 226 (From Fat 65); Fat 7g (Saturated 2g); Cholesterol 8mg; Sodium 653mg; Carbohydrate 31g (Dietary Fiber 7g); Protein 12g.

Baked Italian Fish Packets

PREP TIME: 20 MIN | COOK TIME: 20–25 MIN | YIELD: 4 SERVINGS

INGREDIENTS

2 large red ripe tomatoes, chopped

3 cloves garlic, minced

1 small red onion, minced

2 tablespoons chopped fresh basil

¼ cup balsamic vinegar

¼ cup olive oil

1 tablespoon Dijon mustard

½ teaspoon sea salt

⅛ teaspoon black pepper

Four 4- to 6-ounce red snapper fillets

DIRECTIONS

1 Preheat the oven to 375 degrees. In a medium bowl, combine the tomatoes, garlic, red onion, and basil.

2 In a small bowl, combine the balsamic vinegar, olive oil, mustard, sea salt, and pepper; mix with a whisk until well blended.

3 Cut four 18-x-12-inch sheets of parchment paper and arrange them on your work surface.

4 Place one fish fillet in the center of each sheet of paper. Top each fillet with ¼ of the tomato mixture and drizzle each fillet with ¼ of the olive oil mixture.

5 Lift the short sides of the paper and fold the edges together twice to seal them. Then lift and fold the other sides of the paper to seal them together. Be sure to leave some air space in the packet to allow for heat expansion.

6 Place the fish packets on a cookie sheet. Bake for 20 to 25 minutes, or until the fish flakes when you test it with a fork. (Carefully unwrap one packet and test the fish for doneness.)

7 Place each packet on a plate. Cut a large X across the top of each packet. Serve immediately, making sure to warn diners to be careful of the steam when they open their packets.

PER SERVING: Calories 324 (From Fat 148); Fat 16g (Saturated 2g); Cholesterol 60mg; Sodium 468mg; Carbohydrate 9g (Dietary Fiber 1g); Protein 35g.

NOTE: Baking fish in parchment paper is a wonderful way to keep the fish moist and tender. The paper also helps hold in all the flavors as the fish cooks, and it's a clean way to cook. If you don't mind using foil, though, you can also wrap the fish in foil and grill it over medium coals for 15 to 20 minutes until the fish flakes when you test it with a fork.

Tandoori Pork Tenderloin

PREP TIME: 8 HR 15 MIN | COOK TIME: 40 MIN | YIELD: 6 SERVINGS

INGREDIENTS

1 medium onion, finely chopped

6 cloves garlic, minced

2 tablespoons minced fresh ginger root

3 tablespoons lemon juice

1 tablespoon curry powder

1 teaspoon ground turmeric

1 teaspoon sweet paprika

1 teaspoon grated orange zest

½ teaspoon sea salt

¼ teaspoon white pepper

1 cup Greek lowfat plain yogurt

One 2-pound whole pork tenderloin

DIRECTIONS

1 In a blender or food processor, combine the onion, garlic, ginger root, lemon juice, curry powder, turmeric, paprika, orange zest, sea salt, and white pepper, and blend or process until ground. Stir in the yogurt and transfer to a glass baking dish.

2 Add the tenderloin to the baking dish and turn to coat. Cover and refrigerate for 8 to 24 hours, turning the meat once during marinating time.

3 When ready to eat, preheat the oven to 425 degrees. Remove the pork from the yogurt mixture; discard remaining yogurt mixture. Heat 2 tablespoons olive oil in an ovenproof skillet and add the pork. Brown on all sides, about 5 minutes total.

4 Put the skillet with the pork in the oven and roast the pork for 10 to 12 minutes or until a meat thermometer registers at least 145 degrees.

5 Remove the pork from the oven, cover with foil, and let stand for 5 minutes before slicing to serve.

PER SERVING: Calories 209 (From Fat 30); Fat 3g (Saturated 1g); Cholesterol 100mg; Sodium 292mg; Carbohydrate 7g (Dietary Fiber 1g); Protein 36g.

Spiralized Zucchini with Roasted Veggies

PREP TIME: 20 MIN | COOK TIME: 40 MIN | YIELD: 4 SERVINGS

INGREDIENTS

1 red onion, coarsely chopped

2 cups peeled, seeded, cubed butternut squash

3 tablespoons olive oil, divided

12 cloves garlic, peeled

2 red bell peppers, seeded and chopped

6 plum tomatoes, seeded and coarsely chopped

½ teaspoon sea salt, divided

⅛ teaspoon pepper

1 teaspoon dried marjoram leaves

2 pounds zucchini

2 tablespoons lemon juice

½ cup shredded Parmesan or Romano cheese

DIRECTIONS

1 Preheat the oven to 400 degrees. Combine the onion and squash on a roasting pan and drizzle with 1 tablespoon of the olive oil; toss to coat. Roast for 20 minutes.

2 Remove the pan from the oven and add the garlic, bell peppers, and plum tomatoes. Drizzle with remaining 1 tablespoon of olive oil and sprinkle with ¼ teaspoon salt, pepper, and marjoram. Roast until the vegetables are tender and start to brown, about 15 to 20 minutes longer.

3 While the vegetables are roasting, cut the zucchini into strips using a spiralizer, or cut into long thin strips. Toss with the lemon juice and ¼ teaspoon salt and set aside. Heat 1 tablespoon of the olive oil in a large skillet and add the zucchini; cook for 2 minutes, stirring frequently, until tender. Put into a large serving bowl and cover to keep warm.

4 When the vegetables are done roasting, pour over the zucchini spirals in the serving bowl. Sprinkle with cheese and serve immediately.

PER SERVING: Calories 281 (From Fat 135); Fat 15g (Saturated 4g); Cholesterol 11mg; Sodium 515mg; Carbohydrate 30g (Dietary Fiber 7g); Protein 11g.

TIP: A spiralizer is a specialized tool that cuts vegetables into long, thin, curly strips that resemble pasta. This is an excellent way to serve a "pasta" dish if you're eating Paleo. You can substitute very thin slices of zucchini that you cut by hand. In that case, blanch the zucchini strips for 1 to 2 minutes in boiling water so they'll bend and look like fettuccine.

Salmon Risi Bisi

PREP TIME: 15 MIN | COOK TIME: ABOUT 4 HR | YIELD: 6 SERVINGS

INGREDIENTS

2 tablespoons olive oil

1 large onion, chopped

2 cloves garlic, minced

2 large carrots, cubed

1½ cups brown rice

2 cups water

1¾ cups vegetable broth

1 teaspoon dried thyme

½ teaspoon dried basil

½ teaspoon sea salt

⅛ teaspoon black pepper

Three 6-ounce salmon fillets

2 cups frozen baby peas, thawed

½ cup grated Parmesan cheese

DIRECTIONS

1 In a small skillet, heat the olive oil over medium heat. Add the onion and garlic; cook and stir for 5 minutes, or until tender.

2 Place the onion and garlic mixture in a 4-quart slow cooker with the carrots and brown rice. Add the water, vegetable broth, thyme, basil, sea salt, and pepper. Cover and cook on low for 2½ hours.

3 Stir the mixture and test the rice. If it's still chewy, cover and cook on low for another 30 minutes. When the rice is almost tender, place the salmon fillets on top of the rice and vegetable mixture. Cover the slow cooker and cook for 35 to 45 minutes, or until the salmon flakes when you test it with a fork.

4 Break the salmon up with a fork and stir it into the rice mixture along with the thawed peas. Cover and cook for 15 minutes.

5 Stir in the cheese, turn off the slow cooker, cover, and let stand for 5 minutes. Stir gently and serve immediately.

PER SERVING: Calories 416 (From Fat 103); Fat 12g (Saturated 3g); Cholesterol 54mg; Sodium 568mg; Carbohydrate 49g (Dietary Fiber 7g); Protein 29g.

VARY IT! If you're just getting started eating clean, use white rice instead and reduce the total cooking time to 2½ hours. You can also substitute chicken or pork for the salmon.

Clean Salmon and Fettuccine with Kale Pesto

PREP TIME: 15 MIN | COOK TIME: 30 MIN | YIELD: 4 SERVINGS

INGREDIENTS

2 cups chopped kale

⅓ cup blanched almonds

½ cup fresh basil leaves

2 cloves garlic, chopped

2 tablespoons lemon juice

Salt and pepper, to taste

⅓ cup plus 1 tablespoon olive oil

¼ cup grated Parmesan cheese

Three 6-ounce wild Alaskan salmon filets

½ teaspoon sea salt

⅛ teaspoon white pepper

12 ounces whole-wheat fettuccine

⅓ cup shredded Parmesan cheese

DIRECTIONS

1 In a blender or food processor, combine the kale, almonds, basil, garlic, lemon juice, and salt and pepper to taste. Blend or process until finely chopped. Scrape down the sides. With the blender or food processor running and the cover on, slowly add the ⅓ cup of olive oil and blend until a sauce forms. Scrape into a bowl.

2 Preheat the oven to 400 degrees. Place the salmon filets on a parchment-paper-lined baking sheet and sprinkle with the sea salt and white pepper. Drizzle with the remaining 1 tablespoon of olive oil. Roast for 15 to 20 minutes or until the salmon just flakes when tested with a fork. Remove the salmon from the oven and cover to keep warm.

3 While the fish is roasting, bring a large pot of water to a boil. Cook the fettuccine according to package directions until al dente. Drain, reserving ⅓ cup cooking water. Return the fettuccine to the pot.

4 Add ¾ of the kale pesto and half of the cooking water to the fettuccine and toss with tongs until mixed. Add more cooking water if necessary to make a sauce. Put the fettuccine on a serving plate, top with the salmon fillets, and drizzle with more pesto. Sprinkle with the Parmesan cheese and serve immediately.

PER SERVING: Calories 815 (From Fat 368); Fat 41g (Saturated 7g); Cholesterol 83mg; Sodium 594mg; Carbohydrate 71g (Dietary Fiber 12g); Protein 47g.

Chapter 18

Enjoying the Fun Stuff: Desserts and Snacks

Yes, you can still eat tempting and delicious desserts and snacks on the eating clean plan. But instead of grabbing a packaged cream puff or a carton of double-fudge ice cream to satisfy your sweet tooth, make some of your own homemade snacks. (This chapter provides plenty of ideas to get you started.)

Fortunately, you can find an increasing number of healthful, ready-to-eat snacks at natural food stores, but make sure to read their labels before you buy them. And remember that baking your own snacks and desserts can be fun. After all, few things offer as much satisfaction as enjoying the fruits of your labor.

If you choose to eat six small meals a day as part of your clean eating plan, you get two snacks (see Chapter 2 for details). Those snacks can be anything from air-popped popcorn sprinkled with seasonings to some whole-grain crackers and cheese to any of the delicious recipes in this chapter.

Satisfying the Munchies with Healthy Snacking

Picking out healthy snacks on the clean eating plan requires a bit of skill. But don't worry! We're here to help you gain the skills you need to succeed.

As with all mini-meals, the best snacks and desserts consist of low-calorie, nutrient-dense foods. For the longest-lasting satisfaction (yes, we know this sounds a lot like a chewing gum commercial), combine protein with carbohydrates in all your snacks. For example, the Sweet and Spicy Nuts in this chapter offer carbs and protein in one neat package, and the Rich Chocolate Torte has protein from the eggs and walnuts and carbs from the chocolate.

To help you stick with your six-meal eating plan, try to keep food for snacking available at all times. Take some time every week to prepare small grab bags of fruits, nuts, and veggies that are all ready to eat. That way, when you're hungry, you can satisfy your cravings quickly the healthy way.

Whipping Up Tasty, Clean Desserts and Snacks with Some Easy Recipes

The best part about the recipes we include in this chapter is that you can have fun varying them according to your own taste. For instance, make the Blueberry Cherry Crisp using dried cranberries and cubed apples. Or use your own home-made salsa with the Sweet Potato Chips. Sprinkle some of the Sweet and Spicy Nuts on the Dark Chocolate Bark for added crunch and flavor. You get the idea!

TIP

Don't think that eating clean means you have to leave your favorite dessert and snack recipes in the dust. Instead, adapt your favorite recipes to make them clean. Try the following:

>> **Add fruit purees to baked goods in place of some of the fat.** You can replace up to 30 percent of the fat in most recipes.

>> **Reduce the amount of sugar in baked recipes.** You can usually reduce the sugar by ⅓ to ½ without sacrificing the quality of the recipe.

>> **Substitute dark chocolate for milk or white chocolate.** Dark chocolate is a healthy food that fits into the clean eating plan. Look for dark chocolate with at least 70 percent cacao content.

>> **Look for baked whole-grain chips and dippers rather than the fried or processed varieties.** Make your own pita chips by cutting pita breads into wedges and baking them until crisp.

>> **Choose dessert recipes with lots of fruit in them.** A mixed fruit salad topped with one of the nut mixtures in this chapter makes a great dessert, especially if you add a little honey and lemon juice to the fruit. Poached fruit is also a great snack or dessert.

When you come up with a winning recipe, just be sure to write it down so you can make it again!

WHY CANDY ISN'T A SUITABLE DESSERT

While candy may be an acceptable occasional treat (key word *occasional*), a steady diet of candy isn't healthy (or clean). Most candies contain lots of processed sugar, artificial colors, and artificial flavors. These products (we can't bring ourselves to call them *food*) consist of empty calories, meaning that they provide lots of calories with no nutritive benefit. Too much sugar in your diet can increase the risk of diabetes, heart disease, cancer, high blood pressure, and osteoporosis.

Dark chocolate is the exception. A small square of dark chocolate every day provides many antioxidants, which can help relax blood pressure and protect your body from free radical damage.

Dark Chocolate Bark

PREP TIME: 10 MIN | **COOK TIME: 15 MIN, PLUS STANDING TIME** | **YIELD: 24 SERVINGS**

INGREDIENTS

16 ounces dark or bittersweet chocolate (at least 60 percent cacao), coarsely chopped

water

⅓ cup dried wild blueberries

⅓ cup dried cranberries

⅓ cup coarsely chopped walnuts

⅓ cup coarsely chopped macadamia nuts

DIRECTIONS

1 Line a 13-x-9-inch cake pan with parchment paper and set aside.

2 Place all but ½ cup of the chocolate in the top of a double boiler. Fill the bottom of the double boiler with water and bring it to a simmer.

3 Place the top of the double boiler over the simmering water, making sure the bottom of the double boiler top doesn't touch the water. Heat the chocolate until it's melted and smooth, stirring occasionally.

4 Remove the top of the double boiler from heat. Carefully dry the outside of the pan. Add the reserved chocolate to the melted chocolate and stir constantly in one direction until it's melted and smooth.

5 Stir in the blueberries, cranberries, walnuts, and macadamia nuts. Immediately pour the chocolate mixture into the prepared pan and smooth it out until it's about ⅓ inch thick.

6 Let the bark stand at room temperature until it's firm. Cut the bark into 1-inch squares and store at room temperature in a tightly covered container.

PER SERVING: Calories 137 (From Fat 77); Fat 9g (Saturated 4g); Cholesterol 1mg; Sodium 1mg; Carbohydrate 15g (Dietary Fiber 2g); Protein 2g.

TIP: Dark chocolate is packed full of antioxidants and good fats, so eating one ounce (about the size of one 1-inch square) a day is actually good for you.

Sweet and Spicy Nuts

| PREP TIME: 15 MIN | COOK TIME: 30–40 MIN | YIELD: 16 SERVINGS |

INGREDIENTS

2 egg whites

Pinch of sea salt

2 tablespoons honey, or
½ teaspoon stevia

⅓ cup almond butter

2 tablespoons curry powder

¼ teaspoon cayenne pepper

½ pound raw almonds

½ pound raw pistachios

½ pound raw walnuts

½ pound raw pecans

3 tablespoons butter

DIRECTIONS

1 Preheat the oven to 325 degrees. In a large bowl, beat the egg whites with a pinch of sea salt until soft peaks form. Gradually beat in the honey until the peaks are stiff.

2 Gradually add the almond butter to the egg white mixture, beating until combined. (The egg whites will deflate.)

3 Stir in the curry powder and cayenne pepper. Add the almonds, pistachios, walnuts, and pecans and stir to coat the nuts evenly.

4 Melt the butter and pour it into a 15-x-10-inch jelly roll pan; coat the bottom of the pan. Arrange the nut mixture in a single layer on top of the butter.

5 Bake for 30 to 40 minutes, stirring every 10 minutes, until the nuts are slightly toasted. Cool the nuts completely and store them at room temperature in an airtight container. Serve ⅓ cup per serving.

PER SERVING: Calories 208 (From Fat 172); Fat 19g (Saturated 2g); Cholesterol 3mg; Sodium 13mg; Carbohydrate 7g (Dietary Fiber 3g); Protein 5g.

TIP: You can serve this recipe straight as a snack or sprinkle it over some frozen yogurt or plain yogurt for a quick dessert.

Coconut Balls

PREP TIME: 30 MIN, PLUS CHILLING TIME | COOK TIME: 4 MIN | YIELD: 12 SERVINGS

INGREDIENTS

2½ cups unsweetened shredded coconut

3 tablespoons coconut oil

2 tablespoons coconut milk

2 tablespoons honey

3 tablespoons coconut sugar

2 teaspoons vanilla extract

One 12-ounce package dark chocolate chips (at least 60 percent cacao)

DIRECTIONS

1 In a blender or food processor, combine 1 cup of the shredded coconut with the coconut oil. Blend or process until the mixture is almost smooth. Remove to a medium bowl.

2 Stir the remaining shredded coconut, coconut milk, honey, coconut sugar, and vanilla into the coconut mixture in the bowl, and mix well. Cover and chill for 2 hours.

3 Shape the coconut mixture into 36 balls, pressing firmly with your fingers and the palm of your hand. Place on a wax-paper-lined cookie sheet and chill for another 30 minutes.

4 Place 1½ cups of the chocolate chips in a 2-cup glass measuring cup and microwave on high for 30 seconds. Remove from the microwave and stir. Continue microwaving in 30-second intervals, stirring after each interval, until the mixture is melted and smooth.

5 Stir in the remaining chocolate chips until melted and smooth.

6 Dip the coconut balls into the chocolate mixture and remove with a fork. Tap the fork on the side of the measuring cup to remove excess chocolate. Set the coated balls back on the cookie sheet and let stand until set. Sprinkle with more shredded coconut, if desired. Store covered in the refrigerator.

PER SERVING: Calories 314 (From Fat 223); Fat 25g (Saturated 19g); Cholesterol 0mg; Sodium 11mg; Carbohydrate 27g (Dietary Fiber 5g); Protein 3g.

Garlic Yogurt Cheese Spread

PREP TIME: 15 MIN, PLUS REFRIGERATING TIME	COOK TIME: 45–55 MIN
YIELD: 18 SERVINGS	

INGREDIENTS

4 cups lowfat Greek or regular plain yogurt

1 large head garlic

1 tablespoon olive oil

¼ cup grated Parmesan or Romano cheese

½ teaspoon sea salt

½ teaspoon dried thyme

½ teaspoon dried marjoram

⅛ teaspoon black pepper

DIRECTIONS

1 Line a colander or strainer with four layers of dampened cheesecloth. Place the colander in a large bowl.

2 Place the yogurt in the lined colander, cover it, and place it in the refrigerator for 24 hours.

3 Preheat the oven to 350 degrees. Cut the garlic head across the center into two pieces, exposing the cloves. Drizzle the garlic with the olive oil and wrap it in foil.

4 Place the wrapped garlic on a cookie sheet and bake it for 45 to 55 minutes, or until the cloves are soft when squeezed. Remove the garlic from the oven, unwrap it, and let it cool.

5 Squeeze the garlic cloves out of their papery coating and place them in a medium bowl. Add the yogurt cheese, Parmesan cheese, sea salt, thyme, marjoram, and pepper and stir until blended.

6 Place the yogurt cheese mixture in a serving bowl and chill for 2 to 3 hours before serving. Serve 2 tablespoons per serving.

PER SERVING: Calories 174 (From Fat 68); Fat 8g (Saturated 4g); Cholesterol 15mg; Sodium 358mg; Carbohydrate 10g (Dietary Fiber 0g); Protein 18g.

TIP: If you can find Greek yogurt, use it. It's thicker and has a richer taste than regular yogurt.

TIP: The whey that drains out of the yogurt overnight (see Step 2) works great in soups or casseroles as the liquid.

VARY IT! You can flavor the yogurt cheese any way you'd like for either a dip or a sandwich spread. Omit the garlic and double the Parmesan cheese for a milder spread. For a fruity spread, omit all the ingredients except the yogurt cheese and mash 1 cup of strawberries; stir them into the plain yogurt cheese with ½ teaspoon of cinnamon. For a Tex-Mex spread, use the garlic but omit the Parmesan cheese, thyme, and marjoram; stir in 2 teaspoons of chili powder and 2 tablespoons of chopped jalapeño chiles.

Homemade Nutella

PREP TIME: 15 MIN, PLUS COOLING TIME | **COOK TIME: 10 MIN** | **YIELD: 16 SERVINGS**

INGREDIENTS

1 cup whole hazelnuts

½ cup cashews

1 tablespoon butter, melted, or 1 tablespoon hazelnut oil

¼ cup honey

1½ teaspoons vanilla extract

1 tablespoon cocoa powder

1 tablespoon coconut sugar

⅓ cup hazelnut milk

10 ounces bittersweet chocolate (at least 60 percent cacao), chopped

DIRECTIONS

1   Preheat the oven to 375 degrees. Put the hazelnuts on a rimmed baking sheet. Roast the nuts in the oven for 8 to 10 minutes or until they're slightly darker. Immediately put the nuts on a kitchen towel, wrap, and rub between your hands to remove about half of the skins. Let the nuts cool.

2   Put the cooled nuts in a food processor along with the cashews, melted butter or hazelnut oil, honey, vanilla, cocoa powder, coconut sugar, and hazelnut milk, and process until mostly smooth.

3   Put the chocolate into a microwave-safe bowl and microwave on high for 30 seconds. Remove from the microwave and stir. Continue microwaving on high in 30-second intervals, stirring after each interval, until the chocolate is completely melted and smooth.

4   With the food processor motor running, pour the warm chocolate through the feed tube and process until the mixture is as smooth as possible.

5   Transfer the mixture to a resealable container and refrigerate.

PER SERVING: Calories 206 (From Fat 132); Fat 15g (Saturated 5g); Cholesterol 3mg; Sodium 15mg; Carbohydrate 17g (Dietary Fiber 3g); Protein 3g.

Sweet Potato Chips with Catalan Salsa

PREP TIME: 15 MIN	COOK TIME: 20 MIN	YIELD: 6 SERVINGS

INGREDIENTS

2 large beefsteak tomatoes, seeded and chopped

One 15-ounce can artichoke hearts, drained and chopped

1 jalapeño pepper, minced

2 cloves garlic, minced

½ cup chopped almonds

½ cup chopped fresh flat-leaf parsley

¼ cup olive oil, divided

2 tablespoons lemon juice

1 teaspoon freshly grated lemon zest

2 large unpeeled sweet potatoes, scrubbed

½ teaspoon sea salt

DIRECTIONS

1 In a medium bowl, combine the tomatoes, artichokes, jalapeño pepper, garlic, almonds, parsley, 2 tablespoons of the olive oil, lemon juice, and lemon zest, and mix gently. Set aside while you prepare the chips.

2 Preheat the oven to 425 degrees. Thinly slice the sweet potatoes using a mandolin or a very sharp knife. Toss with the remaining 2 tablespoons of olive oil, spread in a single layer on two cookie sheets that have been lined with parchment paper, and sprinkle with the sea salt.

3 Roast the sweet potatoes for 18 to 22 minutes or until the edges are crisp.

4 Let the chips cool and serve with the salsa.

PER SERVING: Calories 380 (From Fat 289); Fat 32g (Saturated 3g); Cholesterol 0mg; Sodium 365mg; Carbohydrate 21g (Dietary Fiber 5g); Protein 5g.

TIP: A mandolin is the easiest way to make these thin and crispy potato chips. If you don't have one, use a very sharp knife and cut the potatoes into the thinnest slices you can.

Rich Chocolate Torte

PREP TIME: 15 MIN | **COOK TIME: 35 MIN** | **YIELD: 12 SERVINGS**

INGREDIENTS

2 cups walnuts

¼ cup butter, melted

8 ounces dark chocolate (at least 70 percent cacao), chopped

8 ounces semisweet chocolate (at least 60 percent cacao), chopped

⅔ cup butter

2 tablespoons coconut oil

6 eggs

1 tablespoon vanilla extract

Pinch of sea salt

DIRECTIONS

1 Preheat the oven to 325 degrees. Grease a 9-inch springform pan with a bit of butter.

2 Finely chop the walnuts, by hand or in a food processor, and mix with the melted butter. Press this mixture into the bottom of the prepared pan and set aside.

3 Combine the dark chocolate, semisweet chocolate, butter, and coconut oil in a medium microwave-safe bowl and microwave on high for 30 seconds. Remove the bowl from the microwave and stir. Continue microwaving in 30-second intervals on high until the mixture is smooth.

4 In a large bowl, beat the eggs until light and fluffy, about 5 minutes. Reduce the mixer speed to low and blend in the melted chocolate mixture. Stir in the vanilla and sea salt.

5 Pour the chocolate mixture into the pan over the walnut crust.

6 Bake for 45 to 50 minutes or until the torte is just set. Remove the torte from the oven and let cool on a wire rack for 1 hour. Cover and refrigerate for 3 to 4 hours.

7 Run a knife around the cake to loosen then unlatch the pan and remove the sides. Slice into thin wedges to serve.

PER SERVING: Calories 468 (From Fat 377); Fat 42g (Saturated 20g); Cholesterol 143mg; Sodium 43mg; Carbohydrate 20g (Dietary Fiber 4g); Protein 8g.

TIP: For a sweeter cake, you can use increase the amount of semisweet chocolate to 12 ounce and reduce the dark chocolate to 4 ounces. Or you can use all semisweet chocolate.

Clean Edamame Guacamole

PREP TIME: 15 MIN, PLUS REFRIGERATING TIME **COOK TIME: ABOUT 5 MIN**
YIELD: 8 SERVINGS

INGREDIENTS

1½ cups frozen edamame

2 tablespoons lemon juice

2 ripe avocados, pitted

½ teaspoon sea salt

⅓ cup lowfat regular or Greek yogurt

⅛ teaspoon red pepper flakes

½ pint grape tomatoes, chopped

3 green onions, sliced

DIRECTIONS

1 Thaw and cook the edamame according to the package directions. Drain the edamame well and sprinkle with the lemon juice; let cool for 10 minutes.

2 Scoop the flesh of the avocados into a medium bowl. Add the edamame and sprinkle both with the sea salt.

3 Using a potato masher, mash the avocados and edamame together. Make the mixture as smooth or chunky as you like.

4 Stir in the yogurt and red pepper flakes. Add the chopped tomatoes and green onions. Spoon the mixture into a serving bowl.

5 Cover by placing waxed or parchment paper directly on the surface of the guacamole. Chill for 2 to 3 hours to blend flavors. Serve ¼ cup of guacamole per serving.

PER SERVING: Calories 270 (From Fat 137); Fat 15g (Saturated 3g); Cholesterol 1mg; Sodium 340mg; Carbohydrate 26g (Dietary Fiber 14g); Protein 12g.

TIP: You can use this recipe as a sandwich spread, too. Just be sure to store the leftovers in the refrigerator.

Frozen Yogurt Bars

PREP TIME: 15 MIN | **FREEZE TIME: 3 HR** | **YIELD: 12 SERVINGS**

INGREDIENTS

2 cups lowfat Greek or regular yogurt

½ teaspoon stevia

2 cups frozen strawberries

1 cup frozen wild blueberries

1 tablespoon lemon juice

DIRECTIONS

1 Combine the yogurt, stevia, berries, and lemon juice in a food processor. Cover and process until well blended, stopping once to scrape down the sides of the processor.

2 Pour ¼ cup of the mixture into a popsicle form, or fill it according to the package directions. Repeat for a total of 12 popsicle forms. Freeze the bars for at least 3 hours before serving.

3 Remove the yogurt bar from the popsicle form and serve one bar per serving.

PER SERVING: Calories 39 (From Fat 8); Fat 1g (Saturated 1g); Cholesterol 3mg; Sodium 12mg; Carbohydrate 5g (Dietary Fiber 1g); Protein 4g.

TIP: The easiest way to make these bars is to use popsicle forms, which you can find at baking supply stores, hardware stores, and large supermarkets. If you don't have popsicle forms, you can use paper juice cups. Just pour the yogurt mixture into the cups, freeze them for 1 hour, insert a wooden popsicle stick into each cup, and then freeze them until the yogurt mixture is firm. Don't forget to peel the paper cup away before serving!

VARY IT! It's easy to change the flavor of this recipe; just use a different type of fruit! Peaches, raspberries, and bananas all work well and taste delicious!

Apple Pear Cranberry Crumble

PREP TIME: 15 MIN	COOK TIME: 2 HR	YIELD: 6 SERVINGS

INGREDIENTS

2 Haralson or McIntosh apples, chopped

2 firm pears, chopped

2 tablespoons lemon juice

½ cup dried cranberries

1 cup whole-wheat flour

½ cup old-fashioned rolled oats

½ cup chopped pecans

3 tablespoons coconut sugar

3 tablespoons butter

2 tablespoons coconut oil

2 tablespoons honey

½ teaspoon cinnamon

⅛ teaspoon sea salt

DIRECTIONS

1 Preheat the oven to 375 degrees. Grease a 9-x-9-inch glass baking dish with butter.

2 Combine the apples and pears in the prepared baking dish and sprinkle with the lemon juice. Top with the dried cranberries.

3 In a large bowl, combine the whole-wheat flour, rolled oats, pecans, and coconut sugar, and mix.

4 In a small saucepan, combine the butter, coconut oil, honey, cinnamon, and sea salt, and heat over medium-low heat until the fats melt.

5 Pour the butter mixture over the flour mixture and stir until crumbly. Sprinkle evenly over the fruit in the baking dish.

6 Bake for 30 to 40 minutes or until the apples and pears have softened and the topping is browned. Let cool for 25 minutes, then serve.

PER SERVING: Calories 387 (From Fat 162); Fat 18g (Saturated 8g); Cholesterol 15mg; Sodium 55mg; Carbohydrate 58g (Dietary Fiber 9g); Protein 5g.

Chocolate Fruit and Nut Drops

PREP TIME: 35 MIN | COOK TIME: 5 MIN | YIELD: 12 SERVINGS

INGREDIENTS

12 ounces dark chocolate (at least 60 percent cacao), chopped

1 ounce unsweetened chocolate, chopped

2 tablespoons coconut oil

1 cup chopped macadamia nuts

½ cup chopped walnuts

½ cup finely chopped dates

½ cup dried cranberries

½ cup unsweetened coconut

DIRECTIONS

1 Place the dark chocolate, unsweetened chocolate, and coconut oil in a large microwave-safe bowl. Microwave on high for 30 seconds, then remove and stir. Continue microwaving on high in 30-second intervals, stirring after each interval, until the chocolate is melted and smooth.

2 Stir in the remaining ingredients. Drop by spoonfuls onto parchment paper and let stand until set. You can refrigerate the candies if you'd like.

3 Store in an airtight container at room temperature.

PER SERVING: Calories 339 (From Fat 241); Fat 27g (Saturated 12g); Cholesterol 2mg; Sodium 6mg; Carbohydrate 24g (Dietary Fiber 5g); Protein 4g.

TIP: Dates can be purchased either dried or fresh. Any type of whole date works well in this recipe. Do not use the prechopped packaged dates that are covered in sugar, because they will be too dry for this recipe.

Blueberry Cherry Crisp

PREP TIME: 15 MIN	COOK TIME: 33–38 MIN	YIELD: 8 SERVINGS

INGREDIENTS

1 cup old-fashioned oatmeal

⅓ cup whole-wheat flour

½ cup chopped macadamia nuts

2 tablespoons coconut oil

3 tablespoons unsalted butter

2 tablespoons honey

1 teaspoon cinnamon

¼ teaspoon nutmeg

⅛ teaspoon sea salt

4 cups frozen cherries, thawed

2 cups frozen blueberries

1 tablespoon lemon juice

1 teaspoon stevia

DIRECTIONS

1 Preheat the oven to 375 degrees. Grease a 9-x-9-inch glass dish with unsalted butter and set aside.

2 In a large bowl, combine the oatmeal, flour, and macadamia nuts. Set aside.

3 In a small saucepan, combine the coconut oil, butter, honey, cinnamon, nutmeg, and sea salt. Heat the mixture over low heat until the butter melts, about 3 minutes. Stir the oil and butter mixture and pour it over the oatmeal mixture. Stir until the mixture becomes crumbly.

4 Place the thawed cherries and frozen blueberries into the prepared glass dish. In a small bowl, mix the lemon juice and stevia and sprinkle it over the berries.

5 Spoon the oatmeal mixture over the berries. Bake for 30 to 35 minutes, or until the crisp is bubbly and the topping has browned. Serve 1½ cups per serving.

PER SERVING: Calories 276 (From Fat 141); Fat 16g (Saturated 6g); Cholesterol 12mg; Sodium 40mg; Carbohydrate 34g (Dietary Fiber 5g); Protein 4g.

TIP: If you aren't worried about obesity or diabetes, drizzle each serving with a bit of honey. This crisp is just as good cold the next day, so pack some in your lunchbox for a special treat.

6

The Part of Tens

Chapter 19

Ten Ways to Tell If Your Eating Clean Diet Is Working

When you embark on a new diet plan or lifestyle change, you want to see results. Of course you expect to feel better when you eat clean, whole foods. But what kind of specific results can you expect to see on the eating clean diet plan?

In this chapter, we look at ten specific physical (and mental) changes you can look for after you've been eating clean, whole foods for a few weeks or months. Remember that these changes won't happen overnight. But if you've been relying on a diet of heavily processed foods, with refined sugar and flour and lots of additives and preservatives, you may see dramatic results in a short period of time.

Weight Loss

Weight loss is a goal for many people living in the United States. More than 60 percent of the population is overweight or obese, and people continue to gain weight. In the 1970s, only 15 percent of the adult population was obese. So what's changed in that time frame? One of the most radical changes has been in the amount of processed foods Americans eat. Think about what your grandparents ate around the time of World War II. Vegetable gardens were big, family farms were prominent, and soda pop was a special treat. People consumed cakes and cookies only during special occasions. In contrast, junk food is the norm for many families today.

REMEMBER

Eating whole, unprocessed foods, more fruits and vegetables, whole grains, lean meats, and healthy oils and fats can help you lose weight without even trying. Consuming these nutrient-dense foods, which are satisfying as well as healthy, keeps you full longer and naturally reduces your overall caloric intake. And the best part is you don't need to count calories! Eat lower on the food chain, eat when you're hungry, stop eating when you feel full and satisfied, and enjoy every bite.

TIP

If you add exercise to your eating clean plan, you may be able to lose weight even faster. After all, people with more muscles burn more calories, even when they're sleeping or sitting still!

Clearer Skin

Clear skin is one benefit that may get teenagers to jump on the eating clean bandwagon. And because skin problems can persist into adulthood for many people, adults can appreciate this benefit, too. Eating clean provides you with the vitamins, minerals, and phytochemicals your skin needs to be smooth and healthy.

Although foods like chocolate and sugar don't directly cause acne, eating those foods crowds out the healthy foods you need to eat for good skin. As a result, refined carbohydrates may make skin conditions like acne worse. Foods high in sodium and trans fats can increase sebum production in your skin, which causes pores to clog, letting bacteria build up and create acne. Clean eating eliminates added sugar and refined carbs.

Some food allergies can also contribute to skin problems. By eating clean, avoiding foods you're allergic to, and avoiding possible allergenic foods, including additives and preservatives, you can often alleviate or eliminate skin problems.

REMEMBER

The nutrients to focus on for clear skin include essential fatty acids, vitamin A, vitamin B6, and vitamin C.

You find these nutrients in fruits and vegetables, legumes, whole grains, avocados, nuts, seeds, lean meats, and oily fish. Anti-inflammatory nutrients like carotenoids and quercetin, which are found in carrots and apples, may also help reduce skin problems.

Don't forget about wrinkles! The same powerful phytochemicals you eat for clear skin help fight the free radicals that can damage skin cells, making the skin thinner and more prone to wrinkling. The same nutrients that can help keep younger skin clear can help make wrinkle-prone skin look fuller.

TIP

Another way to keep your skin looking young and clear is to drink lots of water. Water helps moisturize your skin from the inside out, maintaining elasticity and keeping the skin supple.

More Energy

Consuming the whole grains and complex carbohydrates on the eating clean plan can help give you more energy and make you stronger. The trick of combining carbohydrates with proteins and fat not only keeps you feeling satisfied longer but also keeps your blood sugar level stable for a longer period of time, which prevents those afternoon slumps.

REMEMBER

All the nutrients in the clean foods on your new diet help increase energy. Vitamins, minerals, and phytochemicals help your cells work more effectively, making your body more efficient overall. Complex carbohydrates take longer for your body to digest, so they provide more fuel over a longer time period.

After you begin your eating clean diet, you'll probably notice that you don't need to nap as often, but do try to get enough sleep. If you feel more energetic, add an exercise program to your daily routine. Doing so gives you even more energy! Soon you'll be leaping tall buildings in a single . . . well, maybe not, but you get the idea.

Healthier Hair and Fingernails

The trick to having healthy, good-looking hair is working from the inside out. While using special shampoos and conditioners can affect your hair's exterior look and feel, eating a good diet of wholesome foods is one of the best ways to keep your hair looking its best.

REMEMBER

Although your hair itself is dead (otherwise you'd be in a lot of pain during your haircuts!), your scalp is alive, and it's actually the basis for healthy hair. Vitamins A, B, and C promote a healthy scalp and can make hair stronger. Iron keeps your hair follicles strong by providing them with oxygen, and zinc can help prevent hair loss. Although healthy hair isn't really a health benefit, it is a sign that your overall health may be improving.

Did you know that many doctors now look at your fingernails for clues about your health? Some nail conditions can indicate chronic health conditions ranging from bronchitis to inflammatory bowel disease and even heart disease. An iron deficiency can cause raised ridges in your fingernails. People with lupus may have blood vessels that show through fingernails, and very pale nails can indicate anemia.

Eating a clean diet with whole foods can help treat or manage these conditions. Healthy nails indicate a healthy body.

Stronger Muscles

If you want to strengthen your muscles, eat five or six small meals a day, and make sure you get plenty of the following:

>> Lean proteins

>> Combination of proteins, complex carbohydrates, and healthy fats

>> Fruits and vegetables

>> Nuts and seeds

Well, that's the eating clean diet plan in a nutshell! All the nutrients in whole foods help build muscle, protect your cells against damage from aging and free radicals, keep your heart muscle (the most important muscle in your body) strong, and keep your veins and arteries strong and healthy so they can pump oxygen to your muscles.

REMEMBER

Good sources of protein include fish, especially fatty fish, lean beef, chicken, pork, nuts, seeds, and whole grains. You find healthy fats in egg yolks, almonds and other nuts, olive oil, and produce like avocados. Whole grains and legumes are the best sources of complex carbohydrates.

For building muscle, a good diet is essential. But you need to exercise regularly, too, combining cardio training with weight lifting and strength training. Lucky for you, the clean diet plan provides more energy so you can work out with ease and get stronger.

Lower Blood Pressure

High blood pressure is troublesome for several reasons. It raises your risk of a heart attack or stroke, it can cause kidney damage and vision loss, and the excess pressure of blood can actually weaken and damage your arteries.

Because diet plays such a significant part in blood pressure, changing your diet can help you lower both the systolic (top) reading and the diastolic (bottom) reading on the blood pressure cuff. Maintaining a healthy weight and improving your overall health can also help lower blood pressure. The eating clean diet is a perfect way to do all three.

REMEMBER

Increasing the nutrients you eat every day helps control blood pressure. Calcium, magnesium, potassium, and zinc, which are important in blood pressure maintenance, are all found in whole foods. In addition, phytochemicals and vitamins can help reduce damage to your arteries by neutralizing free radical damage and preventing oxidation of cholesterol.

Many nutritionists advise people at risk for high blood pressure to lower their sodium intake. Because 70 percent of the sodium you consume is found in processed foods, reducing your consumption of those foods automatically reduces your salt intake.

A Stronger Immune System

A stronger immune system can be a direct result of a healthy diet. After all, phytochemicals like lycopene and quercetin, which you find in clean, whole foods, offer the following benefits:

» They keep your immune system strong.

» They block carcinogens from damaging cells in your body.

» They reduce the inflammation that can cause diseases like cancer and heart disease.

>> They slow the rate of cancer cell growth.

>> They trigger *apoptosis,* which is the natural death of cells when they have lived their normal lifespan. (Cancer cells don't die as they should, which is why tumors form.)

A stronger immune system means that you will catch fewer colds, may be more resistant to flu viruses, and will recover from such illnesses more quickly when you do catch them. Fewer sick days are just one of the benefits of the clean eating lifestyle.

Lower Cholesterol Levels

Lower overall cholesterol numbers, higher HDL cholesterol readings, and lower LDL cholesterol numbers are the goal for many people. The eating clean diet plan helps you improve these numbers by focusing your meals around fruits, vegetables, lean meats, healthy fats, and whole grains.

Your body sends cholesterol to help repair damage in your arteries and to soothe inflammation. So high cholesterol levels are really a sign that your body is under attack from free radicals and other causes of inflammation. Consuming the trans fats, simple carbohydrates, and refined sugars in processed foods can increase your cholesterol levels.

REMEMBER

Eating foods with lots of phytochemicals, like resveratrol and lutein, and vitamins, like the B complex and vitamin D, can help reduce cholesterol levels and improve your HDL/LDL ratio. You find these nutrients in fruits and vegetables. Good fats, like fatty fish, nuts, and seeds, that have high levels of omega-3 fatty acids, are also crucial to high HDL and low LDL cholesterol levels. So throw out the processed foods and turn to natural, wholesome foods for improved test results.

Clearer Thinking

Have you ever binged on junk food and felt woozy and fuzzy afterward? Scientists report that junk food can actually hurt your brain's *synapses,* which are the areas between neurons where chemical messengers communicate with one another. A poor diet can also slow down the production of molecules that improve memory and learning ability.

Nutrients important for clear thinking and good brain health include omega-3 fatty acids, which help keep synapses flexible and plastic and may help protect against brain disorders like depression and dementia. Omega-3 fatty acids are important components of neural membranes and help prevent decline in mental function as you grow older. Essential fatty acids are also important for brain health. Lean protein is essential to making more neurotransmitters that work in your brain's synapses. Other important nutrients for brain health include magnesium, potassium, beta carotene, vitamins C, E, and the B complex, and folate, which helps prevent dementia.

You find all these nutrients in whole, unprocessed, fresh foods like fruits and vegetables . . . you know the drill by now.

A Happy Doctor

One of the most satisfying results of your new eating clean lifestyle is the positive response you'll hear at your annual visit to the doctor. Imagine how surprised and delighted he or she will be when you show up with a healthier weight, a lower blood pressure, lower cholesterol levels, better HDL readings, a stronger heart, and more energy. No need to dread your doctor's visits now! You may even be able to educate your doctor about your new lifestyle and eating plan. Don't be afraid to spread the word because this lifestyle is easy to follow, satisfying to live, and rewarding!

Chapter 20

Ten Foods to Always Put in Your Shopping Cart

When you make out your weekly shopping list, always try to include the ten foods we describe in this chapter. They have many uses in the kitchen, they're inexpensive, and they contain the most potent phytochemicals, vitamins, and minerals your body needs to be at its best.

But even though these foods are the cream of the crop in terms of nutrients, fiber, and good fats, don't limit yourself to these choices. Instead, use them as a jumping off point. Experiment with new foods weekly to help you stay interested in your clean eating plan and to ensure that you're getting as many nutrients as possible in every bite you take. Don't be afraid to try new cuisines and new combinations, too. Combine leafy greens with curry powder, coat your salmon with chopped nuts before baking, and cook broccoli or Brussels sprouts with garlic and olive oil. The possibilities are endless!

Sweet Potatoes

The Center for Science in the Public Interest has ranked sweet potatoes as number one in nutrition, which is no surprise considering that these spuds are loaded with fiber, protein, complex carbohydrates, vitamins, potassium, magnesium, zinc, carotenoids, iron, and calcium. As a matter of fact, sweet potatoes have more than twice the recommended dietary allowance (RDA) of vitamin A, more than 40 percent of the RDA of vitamin C, and four times the RDA for beta carotene. And each sweet potato contains only about 130 calories!

Looking for great meal ideas? Bake your sweet potatoes, slit them open, and stuff them with some low-fat yogurt (or Greek yogurt) mixed with tomatoes and celery. Or cut the sweet potatoes into slender sticks, toss them with olive oil and paprika, and bake them until crisp. If you're looking for a full meal, try the Quinoa Vegetable Soup in Chapter 16 and the Roasted Pork Tenderloin and Veggies in Chapter 17.

REMEMBER

However you decide to cook your sweet potatoes, make sure you always eat the skin! Most of the fiber is located in the skin, and the flesh right under the skin is highest in nutrients.

Wild Salmon

When you're buying salmon, be sure to choose wild salmon rather than farmed salmon because the farmed fish can be high in mercury and toxic chemicals called PCBs, including lead and other heavy metals. Wild salmon contains high amounts of omega-3 fatty acids, magnesium, protein, and vitamin D. It's also a great source of niacin, selenium, and vitamins B12 and B6. Eating salmon also helps prevent heart disease and diseases caused by inflammation.

Scientists have recently found that omega-3 fatty acids can help slow the degenerative effects of Alzheimer's disease and dementia. These fatty acids can also help lower the risk of depression and aggressive behavior.

With all these benefits, it's no wonder that many nutritionists urge people to eat foods like wild salmon twice a week. Putting salmon on the menu twice a week can lower the level of triglycerides in your blood and can improve heart function. Check out the Salmon Salad Sandwich with Peach Salsa in Chapter 16 and the

Curry-Rubbed Salmon and Salmon Risi Bisi in Chapter 17 if you're looking for some new meal ideas.

Olive Oil

You can use olive oil when sautéing foods, as the fat in almost any baking or cooking recipe, in salad dressings, and when frying foods. Most of the fatty acids in olive oil are omega-9 fatty acids, which are healthy monounsaturated fats that can help lower total blood cholesterol levels. Extra-virgin olive oil is made from the first pressing of olives, without heat, so it's high in vitamin E and phenols, both of which are powerful antioxidants. And it has a wonderful flavor. Use it mostly in salad dressings and when briefly sautéing foods.

When cooking with olive oil, remember that unrefined extra-virgin olive oil has a *smoke point* (the point at which the oil begins to break down and emit smoke) of about 375 degrees, which is slightly above the ideal temperature for sautéing or frying food but lower than the smoke points of other oils. So use ordinary (not extra-virgin) olive oil, which has a higher smoke point of up to 430 degrees, for frying and long-sautéed recipes. Save the extra-virgin olive oil for salad dressings and baking! (Many of the recipes in Part 5 call for olive oil, so go there if you're looking for some yummy ideas.)

Cruciferous Vegetables

Cruciferous vegetables include broccoli, cauliflower, Brussels sprouts, kohlrabi, cabbage, kale, and bok choy. What makes them so great? Many studies have found a link between eating these veggies and protecting the body from cancer. Specifically, phytochemicals in these foods, including sulforaphane, indole-3-carbinol, and crambene, help the enzymes in your body that destroy carcinogens before they can damage your cells. As an added bonus, these veggies are high in antioxidants, which help prevent oxidation and damage from free radicals.

REMEMBER

The key to preparing these vegetables is not to overcook them. Because they have a high sulfur content, overcooking them releases that chemical and gives them a very unappealing taste. Steam them lightly or eat them raw to keep your body (and your tongue) happy. (Check out the Fruity Coleslaw in Chapter 16, the Kale Chips with Spanish Salsa in Chapter 18, or any of the tasty veggie meals in Chapter 17.)

Nuts

Did you know that nuts are actually seeds? Well, it's true; any one nut contains every nutrient needed to support the sprouting and growth of an entire young tree! The many nutrients that nuts provide offer plenty of benefits to you, too:

>> **Essential fatty acids and monounsaturated fats:** Help lower LDL cholesterol and reduce the risk of blood clots

>> **Vitamin E:** Helps reduce plaque development in your arteries

>> **Fiber:** Lowers blood cholesterol levels

>> **Plant sterols:** Lower blood cholesterol levels

Because nuts have so many health benefits and are so satisfying to eat, they're a great choice for a healthy snack on the eating clean plan. The healthiest nuts include walnuts, almonds, macadamia nuts, hazelnuts, and pecans. This may surprise you: Peanuts aren't technically nuts! They're legumes, just like peas and beans.

REMEMBER

Keep in mind that nuts lose many of their nonmineral nutrients to oxidation when they're roasted, so eat nuts raw whenever possible.

TIP

If you're looking for new ways to enjoy nuts, try the Nut Butter Granola, Pear Banana Nut Muffins, and Fruit and Nut Muesli in Chapter 15, the Clean Cobb Salad, Fruity Coleslaw, Fruity Chicken Pasta Salad, and Fruit and Grains Salad in Chapter 16, and the Dark Chocolate Bark, Sweet and Spicy Nuts, Apricot Pistachio Laraballs, Stuffed Dates, Granola Berry Parfaits, Slow Cooker Stuffed Apples, Chile-Spiced Nuts and Fruit, and Blueberry Cherry Crisp in Chapter 18.

Avocados

Avocados are a rich and buttery treat, and — as surprising as it may be — they're very good for you! These fruits are high in vitamins E, C, and K, potassium, oleic acid, folate, antioxidants, and phytochemicals (which stop free radical damage). The fat in avocados is monounsaturated, which means it lowers blood cholesterol levels. Plus, avocados contain beta-sitosterol, which is a phytochemical that also reduces cholesterol.

Use avocados as a sandwich spread in place of mayonnaise or butter. Just mash up an avocado with a little lemon or lime juice and spread it on whole-wheat rolls or bread. Include avocados in your green salads, eat them plain as a snack, and use them to top burgers and grilled sandwiches. Plus, check out the Clean Cobb Salad in Chapter 16 and the Clean Edamame Guacamole in Chapter 18.

Leafy Greens

To get the most nutrients for the fewest calories, always put foods like kale, collard greens, romaine lettuce, spinach, Swiss chard, and escarole in your shopping cart. These greens are rich in vitamins and minerals, especially vitamins C, K, E, the B complex, potassium, and magnesium, as well as phytonutrients, including lutein, quercetin, zeaxanthin, and beta carotene.

A diet rich in dark leafy greens can help reduce the risk of atherosclerosis and heart disease, prevent diabetes and osteoporosis, and reduce the risk of developing cancer. Eat the greens raw, or cook them in soups and stews. Sturdy leafy greens are delicious in stir-fry recipes, too. In fact, you can add leafy greens to just about any of the lunch and dinner recipes we include in Chapters 16 and 17.

Curry Powder

Curry powder is a blend of several different spices, all of which are high in antioxidants and phytochemicals. But the most important spice in curry powder is turmeric, which provides a yellow color and subtle rich flavor. Turmeric contains curcumin, which is a powerful phytochemical.

People who consume a lot of turmeric-containing curry powder have lower cancer rates, lower rates of Alzheimer's disease, less inflammation, and improved memory. Curcumin has also been shown to slow the progress of prostate cancer.

Sprinkle curry powder on salads, use it in salad dressings, and add it to stir-fries and even your breakfast smoothie. You can find curry powder in mild and spicy blends, or you can make your own (just be sure to include plenty of turmeric!). If you're new to curry powder, try the Wild Rice Egg Roll Ups in Chapter 15, the Curry-Rubbed Salmon in Chapter 17, and the Sweet and Spicy Nuts in Chapter 18.

Berries (Especially Blueberries)

Berries are a wonderful sweet treat, and they make a delicious dessert all by themselves. Plus, they're very good for you. Strawberries are an excellent source of vitamin C and contain phytochemicals that can help fight cancer. Blueberries, especially wild blueberries, are one of the healthiest foods on earth, with the highest antioxidant content of all fresh fruit.

Dried berries have just as many nutrients as fresh. They're higher in calories, though, because they have less water. Still, they make a wonderful snack when eaten in moderation. And don't forget about frozen berries! These fruits are harvested at their peak and are often processed right in the field. Frozen berries can have more nutrients than fresh berries which may have been shipped for miles.

These fruits are also high in fiber, which can help you feel full longer and can reduce blood cholesterol levels. Add berries to green salads, fruit salads, use them to top your morning cereal, and eat them out of your hand as a tasty, sweet snack. Or try the Fruit and Nut Muesli in Chapter 15, the Fruity Chicken Pasta Salad and Salmon Salad Sandwich with Peach Salsa in Chapter 16, and the Granola Berry Parfaits, Frozen Yogurt Bars, and Blueberry Cherry Crisp in Chapter 18.

Garlic and Onions

These pungent root vegetables are good sources of allyl sulfides, which are phytochemicals that can help reduce the risk of cancer and calm inflammation in the body. These veggies are also high in polyphenols and flavonoids, which prevent oxidation and stop free radical damage. Garlic can help lower cholesterol levels, too.

TIP

To get the most benefit from garlic, chop or crush it and let it sit for a few minutes at room temperature before cooking it. Doing so helps preserve the allicin content, even after the garlic is cooked. Because the flavonoids in onions are concentrated near the skin, peel your onions as little as possible to get the most health benefits. Turn to Part 5 to find plenty of recipes that call for garlic and onions.

Chapter 21

Ten Ways to a Cleaner World

Eating clean not only helps make you healthier and improve your life; it can also help improve the world. When you buy lower on the food chain by buying whole foods, you avoid packaged and processed foods that take a lot of energy to produce. And you're not contributing to the facilities and transport methods that cause pollution. The amount of garbage you produce will be less, too, because there will be less to throw away.

In this chapter, we look at ten ways you can help the environment by eating clean. We'll talk about buying local and hyper-local foods, as well as how to support sustainability, grow your own foods, reduce waste, recycle, and compost.

REMEMBER

Every little bit helps. If you aren't completely avoiding processed and packaged food, any changes you make will help. And when more people start the eating clean lifestyle, the changes can be dramatic!

Buying Local and Hyper-Local

The local food movement has been growing since the 1970s. When you buy your food from local, independent farmers and businesses, you support your local town economy. This helps reduce the environmental impact of your diet because less transportation is needed, which means less pollution and wild animal habitat loss. In addition, you'll help create more good jobs in your community.

In addition, buying locally produced and sourced foods means the food you eat will contain more nutrients. Most produce sold in the United States is picked about a week before you buy it and travels 1,500 miles. During that time, nutrients are depleted.

Buying *hyper-local* means you do most of your shopping in your own neighborhood, and help farmers and businesses connect into a well-defined community. For instance, if you support your neighborhood farmer's market you may find cheese from a local producer, eggs from a family farm, fruits and vegetables from a truck garden, new curtains for your kitchen, and plants for your garden, all in one stop.

TIP

Community supported agriculture (CSA) is a great way to buy local. You pay a fixed amount to a local farmer at the beginning of a season, and then you're entitled to take some of the harvest home during the growing season. You'll find that the taste and nutrition of the food grown and purchased locally is much better than anything you can buy in a grocery store. Plus, it's fun to visit a farm and get your food right at the source.

Supporting Sustainability

Sustainability is the ability to endure and prosper over a long period of time. Long-lived ecosystems that are healthy and pollution-free benefit everyone. Buildings, farms, and communities that are sustainable help future generations by minimizing their environmental impact. With a little research and comparison-shopping, you can support sustainability with every purchase you make.

For instance, when you buy meat, look for animals that are raised in the pasture, not on large factory farms or concentrated animal feeding operations (CAFOs). The animals live better lives when they graze in a pasture, there is less harm done to the environment, and you'll be healthier, too. And the meat from pasture-raised animals has a better balance of omega-3 and omega-6 fatty acids than conventionally raised meats.

Sustainable crops are grown differently from conventional crops. Multiple species are planted on the same land every crop cycle, which minimizes soil depletion and increases yields. Farmers don't have to use as many pesticides and herbicides because this type of farming can reduce insect infestation and discourage weeds.

TIP

Sustainable crops may be higher in nutrients. Crops grown on industrial farms are bred for high yield and fast growth instead of nutrient content, and animals raised for meat are bred for fast growth. These factors may reduce the macronutrients and micronutrients available in produce and meat.

Spending Money on the Best Food

If you're like most people, you're concerned about budgets, overspending, and getting the most for your money. By eating clean, you may find your budget improving along with your health! Let's face it: Junk food is expensive in more ways than one.

When you want to get the most for your money, buying foods low on the food chain — such as fresh tomatoes instead of canned tomatoes, dried beans for homemade soup instead of canned soup, or fresh spinach instead of frozen spinach — can help your budget and your health. Whenever food is processed, nutrients are lost and cost is added.

REMEMBER

Buying in season can help you get the most for your money. When you buy peaches in January imported from Mexico, you're paying a premium for the cost of transportation, and the fruit won't taste as good as peaches grown in your own backyard. But when you buy peaches in August from a local farmer, the cost will be less and the taste and the nutrition of those peaches will be far superior.

It's true that some junk food or fast food is cheaper and can be more filling than whole, nutritious foods, but the price of junk food is far higher in the long run. A steady diet of fast food hamburgers, potato chips, and snack foods will cost you in healthcare dollars later on. It does take more work and effort to cook at home with whole foods, but that effort may pay off in a longer, healthier life!

Factory Farms and Antibiotic Resistance

Not only is staying away from any meat or produce produced by factory farms a good idea nutritionally, but it's better for the health of everyone in the world. On many factory farms, livestock crowded into filthy stalls are given subtherapeutic doses of antibiotics to prevent disease and to spur growth. This practice helps bacteria develop resistance to antibiotics. And now we're looking at superbugs that won't respond to medical treatment.

The FDA and USDA have asked manufacturers of veterinary drugs to stop labeling them for the use of disease prevention, but the antibiotics can still be used for growth promotion. It's possible that those drugs get into the meat, and then into you when you eat that steak.

Large feedlots also contribute to air and water pollution, and indirectly to food poisoning outbreaks. Runoff from these farms, which can contain pathogenic bacteria, gets into the groundwater and pollutes it. When that water is used to irrigate farm fields, crops can become contaminated and cause foodborne illness outbreaks.

The USDA estimates that confirmed farm animals generate more than 450 million tons of manure every year. And these facilities generate huge amounts of greenhouse gases that contribute to climate change. Factory farms contribute 37 percent of methane emissions into the environment. That gas has 20 times the global warming potential of carbon dioxide.

Raw Foods Caution

Whole foods are good for you, and gentle cooking methods such as the slow cooker may be best, but eating *raw* (uncooked) foods can be problematic, especially if you have a serious health condition or are at risk for food poisoning (young children, the elderly, those with compromised immune systems or chronic illnesses, and pregnant women). Outbreaks of foodborne illness have been linked to everything from ice cream to spinach to ground beef.

In fact, the FDA says that the food that causes the most food poisoning outbreaks is fresh produce. Outbreaks have been linked to raw nuts, fresh spinach, fresh cilantro, tomatoes, raspberries, and raw sprouts. The raw food movement encourages whole food consumption, but it also disallows any food that has been heated above 104 degrees. The problem is that bacteria are only killed when food is heated to 160 degrees.

TIP

Eating some foods raw is good for you, but you'll get more nutrients out of other foods when they're cooked. For instance, your body can absorb more vitamin A precursor from carrots when they're cooked. When mushrooms are cooked, potassium is more available.

WARNING

Anyone who follows a raw food diet could be lacking in vitamin B12, which can cause anemia and damage to the nervous system. Meat is one of the best sources of this vitamin. If you're eating a raw diet, you shouldn't be eating meat, which means you may be deficient in vitamin B12. Check with your doctor and ask about supplementation if you're interested in this plan.

Your Own Garden

Growing your own food is rewarding, inexpensive, and really the best way to ensure that your food is as fresh as possible. If you have a backyard garden, you won't be contributing to pollution through food transportation or packaging, and you're living the ultimate local lifestyle!

Try to get your family involved when you plant a garden. You don't have to have a huge plot of land to grow a significant part of your diet in the summer. A few raised beds or half a dozen large pots can provide lots of tomatoes, bell peppers, herbs, peas, beans, and fruit throughout the growing season.

TIP

If you start your garden from seed, look for heirloom varieties. These are seeds that have not been subject to genetic engineering and are often open pollinated. Plus, heirloom seeds usually aren't treated with pesticides.

Reducing Waste

Another great way to help the planet is to reduce the waste you produce. There are several easy ways to do this that are cheap or free. This can become a family project, too. Challenge each other to find ways to reuse materials and avoid one-use containers. You can

>> Bring your own reusable bags to the store.

>> Use a thermos for water instead of buying bottles.

>> Use reusable containers for leftovers instead of plastic, wax paper, and foil.

>> Use kitchen towels that you keep scrupulously clean instead of paper towels.

>> Shop in bulk when you buy products such as dried beans, flour, or seasonings.

>> Keep track of food in your fridge and freezer to avoid waste. Americans throw away at least 15 percent of the food they buy because it goes bad before they can use it.

REMEMBER

If you do have some canned or boxed foods in your kitchen, the expiration date printed on them is not an indicator of safety, but of quality. A can with an expiration date of last week will still be safe to eat, but the flavor may be reduced. An exception to this rule is bagged salads. Those products have been linked to food poisoning outbreaks and should never be used past their expiration date.

Recycling and Composting

Recycling and composting have been part of the green environmental movement for decades. In many communities, glass, metal, plastic, and paper must be recycled, or you'll pay a fine.

Trash can cause garbage pollution that dirties the land, air, and water. Anything that is discarded can eventually enter the groundwater and pollute the water we drink. Trash that is burned causes air pollution. Reducing the amount that you throw away helps protect the Earth. Always recycle everything you can and make a conscious effort to use less.

REMEMBER

Our oceans are becoming overloaded with discarded plastic. In fact, researchers say that plastic bottles take 450 years to break down, and when they do, they release chemicals that cause even more pollution. The "Great Pacific Garbage Patch" is a huge area of plastic debris in the ocean formed by ocean currents. Some estimates say that it is about the size of the state of Texas.

Backyard composting is a great way to help reduce waste. You can compost by buying a composting bin or making one from untreated wood. Mix dry leaves, twigs, and straw with kitchen scraps and grass clippings. Wet the pile just until it's damp. Turn the compost with a large fork to help speed decomposition and eliminate odors. Don't compost meat, bones, whole eggs, or dairy products.

Buying Organic

Organic foods can be cleaner for your body in terms of fewer pesticides and herbicides. Buying organic can also help the environment because you're encouraging farmers to work without harmful chemicals.

Organic farming keeps these chemicals, which are persistent and can last for years in the soil, out of the environment. When you're shopping, look for the organic seal which indicates the food is certified organic by the USDA. Foods produced without harmful chemicals will be labeled 100 percent organic. Foods with the label "made with organic ingredients" means at least 70 percent of the ingredients are organic. But beware of the term *natural*, which may only mean that the food doesn't have artificial ingredients or added colors.

WARNING

One herbicide, Roundup, contains a compound called glyphosate that scientists believed did not harm animals. The chemical affects the shikimate pathway in plants, which is missing in mammals. But we now know that the bacteria in our guts use the shikimate pathway, so glyphosate will harm animals and people.

Conserving Water

Clean drinking water is a resource necessary to life, but that resource is threatened by pollution and waste. You can make a difference by how you use it. You can

>> Turn off the water while you brush your teeth and take shorter showers.

>> Drink filtered tap water instead of buying bottled water.

>> Save rain water in barrels if your community allows it, and use it to water your gardens or wash your car.

>> Only use the dishwasher and clothes washer when they're fully loaded, and make sure those appliances are efficient.

>> While running the water and waiting for it to get hot, capture the cold water and use it for cleaning or watering plants.

Index

organic, 207–208

reading, 90, 265

Lactobacillus, 79–80, 81

lapses, 33–34

large intestine, role in digestive system, 41

Larsen, Linda (author)

  Gluten-Free Baking For Dummies, 276

Layton, Jean (author)

  Gluten-Free Baking For Dummies, 276

L-carnitine, 113, 163

leafy dark-green vegetables

  eating raw, 221

  for energy, 113

  on filthy fifteen list, 212

  in Paleo diet, 96

  for preventing diabetes, 150

  purchasing, 361

learning ability, 354–355

leftovers, 226–228

legumes

  for diabetes management, 166

  eating raw, 222

  for heart health, 126

  as incomplete proteins, 51

  for irritable bowel syndrome, 178

  as a protein source for vegetarians, 279

  for reducing cancer risk, 144

Leuconostoc, 79–80

lifestyle

  about, 21–22

  cravings, 29–34

  deprivation, 29–34

  environment, 34–38

  principles of clean eating, 22–29

lignans

  cancer and, 140

  diabetes and, 148

linolenic acid (LA), 54

'live and active cultures,' 81

liver, role in digestive system, 41

Living Gluten-Free For Dummies (Korn), 276

local, buying, 363–364

Local Harvest (website), 200

longevity

  about, 101–102

  as a benefit of eating clean, 19

  detoxification, 115–120

  energy, 111–115

  immune system, 105–107

  inflammation, 102–104

  weight loss, 107–111

lowering

  inflammation, 102–104

  packaging, 35–37

  waste, 35–37, 367

low-fat dairy, 23

lunch

  about, 301

  optimizing, 302

  packing, 239–241

  recipes, 303–315

lupus, 173–174

lutein, 137, 354

lycopene

  for disease management, 157

  for immune system, 353–354

  for lupus, 173

M

macronutrients

  about, 70

  excess, 45–48

  of food, 41–42

"Made with organic ingredients," 14

"Made with whole wheat," 15

magnesium

  for blood pressure, 353

  for brain health, 355

  cholesterol and, 138

  for heart health, 124, 126

  for immune system, 106–107

  in leafy greens, 361

  for preventing diabetes, 149

  role of, 61

  in sweet potatoes, 358

T

Tahoma Clinic Dispensary (website), 132
Tandoori Pork Tenderloin recipe, 327
tannins, 73
tap water, 77–78
taste receptors, 26
teas
  for inflammation, 103
  for reducing cancer risk, 144
temperature, 28
Tex-Mex Bison Chili recipe, 322
texture, 28
TGFs (triple-fat-gainers), 96
thickeners, 188
thirst cues, 86–87
thyroid, 113–115
Tip icon, 4
Toasted Oat and Barley Hot Cereal recipe, 291
tomatoes
  combining with cruciferous vegetables, 224
  on filthy fifteen list, 212
  managing heart disease with, 161
  for preventing diabetes, 150
  for reducing cancer risk, 143
toxins, 116
tracking hunger, 85
trans fats
  about, 23, 66
  avoiding at lunch, 303
  cancer and, 170
  chronic inflammation and, 134
  heart health and, 127
  inflammation and, 104
  used in processed foods, 45
transitioning, to clean eating, 247–252
tree nuts, allergies to, 269
triglycerides, 273
triple-fat-gainers (TGFs), 96
triticale, 276
Turkey with Caramelized Onion Apple Pecan Stuffing recipe, 320

turmeric
  for cancer fighting, 172
  for detoxification, 118
2-hydroxyestrogen:16-hydroxyestrogen ratio, 177
type-1 diabetes, 152, 164. *See also* diabetes
type-2 diabetes, 46–47, 52, 129, 135, 136, 145–146, 164. *See also* diabetes

U

udorn, 276
ulcerative colitis, 174–175
umami/meaty taste receptor, 26
unprocessed foods, 23
unrefined foods, 23
U.S. Department of Agriculture (USDA), 12
U.S. Environmental Protection Agency (EPA), 37, 210
U.S. Food and Drug Administration (FDA), 12
USDA (U.S. Department of Agriculture), 12
use-by date, 187

V

vegans, 277, 280–281
vegetable oils, 104
vegetables. *See also specific vegetables*
  brassica, 96, 171
  for cancer fighting, 172
  combining with fats, 225
  cruciferous, 117, 143, 224, 359
  in detox diet, 117
  for diabetes management, 165
  for energy, 112
  growing, 257, 367
  heart disease and, 122–127
  for heart health, 125
  in Paleo diet, 96–97
  for preventing autoimmune diseases, 153
  for snacks, 237
vegetarian diets, 277–279
veggie chips, 237
vinegar, 150

Violet #1, 13

viral fighters, phytochemicals as, 70

vitamin A
  about, 59, 72
  cancer and, 141
  for clear skin, 350
  for hair health, 352
  in sweet potatoes, 358

vitamin B complex
  about, 58–59, 114
  for brain health, 355
  for cholesterol, 354
  for hair health, 352
  for heart health, 124
  for immune system, 106
  in leafy greens, 361

vitamin B6
  for clear skin, 350
  for lupus, 173

vitamin B12
  raw food diet and, 366
  for vegans, 280–281
  for vegetarians, 279

vitamin C
  about, 49, 58
  in avocados, 360
  in berries, 362
  for brain health, 355
  cancer and, 141
  for clear skin, 350
  combining with iron-rich nonmeat foods, 224
  combining with protein, 225
  for detoxification, 119
  for disease management, 158
  for hair health, 352
  for heart health, 124
  for immune system, 106
  in leafy greens, 361
  as a nutrient, 157
  for preventing autoimmune diseases, 153, 154
  for rheumatoid arthritis (RA), 177

in sweet potatoes, 358
  for weight loss, 108

vitamin D
  about, 59–60, 115
  for cholesterol, 138, 354
  for disease management, 158
  for heart disease, 160
  for heart health, 124
  for immune system, 106
  for lupus, 173
  for rheumatoid arthritis (RA), 177
  for type-1 diabetes, 164
  for ulcerative colitis, 175
  for vegans, 280
  for weight loss, 108

vitamin E
  about, 60
  in avocados, 360
  for brain health, 355
  combining with fats, 225
  for heart health, 123
  for immune system, 106
  in leafy greens, 361
  as a nutrient, 157
  in nuts, 360
  in olive oil, 359
  for preventing autoimmune diseases, 154
  for preventing diabetes, 149
  for rheumatoid arthritis (RA), 177

vitamin K
  about, 60
  in avocados, 360
  in leafy greens, 361
  for preventing diabetes, 149

vitamins
  about, 56–64
  for blood pressure, 353
  cancer and, 139
  fat-soluble, 59–60
  role of, 57–60
  in sweet potatoes, 358
  water-soluble, 58–59

W

walking, as exercise, 31
Warning icon, 4
waste, reducing, 35–37, 367
water
  about, 76
  after sugar binge, 118
  bottled, 78–79
  for cancer fighting, 172
  conserving, 369
  for energy, 113
  fiber and, 75
  requirements for, 24, 76–77
  tap, 77–78
  thirst cues and, 86–87
watermelon, 216
water-soluble vitamins, 58–59
websites
  Cheat Sheet, 4
  Consumer Confidence Report (CCR), 77
  coupons, 197
  Dummies, 4
  Local Harvest, 200
  portion sizes, 24
  Tahoma Clinic Dispensary, 132
  vitamins, 158
weight gain, calories and, 47–48
weight loss
  about, 349–350
  awareness of calorie consumption,
    108–109
  as a benefit of eating clean,
    18–19
  eating clean for, 107–111
  energy and, 24
  fiber and, 76
  habits and, 110–111
  strengthening willpower, 109
  supplements for, 108
Weissella, 79–80

wheat products
  allergies to, 270
  celiac disease/non-celiac gluten sensitivity
    and, 276
  in detox diet, 116
  irritable bowel syndrome and, 178
whole foods
  about, 23
  compared with processed food, 9–10
  for managing diabetes, 165–167
Whole Grain and Nut Bread recipe, 295
whole grains
  for diabetes management, 165
  for heart health, 125
  managing heart disease with, 161
Whole-Grain Waffles recipe, 299
wild game, in Paleo diet, 96
Wild Rice Egg Roll-Ups recipe, 289
willpower, strengthening, 109
Wright, Johnathan (author), 265

Y

yeast, in detox diet, 116
yellow fruits/vegetables, for inflammation, 103
Yudkin, John (professor), 146

Z

"Zero trans fats," 14
zinc
  about, 115
  for blood pressure, 353
  cancer and, 142
  for hair health, 352
  for immune system, 106
  as a nutrient, 157
  for preventing autoimmune diseases, 154
  for rheumatoid arthritis (RA), 176
  role of, 62
  in sweet potatoes, 358

About the Authors

A Harvard University and University of Michigan graduate, **Dr. Jonathan Wright** is a fore-runner in research and application of natural treatments for healthy aging and illness. Along with Alan Gaby, MD, he has since 1976 accumulated a file of over 50,000 research papers about diet, vitamins, minerals, botanicals, and other natural substances from which he has developed all-natural treatments for health problems. Since 1983, Drs. Wright and Gaby have regularly taught seminars about these methods to tens of thousands of physicians in the United States and overseas.

He was the first to develop and introduce the use of comprehensive patterns of bio-identical hormones (including estrogens, progesterone, DHEA, and testosterone) in 1982 and (at Meridian Valley Laboratory) directed the development of tests to ensure their safe use. He teaches use and laboratory monitoring of bio-identical hormones at several seminars each year.

He also originated successful natural treatment for elimination of childhood asthma, popularized the use of D-mannose treatment for E. coli urinary tract infection, developed effective natural treatment for seborrheic dermatitis, allergic and viral conjunctivitis, and Osgood-Schlatter's disease, and discovered the effect of cobalt and iodine on estrogen and other steroid detoxification.

Dr. Wright founded the Tahoma Clinic (1973), Meridian Valley Laboratory (1976), and the Tahoma Clinic Foundation (1996). Tahoma Clinic was established to prevent and treat disease and help us stay healthy and live longer with the use of natural substances and natural energies. The infamous 1992 FDA Tahoma Clinic "raid" ("The Great B-Vitamin Bust") was a major impetus for Congressional reform of vitamin/mineral regulation. Dr. Wright continues to be an advocate for patient freedom of choice in healthcare.

Internationally known for his books and medical articles, Dr. Wright has authored or coauthored 11 books, selling over 1.5 million copies, with two texts achieving best-selling status: *Book of Nutritional Therapy* and *Guide to Healing with Nutrition.* He authors *Nutrition and Healing,* a monthly newsletter emphasizing nutritional medicine that reaches over 100,000 in the United States and another 7,000 or more worldwide.

Linda Larsen is an author and journalist who has written 34 books, many of which are about food and nutrition. She earned a BA degree in Biology from St. Olaf College and a BS with High Distinction in Food Science and Nutrition from the University of Minnesota.

Linda worked for the Pillsbury Company for many years, creating and testing recipes. She was a member of the Pillsbury Bake-Off staff five times, acting as

Manager of the Search Team and working in the test kitchens. Linda is the Busy Cooks Guide for About.com and writes about food, recipes, and nutrition. She is also the editor of Food Poisoning Bulletin, a Google News site, which reports on outbreaks, food safety issues, and food recalls. She has written articles for *Woman's Day* magazine, *Quick and Simple* magazine, and *First* magazine. Her books include *Medical Ethics For Dummies, Gluten-Free Baking For Dummies, Knack Grilling Basics: A Step-by-Step Guide to Delicious Recipes, The Starter Cook: A Beginner Home Cook's Guide to Basic Kitchen Skills & Techniques, The $7 Meal Cookbook: 301 Delicious, Nutritious Recipes the Whole Family Will Love, The Big Book of Paleo Recipes,* and *The Everything Healthy Cooking for Parties Book.*

Dedication

From Dr. Wright: For Holly, my wife and very best friend.

From Linda: I dedicate this book first and foremost to my husband Doug. Throughout the last 35 years, we've had many adventures in food. Good food got us through a cancer diagnosis (he gained 70 pounds on chemotherapy with my cooking!), and we've turned to a clean diet in the last year. Through it all, he's been by my side and is my biggest cheerleader and confidant. I'd also like to dedicate the book to my parents, Duane and Marlene Johnson, for their support and encouragement. They always told me I could do anything I attempted and let me cook and bake anything I wanted to.

Authors' Acknowledgments

From Dr. Wright: Two real pioneers in staying well and healing disease:

Adelle Davis (1904–1974), whose book *Let's Eat Right to Keep Fit* — with hundreds of citations to medical research never taught at medical schools — put me on a path to help those I worked with regain health, prevent disease, and stay healthy with the natural substances and natural energies of our planet Earth. Adelle Davis wrote: "As I see it, every day you do one of two things: build health or produce disease in yourself."

Roger J. Williams (1893–1988), whose books *Biochemical Individuality* and *Free and Unequal: The Biological Basis of Individual Liberty* established the scientific basis for an individualized and entirely natural approach to preventing and treating disease and also established the scientific and biological basis for individual freedom, which was previously viewed only as a philosophical concept and not as a concept based on our biological and biochemical heritage. As Professor at the University of

Texas and Founder of the Clayton Foundation Biochemical Institute (now called the Biochemical Institute) from 1940 to 1963, he supervised the discovery of more vitamins and their variants than discovered at any other laboratory in the world.

On a practical level, the two people who made this book possible: Linda Larsen — who wrote most of it and let me kibbitz about the science — and Barb Doyen, who put the project together. And of course, the editors who rearrange everything for publication, and the publishers who make it available to you!

From Linda: I'd like to thank my coauthor, Dr. Wright, first of all, for being such a wonderful friend and guide while working on this book. We have the same sense of humor and the same desire to share this information with the world. He is such a valuable resource for nutrition and medical information. I'd also like to thank the Department of Food Science at the University of Minnesota for giving me such a strong foundation in science. Thanks to our agent Barb Doyen. She had such confidence in my ability to write this book and encouraged me every step of the way. Thanks to our wonderful editors for their support, suggestions, and guidance. And thanks to my friends, especially my Facebook friends, and my faithful family for their support and love as I worked on this book.

Publisher's Acknowledgments

Senior Acquisitions Editor: Tracy Boggier
Project Editor: Elizabeth Kuball
Copy Editor: Elizabeth Kuball
Technical Editor: Rachel Nix, RDN

Production Editor: Kumar Chellappan
Nutrition Analyst: Rachel Nix, RDN
Recipe Tester: Emily Nolan
Cover Image: ©Nataliia Melnychuk/Shutterstock